Primer of Dermatopathology

Antoinette F. Hood, M.D.
Assistant Professor of Dermatology,
The Johns Hopkins University, School of Medicine;
Active Staff, Department of Dermatology,
The Johns Hopkins Hospital,
Baltimore

Theodore H. Kwan, M.D.
Instructor, Harvard Medical School;
Assistant in Pathology,
Beth Israel Hospital,
Boston

Daniel C. Burnes, M.D.
Special Assistant to the President,
Harvard Community Health Plan,
Boston

Martin C. Mihm, Jr., M.D.
Professor of Pathology, Harvard Medical School;
Associate Pathologist and Dermatologist,
Massachusetts General Hospital,
Boston

Little, Brown and Company
Boston/Toronto

To Wallace H. Clark, Jr., M.D.

Contents

Preface

Looking at a skin biopsy under the microscope can be a bewildering and frustrating experience for inexperienced dermatology and pathology residents and practioners alike. This book was conceived from that frustration. When Dan Burnes was rotating through dermatopathology as a dermatology resident at the Massachusetts General Hospital, he frequently complained that there should be a logical and systematic way to look at and evaluate a skin biopsy. The textbooks available at that time were all traditionally organized by pathogenesis, which was useful only if you knew the answer in advance. Challenged by the problem, Dan sat down and outlined dermatopathologic disorders according to (1) their location in the skin—from the stratum corneum to the panniculus—and (2) "reaction patterns" of disease. The latter organization he had learned from Martin Mihm, who had learned it from Wally Clark, who learned it from heaven knows whom. Encouraged by Dr. Thomas Fitzpatrick, who loves a logical approach to disease, Dan's outline was filled in and expanded, and line drawings and photographs were added. Many revisions later, *Primer of Dermatopathology* became a functional entity.

We deliberately called this book a primer to identify its purpose. It is an introduction to dermatopathology, an expanded outline of diseases according to the anatomic location and the pattern of changes observed. It attempts to simplify and clarify a complex situation in order to get people involved in making a (differential) diagnosis from a piece of tissue on a slide.

This book includes most of the diseases seen by dermatology or pathology residents during their years of training. It is not, however, all-inclusive, and for completeness, the reader should have ready access to at least one (inclusive) major textbook, such as those written by Walter Lever, James Graham and Elson Helwig, and, for inflammatory disorders, that of A. Bernard Ackerman.

A.F.H.
T.H.K.
D.C.B.
M.C.M.

Acknowledgments

It is impossible to adequately thank everyone who contributed to *Primer of Dermatopathology*; however, certain people must be mentioned. We voice our appreciation to Dr. Thomas B. Fitzpatrick, Department of Dermatology, Harvard Medical School; Dr. Irwin M. Freedberg, Department of Dermatology, New York University School of Medicine; Dr. Thomas T. Provost and Dr. Evan R. Farmer, Department of Dermatology, The Johns Hopkins University, School of Medicine; and Dr. Harold F. Dvorak, Department of Pathology, Harvard Medical School. Their continued encouragement and gentle prodding kept the project going. Appreciation is also extended to Otto Coontz for his beautiful drawings, to Ben Bronstein of the Massachusetts General Hospital Dermatopathology Unit, and to the dermatology residents at Johns Hopkins, who reviewed the manuscript in its various stages of evolution and offered constructive criticism and helpful suggestions.

We owe special thanks to Marletta Winston, Linda Pottillo, Denise Fritter, and Bonnie Weissfeld, who patiently turned illegible squiggles into final copy. We are ever grateful to histology technologists such as Norma King and Obdula Morales, who maintain such standards that our work at the microscope is not only possible but esthetically delightful. The photomicrographs in this primer were made possible by Beth Israel Hospital Photographic Services, the Massachusetts General Hospital Pathology Photography Laboratory, Steven Halpern of the Tufts University Medical School Department of Pathology, and Rita Ann Monahan of the Beth Israel Hospital Department of Pathology.

Finally, we acknowledge our debt to patients, residents, and associates, from whom we learn daily.

A.F.H.
T.H.K.
D.C.B.
M.C.M.

Guide to the Use of this Book

Primer of Dermatopathology is designed to assist dermatologists and pathologists (in training or in practice) in the microscopic diagnosis of skin disease. By emphasizing a systematic approach to the examination of a skin biopsy, we hope to enable even the relatively uninitiated individual to locate and identify the abnormal histologic features present in a given lesion and to establish either a diagnosis or a differential diagnosis.

To use this book most effectively, we recommend an initial reading of the introductory section. The normal histology of the skin is briefly reviewed, and the illustrated glossary provides an introduction to common pathologic alterations (parakeratosis, basal vacuolation, etc.) and to the terminology used in dermatopathology.

A skin biopsy should be examined first with the unaided eye and then with the lowest-power objective on the microscope. Simple appreciation of the *type* of biopsy submitted can give valuable insight into the questions being asked by the referring physician. For example, trephine (punch) biopsies are usually obtained from inflammatory lesions while shave biopsies and elliptical excisions are usually from neoplastic lesions. Inked margins indicate the surgeon's concern about the extension of a malignant tumor.

While still using low power, identify the anatomic site of the major pathologic change (i.e., the epidermis, basement membrane zone, dermis, appendages, or panniculus), turn to that section of the book, and note the chapter headings. At higher power, determine the predominant abnormality and match it with the corresponding chapter. Some chapters (e.g., Chapter 21, Cysts in the Dermis) will require perusal of the entire contents to generate a diagnosis, while others (e.g., Chapter 8, Disorders of the Melanocyte) are further subdivided. For example, examination of a skin biopsy reveals that the most prominent change is a perivascular infiltrate in the reticular dermis. Turn to Part IV (Reticular Dermis), Chapter 14 (Predominantly Perivascular Infiltrate). To further classify the lesion, determine the cellular composition of the infiltrate and whether there is vascular damage or thrombosis. Accordingly, a subdivision can be selected and a differential diagnosis generated. Histologic differential diagnoses are given in the right-hand column. The differential diagnoses of specific histologic findings, such as Pautrier microabscesses or hypogranulosis, are also in the right-hand column but are boxed for emphasis.

Skin biopsies, especially when taken from inflammatory lesions, often show histologic changes in more than one anatomic area. A lesion of lupus erythematosus, for example, may exhibit epidermal atrophy, basal vacuolation, and a perivascular mononuclear cell infiltrate. The diagnosis may be established by looking at any one of those features in Chapter 7 (Atrophic Processes of the Epidermis), Chapter 9 (Vacuolation of the Basement Membrane Zone), or Chapter 14 (Predominantly Perivascular Infiltrate).

Characteristic histologic features of the individual disorders are enumerated in the text and illustrated wherever possible with schematic drawings and/or photomicrographs. The most important or distinguishing histologic features are emphasized with bold type.

Suggested readings are given at the end of each chapter to provide additional information to the curious and inquiring student of dermatopathology.

Part **I**

Introduction

Chapter 1

Normal Histology of
the Skin

A basic knowledge of cutaneous histology is easily attained by a systematic approach. The skin can be considered by anatomic levels: epidermis, dermoepidermal junction, dermis, and subcutis (Fig. 1-1). Traversing the dermis and subcutis are the peripheral branches of the vascular and nervous systems as well as the epidermal appendages (pilosebaceous, apocrine, and eccrine units). Regional variations in the skin account for marked differences in epidermal thickness, dermal thickness, elastic fiber content, and the presence or absence of hair follicles and sebaceous, apocrine, or eccrine glands.

Epidermis

The epidermis is composed of four types of cells—keratinocytes, melanocytes, Langerhans cells, and Merkel cells. These cells vary markedly in structure, function, and place of origin. *Keratinocytes* comprise the major cell population of the epidermis (80%). Keratinocytes are subclassified by their location in the epidermis (Fig. 1-2). The *basal layer* (stratum basale) consists of a single layer of cuboidal cells located next to the dermoepidermal junction. These cells have a relatively large nuclear-cytoplasmic ratio and slightly basophilic cytoplasm. The *spinous layer* (stratum spinosum), named for its prominent intercellular connections, which allegedly resemble spines, is located above the basal layer. Usually several cells thick, the spinous layer consists of polygonal cells, which exhibit cytoplasmic eosinophilia reflecting increased keratinization. The *granular layer* (stratum granulosum) is one to five cells thick, and consists of flattened cells with coarse, deeply basophilic cytoplasmic granules. These are called *keratohyaline granules*. The *cornified layer* (stratum corneum), the most superficial layer of the epidermis, is composed of extremely flattened, anucleate keratinocytes arranged in a pattern sometimes described as "basketweave." The cornified layer appears dense and thickened on surfaces subject to friction, such as the palms and soles. Keratinocytes—particularly basal cells—also may contain small, brown pigment (melanin) granules. The degree of epidermal melanization varies with genetic and environmental factors.

Melanocytes have a variable appearance, which sometimes makes definitive identification difficult in routine hematoxylin-eosin (H&E) stained sections. Melanocytes are located in the basal layer and usually appear as cuboidal cells with clear cytoplasm and eccentrically placed, crescent-shaped nuclei. The function of these neural crest–derived cells is to synthesize melanin, which is then transferred to adjacent keratinocytes via dendritic projections. Pigment production in these cells and their true dendritic shape are infrequently appreciated without special stains. The ratio of melanocytes to basal cells is 1:4 to 1:9 and varies with anatomic location on the body (but not with race).

Langerhans cells have an appearance similar to that of melanocytes but are located at any level of the epidermis. Reliable identification can be made with gold chloride–stained sections or by electron microscopy. Ultrastructural cytoplasmic organelles called *Birbeck granules* (said to resemble tennis rackets) are characteristic of Langerhans cells. Langerhans cells have many features of monocytes and macrophages and probably migrate to the skin from the bone marrow.

Merkel cells, located in the basal layer, are also difficult to visualize in hematoxylin-eosin stained sections. They are identified by distinctive ultrastructural membrane-bound granules similar to those found in neuroendocrine tissues. The function of Merkel cells is not understood.

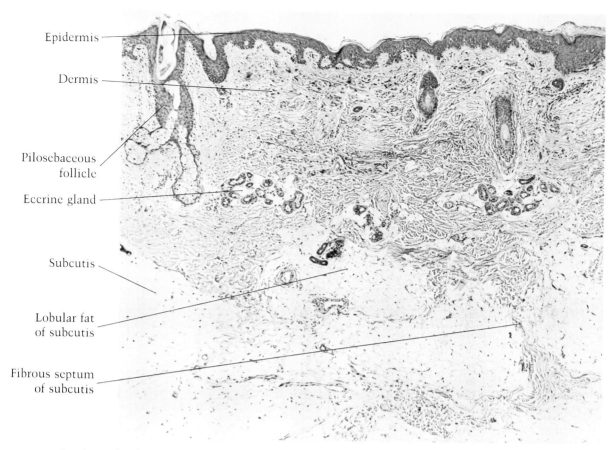

Epidermis

Dermis

Pilosebaceous
follicle

Eccrine gland

Subcutis

Lobular fat
of subcutis

Fibrous septum
of subcutis

Fig. **1-1.** *The skin. The three
anatomic layers of the skin are
the epidermis, dermis, and subcutis. The epidermal appendages,
including pilosebaceous follicles
and eccrine glands, extend into
the dermis. The subcutis is subdivided into lobular and septal
areas. (approximately ×64)*

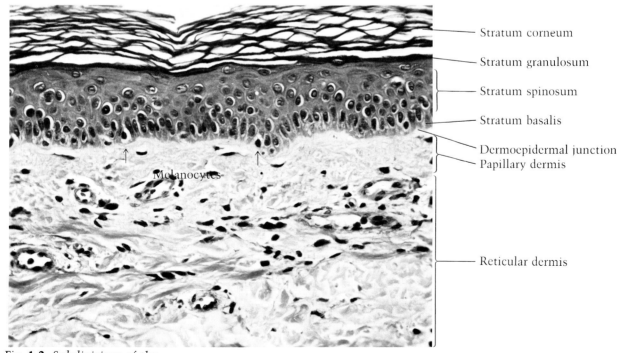

Stratum corneum

Stratum granulosum

Stratum spinosum

Stratum basalis

Dermoepidermal junction
Papillary dermis

Melanocytes

Reticular dermis

Fig. **1-2.** *Subdivisions of the
epidermis and dermis. (×256)*

Dermoepidermal Junction

The dermoepidermal junction in hematoxylin-eosin stained sections appears as a fine (1–2 μm) band of slightly condensed eosinophilic material (Fig. 1-2). This basement membrane zone consists of a glycoprotein matrix in which are embedded collagen, reticulin, and elastic fibers. Periodic acid Schiff (PAS) stain highlights this area. The basement membrane zone continues around all the epidermal appendages.

The lower border of the epidermis on most parts of the body has numerous undulating downward projections called *rete ridges* (when seen in three dimensions, these form a netlike, or rete, pattern). The corresponding and interdigitating upward elevations of the dermis are called *dermal papillae.*

Dermis

The dermis is divided into two parts: a thin superficial portion known as the *papillary dermis* and a wider, deep area known as the *reticular dermis* (Fig. 1-2). Both the papillary and reticular dermis contain collagen, reticulin, and elastic fibers embedded within a matrix of glycoproteins. Collagen, the major component of the dermis, is readily visualized in hematoxylin-eosin stained sections as eosinophilic fibers of regular diameter which are gathered into bundles of varying size. Collagen fibers are birefringent in polarized light. Reticulin fibers are small, possibly young, collagen fibers and are best visualized with special reticulin stains. Elastic fibers are wavy, eosinophilic, and slightly refractile, and they vary markedly in their diameter and length. They are easily visualized with stains such as the Verhoeff–van Giesen. The glycoprotein matrix of the dermis cannot be visualized in hematoxylin-eosin stained sections. In certain pathologic states characterized by excessive production of acid mucopolysaccharides, these materials can be identified by alcian blue stain.

The papillary dermis is recognized microscopically as a thin (40–100 μm) zone of connective tissue located below the dermoepidermal junction and above the reticular dermis. The small collagen bundles of the papillary dermis are easily distinguished from the larger collagen bundles of the reticular dermis. The papillary dermis surrounds all the appendageal structures as they plunge downward into the dermis and subcutis. This periadnexal papillary dermis is called the *adventitial* (outermost) *dermis.*

The reticular (netlike) dermis is easily distinguished from the papillary dermis by the presence of large (12–25 μm) collagen bundles. These bundles, which appear to be oriented in every possible plane, are mingled with reticulin and elastic fibers to form a closely knit net.

Subcutis

The subcutis (panniculus adiposus, subcutaneous fat) is composed of lobules of lipocytes separated by fibrous connective-tissue septa. The thickness of the subcutis varies with the sex and nutritional status of the individual and with anatomic location. Vessels, nerves, and appendages pass into and through the subcutis. Below the subcutis, muscle and/or fascia can be found.

Vessels: Arteriovenous and Lymphatic

The arteriovenous framework of the skin can be visualized as follows. Arteries traverse the septa of the subcutis and form a *deep plexus* in the region of the junction of the subcutis and dermis. From this deep plexus, smaller arteries pass upward to the junction of the reticular and papillary dermis, where they form the *superficial plexus*. From these arterioles, capillary-venules form superficial vascular loops, which ascend into and descend from the dermal papillae. Capillary-venules are so named because the flow of blood may be arterial to venous or vice versa. The venous return in the skin follows a reverse, and frequently more variable, course. The arteriovenous system of the skin, therefore, consists of deep and superficial plexuses with communicating vessels and, most distally, capillary venular loops (Fig. 1-3).

Given this framework, note that considerable regional variation exists with regard to the density and caliber of these vessels. Furthermore, there are numerous arteriovenous shunts, particularly on distal extremities. These arteriovenous shunts are controlled by *glomus cells*, abundantly innervated by adrenergic fibers. Glomus cells are

Fig. **1-3.** *Arteriovenous system. ART, artery; SM ART/A, small artery/arteriole; SAP, superficial arterial plexus; SCV, superficial capillary venule; SVP₁ and SVP₂, components of superficial venular plexus. (Reprinted with permission from M. C. Mihm., et al., J. Invest. Dermatol. 67:306, 1976. Copyright © 1976, The Williams & Wilkins Co., Baltimore.)*

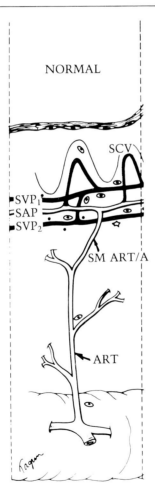

NORMAL

SCV

SVP₁
SAP
SVP₂

SM ART/A

ART

recognized by their round nuclei, polygonal shape, and tendency to group around vessels (Fig. 1-4).

The microscopic structure of cutaneous vessels is similar to that of visceral vessels. Surrounding a lumen, endothelial cells rest on a PAS-positive basement membrane zone, which in turn is surrounded by smooth muscle cells, pericytes, and/or connective tissue. The latter layers vary with the size and type of vessel.

Mast cells in varying numbers (up to five per sectioned vessel) are present almost always about superficial vessels and to a lesser extent throughout the dermis. In hematoxylin-eosin stained sections, mast cells have densely basophilic nuclei and opaque, violet cytoplasm. Their characteristic and identifying cytoplasmic granules are metachromatic blue-purple when stained with Giemsa.

The lymphatics of the skin consist of a blind-ended vascular system that flows from the superficial dermis to the subcutis and then more centrally. The most distal tributaries in the papillary dermis are lined by endothelial cells without a basal lamina. The thicker-walled, more proximal portions of the system contain valves. Thin walls and valves are the features that distinguish lymphatics from other vessels. Probably because they are collapsed, lymphatic channels are observed infrequently in the skin of normal individuals.

Nerves

The cutaneous nerves comprise a system of nerve plexuses and branches that roughly parallels the vascular system. Cutaneous nerves function in sensory (afferent) and autonomic (efferent) modes. Sensory impulses, generated from encapsulated (Meissner and Vater-Pacini corpuscles) and nonencapsulated ("end organs" ramifying about hair follicles and in dermal papillae and ending in Merkel cell–neurite complexes) receptors, pass to the dorsal root ganglia and centrally. By a presumed process of summation and integration there is perception of particular sensations described as touch, pressure, temperature, pain, itch, and location. Motor impulses, which in the skin are autonomic, originate in the sympathetic nervous system and pass to glomus bodies and smooth muscles of vessels (affecting peripheral flow), to hair follicle–associated smooth muscle (causing gooseflesh), and to apocrine and eccrine glands (causing sweating).

In hematoxylin-eosin stained sections, sensory fibers cannot be distinguished from autonomic fibers, and one appreciates little more than small nerve branches and Meissner and Vater-Pacini corpuscles. Nerve branches have the same structure as elsewhere in the peripheral nervous system. Larger nerves of the subcutis exhibit epineurium, perineurium, and endoneurium (Fig. 1-5). Small nerve branches in the superficial dermis lack these layers. Individual nerve fibers with Schwann cells measure 3 to 5 μm in diameter. The small size of these fibers helps one to distinguish them from smooth muscle. Meissner corpuscles are said to play a role in mediation of the sensation of touch. Located in the dermal papillae, each of these encapsulated ellipsoid structures (20–50 μm) has the appearance of string wound about a spindle (Fig. 1-6). The Vater-Pacini corpuscles, which mediate the sensation of pressure, are located in the subcutis, each appearing as a large (up to 1 mm) oval encapsulated body with a distinctive internal structure of concentric lamellae (Fig. 1-7). Vater-Pacini bodies are most numerous on the palms and soles.

Special stains are necessary to demonstrate nonencapsulated receptors and autonomic innervation.

Fig. **1-4.** *Glomus body. Numerous glomus cells surround arteriovenous anastomoses. Glomus bodies are numerous in nailfolds, toes, fingerpads, and the pinnae. (×256)*

Glomus cells —

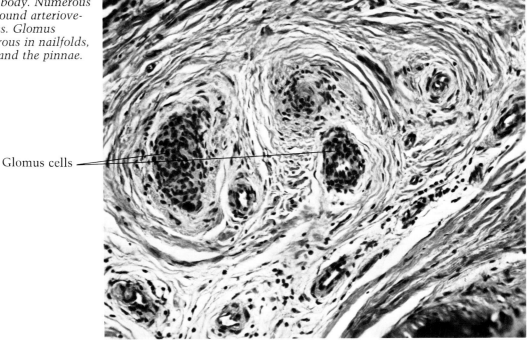

Fig. **1-5.** *Peripheral nerve. A thin fibrous capsule, the perineurium, surrounds the bundle of myelinated nerve axons.* Endoneurium *refers to the delicate collagen fibers surrounding nerve trunks within the perineurium. Schwann cell nuclei can be identified, but nerve axons are difficult to visualize. Two capillaries also are present in this field. (×640)*

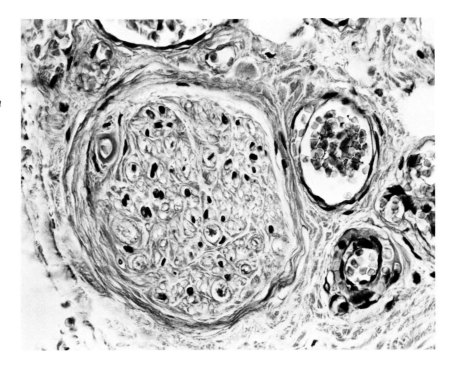

Fig. **1-6.** *Meissner corpuscle. Tucked within the dermal papilla, this neuroreceptor resembles a ball of string wound about a spindle. Portions of an intraepidermal eccrine duct are present at left. (×400)*

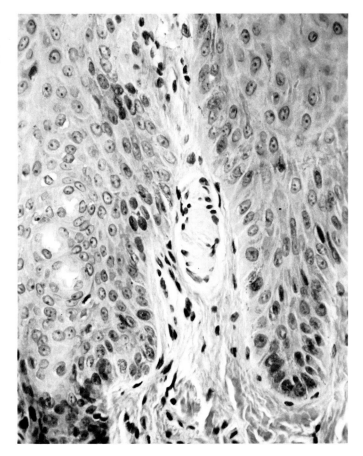

Fig. **1-7.** *Pacinian corpuscles. The rounded forms of these concentric lamellated structures in the subcutis are characteristic. (×64)*

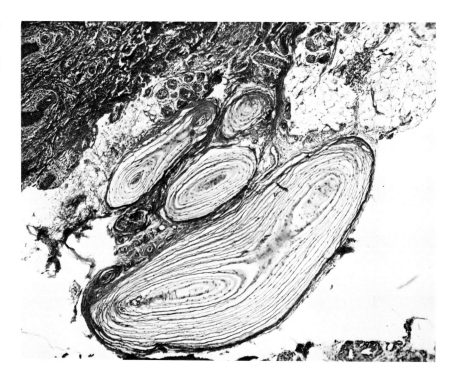

Pilosebaceous Unit

Hair is present everywhere on the body except the palms, soles, and mucocutaneous junctions. The fine, almost imperceptible hairs that cover most of the body are called *lanugo,* or *vellus hairs.* The larger hairs such as those of the scalp and eyebrows are called *terminal hairs.* The pilosebaceous unit makes hair and an oily, fatty emollient; moreover, it is equipped for sensory and motor functions. The components of the pilosebaceous follicle include the hair and hair follicle, sebaceous gland, sensory end organ, and arrector pili.

The Hair and Hair Follicle

Hair, composed of a shaft of densely layered keratinized material, is the product of cellular differentiation occurring within the follicle. The hair and hair follicle are first described longitudinally and then in cross section. Finally, the histologic changes associated with phases of growth, involution, and rest are described briefly.

Viewed in its long axis, the hair follicle can be divided into three parts:

1. The *infundibulum* (funnel) extends from the surface to the opening of the sebaceous duct into the follicle. On certain areas of the body, the duct of the apocrine gland also opens into the infundibulum.
2. The *isthmus* (by definition, a contracted anatomic part connecting two larger structures) joins the portion from the opening of the sebaceous duct to the insertion of the arrector pili.
3. The *inferior portion* consists of the hair follicle below the insertion of the arrector pili.

Hair formation begins within the bulb, or rounded extremity of the inferior portion. The bulb contains the hair *matrix,* a group of undifferentiated cells with vesicular nuclei and intensely basophilic cytoplasm. The matrix cells in association with melanocytes sit astride the dermal *papilla* of the hair, a specialized mesenchymal tissue continuous with the papillary dermis. Under the influence of the dermal hair papilla, matrix cells give rise to the hair shaft as well as the inner and outer root sheaths. The hair shaft forms by keratinization of matrix cells and derives its pigment from the melanocytes of the matrix. The mature hair shaft in cross section exhibits a central *medulla* (absent in vellus hairs) surrounded by *cortex* and covered by a cuticle, which somewhat resembles overlapping shingles. Concentric and superior to the matrix are the *inner and outer root sheaths* (Fig. 1-8); these two keratinizing layers form a support for the growing hair. Surrounding the outer root sheath are the *vitreous,* an eosinophilic band continuous with but thicker than the epidermal basement membrane zone; the *fibrous root sheath;* and the *periadnexal adventitial dermis.*

In the hair follicle cycles of growth, involution, and rest (anagen, catagen, and telogen, respectively) correlate with the following histologic features. During telogen the inferior portion of the hair follicle is absent. With the onset of anagen the inferior portion, apparently under the influence of the dermal papilla of the hair, elongates and forms a bulb which contains matrix and papilla. The papilla during anagen exhibits metachromasia. Loss of metachromasia signals the onset of catagen, and the inferior portion retreats to the region of attachment of the arrector pili, leaving in its wake a pleated collagen streamer.

Fig. **1-8.** *Hair follicle. (approximately ×256)*

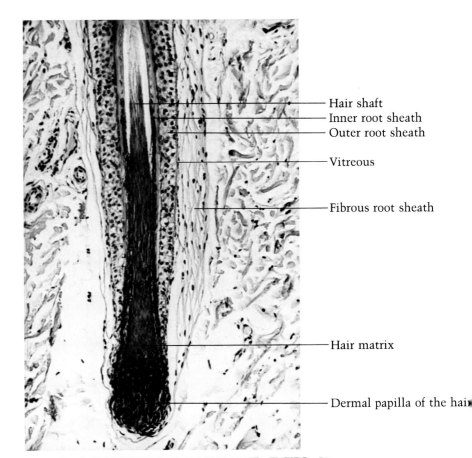

— Hair shaft
— Inner root sheath
— Outer root sheath

— Vitreous

— Fibrous root sheath

— Hair matrix

— Dermal papilla of the hair

Fig. **1-9.** *Sebaceous glands. Basophilic cells at the periphery of each lobule give rise to the central cell with foamy cytoplasm. These glands are usually associated with a hair. (×400)*

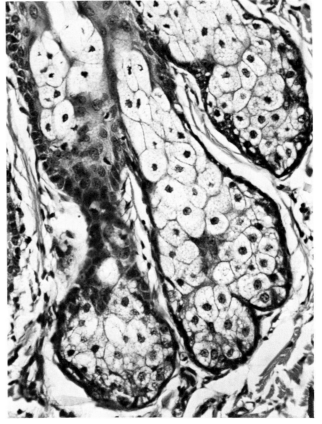

Sensory End Organ and Arrector Pili

The sensory end organ consists of distal, apparently unencapsulated, ramifications of sensory nerves present about the isthmus and inferior portions of the follicle. These receptors and nerves apparently convey information about the movement of hair follicles. As noted earlier, these sensory end organs are not apparent in hematoxylin-eosin stained sections but can be demonstrated by special techniques.

Arrector pili muscles are associated with hair follicles and are composed of bundles of smooth-muscle fibers. The arrector pili, which inserts into the follicle below the sebaceous gland duct, extends obliquely upward to the superficial dermis. Contraction of the arrector pili (mediated by autonomic nerves) causes the hair to be pulled from its normally angled position to a more perpendicular position. This results in cutis anserina, or goosebumps.

Sebaceous Gland

Sebaceous glands produce oily, fatty secretions that function as emollients for the hair and skin. These glands frequently are associated with hairs, but the hairs may be so vestigial as to be inapparent. Present everywhere except on the palms and soles, sebaceous glands are most numerous on the face, chest, and back; also they are found frequently on the lip (Fordyce spots), areola (Montgomery's tubercles), labia minora, prepuce (Tyson's glands), and even in the parotids and on the tongue and cervix. The Meibomian glands of the eyelid are also sebaceous. Hormonal factors probably regulate the holocrine secretions of these glands.

The sebaceous gland can be multilobular or unilobular. Cuboidal cells with basophilic cytoplasm located at the periphery of the lobule differentiate into large, vacuolated lipid-laden cells (Fig. 1-9), which disintegrate as they reach the sebaceous duct. This short duct, composed of squamous epithelium, conveys the cellular contents to the infundibulum of the follicle or, less frequently, directly to the skin surface. As with all appendages, a basement membrane zone and periadnexal dermis surround the sebaceous gland.

Eccrine Glands and Ducts

Eccrine glands produce a watery substance that is modified by the ducts and emerges on the skin surface as sweat. Especially numerous on the palms, soles, and forehead and in the axillae, eccrine glands are found everywhere on the skin except the mucocutaneous junctions, earlobes, and nailbeds.

The eccrine unit can be divided into the secretory gland, intradermal duct, and intraepidermal duct (Fig. 1-10A). The coiled secretory gland is located in the area of the deep dermis and subcutis (Fig. 1-10B). Adjacent to the lumen (20-μm diameter) are two types of cells: cells with clear cytoplasm that contain glycogen and cells with dark (basophilic) cytoplasm that contain mucopolysaccharides. These secretory cells overlie a basal lamina that is surrounded by myoepithelial cells and periadnexal dermis (Fig. 1-10C). Nonmyelinated cholinergic and adrenergic fibers innervate the gland. The intradermal duct coils just before beginning its relatively direct ascent through the dermis. Adjacent to the duct lumen is a PAS-positive eosinophilic cuticle that is produced by the basophilic duct cells. The duct is surrounded also by myoepithelial cells and periadnexal dermis. The intraepidermal duct follows a spiral course through the epidermis to the surface (Fig. 1-10C). The lumen in this portion of the duct is lined by cells that undergo keratinization independently of adjacent epidermal keratinocytes. The intraepidermal duct cells do not contain melanin granules.

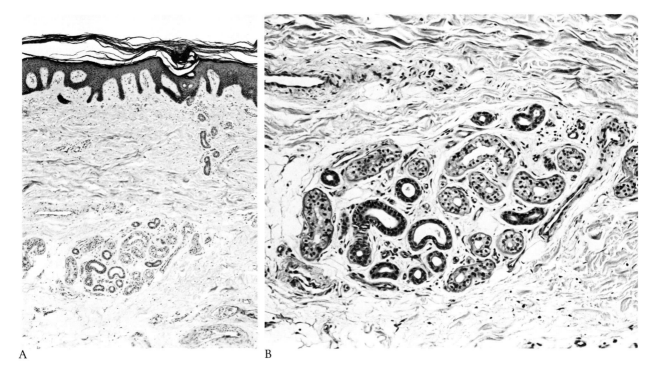

A

B

Fig. **1-10.**

A. *Eccrine gland and duct (with overlying lentigo). Two cell layers line the entire system; an inner secretory cell adjacent to the lumen is ensheathed by an outer myoepithelial cell. (×64)*

B. *Eccrine gland. Note the normal investment of the gland by loose connective tissue and lipocytes. The cytoplasm of these cells is clear to amphophilic. (×160)*

C. *Eccrine duct within the dermis and epidermis. Two cell layers with a PAS-positive cuticle lining the lumen are characteristic. (×400)*

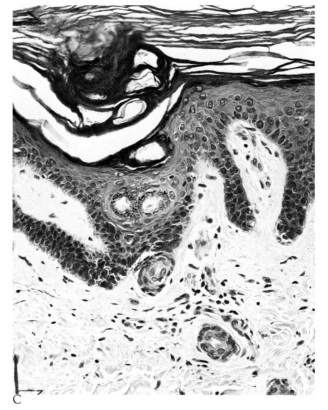

C

Apocrine Glands and Ducts

Apocrine glands produce secretions that are rendered odoriferous by bacteria. They are most numerous in the axillae and groin, but can also be found on the scalp, forehead, and areolae as well as in the periumbilical region. Also considered to be of apocrine derivation are the mammary glands of the breast, the ceruminous glands of the external auditory canal, and Moll's glands in the eyelid. Apocrine secretions have been difficult to isolate and study because of the proximity of their duct openings to those of sebaceous glands. In animals, apocrine secretions act as pheromones and in thermoregulation, but their function in humans is unclear.

The apocrine unit consists of a secretory coil, an intradermal duct, and an intraepidermal duct. The secretory coil is located in the subcutis and has a large (up to 200-μm) lumen surrounded by columnar to cuboidal cells with eosinophilic cytoplasm. The latter often show apical budding, for which the glands are named (apocrine means "to separate") (Fig. 1-11). Cytoplasmic granules are present which are best visualized with PAS or iron stains. These secretory cells rest on a basal lamina and are surrounded by elongated myoepithelial cells and periadnexal dermis. Response to cholinergic and adrenergic stimulation as well as to circulating catecholamines has been proposed. The intradermal duct ascends in a relatively straight course to the hair follicle, where it opens above the sebaceous duct orifice. The duct also may open directly to the skin surface. The intradermal duct closely resembles its eccrine counterpart. Surrounding the lumen is a double layer of cells with basophilic cytoplasm resting on a basal lamina. The basal lamina is surrounded by myoepithelial cells and periadnexal dermis. The portion of the apocrine duct that traverses the epithelium of the follicle or of the epidermis is less well characterized than that of the eccrine unit.

Fig. **1-11.** *Apocrine gland. The cells appear larger and more eosinophilic than eccrine gland cells (which have clear or amphophilic cytoplasm). Note the appearance of apical budding in some of these cells as well as the underlying myoepithelial cells. ($\times$400)*

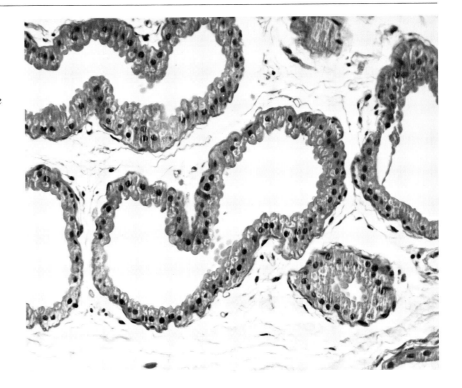

Examples of specialized epidermal structures and regional variation are given in Figure 1-12.

Some disorders exhibit such subtle histologic changes that at first inspection they appear normal (see table, inside back cover). Closer examination and/or special stains in light of the clinical history often yield diagnostic clues.

Fig. **1-12.**

A. *Nail. The nailplate is formed within the nail matrix, the area of indentation. The nailfold lies above the matrix and nail. The structure at the lower left portion of the field is bone with artifactual loss of medulla. (×9)*

B. *Nipple. Primary as well as accessory nipple tissue contains numerous smooth-muscle bundles within the dermis. (×400)*

C. *Scrotal tissue. Many small smooth-muscle bundles and numerous thin-walled vessels are typical of genital skin. (×100)*

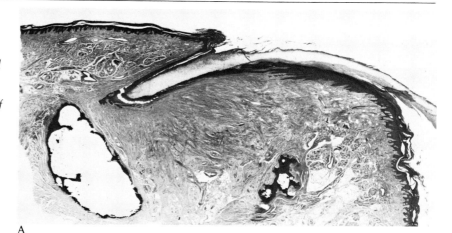

A

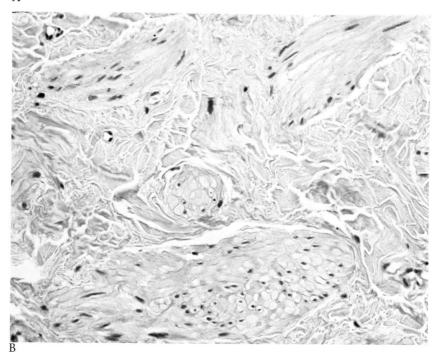

B

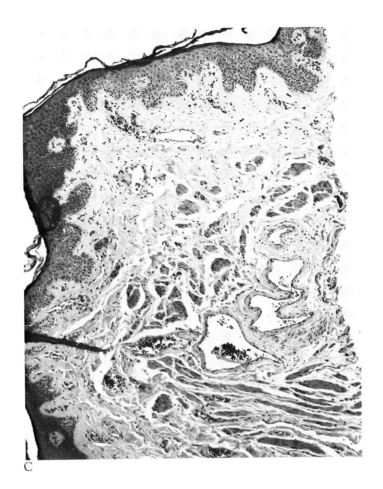

C

Suggested Reading	*Keratinocytes*
Epidermis	Brody, I. The Epidermis. In O. Gans and G. K. Steigleder (Eds.), *Handbuch der Haut-und Geschlechtskrankheiten.* Vol. 1. Berlin: Springer-Verlag, 1968. Pp. 1–142.

Keratinocytes

Brody, I. The Epidermis. In O. Gans and G. K. Steigleder (Eds.), *Handbuch der Haut-und Geschlechtskrankheiten.* Vol. 1. Berlin: Springer-Verlag, 1968. Pp. 1–142.

Fukuyama, K., Inone, N., Suzuki, H., et al. Keratinization. *Int. J. Dermatol.* 15:474, 1976.

Montagna, W., and Lobiz, W. C., Jr. (Eds.). *The Epidermis.* New York: Academic, 1964.

Wessels, W. K. Differentiation of epidermis and epidermal derivatives. *N. Engl. J. Med.* 277:21, 1967.

Melanocytes

Montagna, W., and Hu, F. (Eds.). *Advances in Biology of Skin.* Vol. VIII. *The Pigmentary System.* Oxford, New York: Pergamon, 1967.

Szabo, G. Quantitative Histological Investigations on the Melanocyte System of the Human Epidermis. In M. Gordon (Ed.), *Pigment Cell Biology.* New York: Academic, 1959. P. 99.

Langerhans Cells

Breathnach, A. S. The cell of Langerhans. *Int. Rev. Cytol.* 18:1, 1965.

Katz, S. I., Tamaki, K., and Sachs, D. H. Epidermal Langerhans cells are derived from cells originating in bone marrow. *Nature* 282:324, 1979.

Stingl, G., Katz, S. I., Clement, L., et al. Immunologic functions of Ia-bearing epidermal Langerhans cells. *J. Immunol.* 121:2005, 1978.

Streilein, J. W., Toews, G. B., and Bergstresser, P. R. Langerhans cells: Functional aspects revealed by in vivo grafting studies. *J. Invest. Dermatol.* 75:17, 1980.

Merkel Cells

Winkelmann, R. K. The Merkel cell system and a comparison between it and the neurosecretory or APUD cell system. *J. Invest. Dermatol.* 69:41, 1977.

Dermoepidermal Junction

Briggaman, R. A., and Wheeler, C. E. The epidermal-dermal junction. *J. Invest. Dermatol.* 66:71, 1975.

Hodge, S., and Freeman, R. G. The basal lamina in skin disease. *Int. J. Dermatol.* 17:261, 1978.

Murray, J. C., Stingl, G., Kleinman, H. K., et al. Epidermal cells adhere preferentially to type IV (basement membrane) collagen. *J. Cell Biol.* 80:197, 1979.

Vracko, R. Basal lamina scaffold—Anatomy and significance for maintenance of orderly tissue structure. *Am. J. Pathol.* 77:314, 1974.

Dermis

Jarrett, A. (Ed.). *The Physiology and Pathophysiology of the Skin.* Vol. 3. *The Dermis and the Dendrocytes.* New York: Academic, 1974.

Montagna, W., Bentley, J. P., and Dobson, R. L. (Eds.). *Advances in Biology of Skin.* Vol. 10. *The Dermis.* Publication No. 396 from the Oregon Regional Primate Research Center. New York: Appleton-Century-Crofts, 1970.

Prockop, D. J., Kivirikko, K. I., Tuderman, L., et al. The biosynthesis of collagen and its disorders. *N. Engl. J. Med.* 301:13 and 77, 1979.

Sandberg, L. B., Suskel, N. T., and Leslie, J. G. Elastin structure, biosynthesis and relation to disease states. *N. Engl. J. Med.* 304:566, 1981.

Blood Vessels

Montagna, W., and Ellis, R. A. (Eds.). *Advances in Biology of Skin.* Vol. II. *Blood Vessels and Circulation.* New York: Pergamon, 1961.

Moretti, G. The blood vessels of the skin. In O. Gans and G. K. Steigleder (Eds.), *Handbuch der Haut-und Geschlechtskrankheiten.* Vol. 1. Berlin: Springer-Verlag, 1968. Pp. 491–623.

Ryan, T. J. Structure, pattern and shape of the blood vessels of the skin. In A. Jarrett (Ed.), *The Physiology and Pathophysiology of the Skin,* Vol. 2. London: Academic, 1973.

Mast Cells

Bloom, G. D. Structural and biochemical characteristics of mast cells. In B. W. Q. Zwerbach, L. Grant, and R. J. McCluskey (Eds.), *The Inflammatory Process.* New York: Academic, 1965.

Eady, R. A. J. The mast cells: distribution and morphology. *Clin. Exp. Dermatol.* 1:313, 1976.

Lagunoff, D., and Chi, E. Y. Mast cell secretion: membrane events. *J. Invest. Dermatol.* 71:81, 1978.

Nerves

Kenshalo, D. R. (Ed.). *International Symposium on the Skin Senses,* Second, Florida State University, 1978. New York: Plenum, 1979.

Montagna, W. (Ed.). *Advances in Biology of Skin.* Vol. I. *Cutaneous Innervation.* New York: Pergamon, 1960.

Montagna, W., and Brookhart, J. M. (Eds.). Proceedings of the 26th Annual Symposium on the Biology of Skin: Cutaneous innervation and modalities of cutaneous sensibility. *J. Invest. Dermatol.* 69:3, 1981.

Pilosebaceous Unit

Hair

Johnson, E. Cycles and Patterns of Hair Growth. In A. Jarrett (Ed.), *The Physiology and Pathophysiology of the Skin.* Vol. 4. New York: Academic, 1977.

Montagna, W., and Dobson, R. L. (Eds.). *Advances in Biology of Skin.* Vol. IX. *Hair Growth.* Research Publication No. 277 from the Oregon Regional Primate Research Center. New York: Pergamon, 1967.

Morretti, G., Rampini, E., and Rebora, A. The hair cycle re-evaluated. *Int. J. Dermatol.* 15:277, 1976.

Snell, B. S. An electron microscopic study of melanin in the hair and hair follicles. *J. Invest. Dermatol.* 38:218, 1972.

Spearman, R. I. C. Hair Follicle Development, Cyclical Changes and Hair Form. In A. Jarrett (Ed.), *The Physiology and Pathophysiology of the Skin.* Vol. 4. New York: Academic, 1977.

Spearman R. I. C. The Structure and Function of the Fully Developed Follicle. In A. Jarrett (Ed.), *The Physiology and Pathophysiology of the Skin.* Vol. 4. New York: Academic, 1977.

Sebaceous Gland

Montagna, W., Ellis, R. A., and Silver, A. F. (Eds.). *Adances in Biology of Skin.* Vol. IV. *The Sebaceous Glands.* New York: Pergamon, 1963.

Strauss, J. S., and Pochi, P. E. Histology, Histochemistry, and Electron Microscopy of Sebaceous Glands in Man. In O. Gans and G. K. Steigleder (Eds.). *Handbuch der Haut-und Geschlechtskrankheiten.* Berlin: Springer-Verlag, 1968.

Eccrine Glands

Dobson, R. L., and Sato, K. The secretion of salt and water by the eccrine sweat gland. *Arch. Dermatol.* 105:366, 1972.

Ellis, R. A. Eccrine Sweat Glands: Elektron [sic] Microscopy; Cytochemistry and Anatomy. In O. Gans and G. K. Steigleder (Eds.), *Handbuch der Haut-und Geschlechtskrankheiten.* Vol. 1. Berlin: Springer-Verlag, 1968. Pp. 224–266.

Munger, B. L. The ultrastructure and histophysiology of human eccrine sweat glands. *J. Biophys. Biochem. Cytol.* 11:385, 1961.

Apocrine Glands

Hurley, H. J., and Shelley, W. B. *The Human Apocrine Gland in Health and Disease.* Springfield, Ill.: Thomas, 1960.

Shehadeh, N. H., and Kligman, A. M. Bacteria responsible for axillary odor. II. *J. Invest. Dermatol.* 41:3, 1963.

General

Ackerman, A. B. Skin: Structure and Function. In *Histologic Diagnosis of Inflammatory Skin Diseases.* Philadelphia: Lea & Febiger, 1978.

Bloom, W., and Fawcett, D. W. Skin. In *A Textbook of Histology* (10th ed.). Philadelphia: Saunders, 1975.

Lever, W. F., and Schaumberg-Lever, G. Histology of the Skin. In *Histopathology of the Skin* (6th ed.). Philadelphia: Lippincott, 1983.

Mihm, M. C., Soter, N. A., Dvorak, H. F., et al. The structure of normal skin and the morphology of atopic eczema. *J. Invest. Dermatol.* 67:305, 1976.

Montagna, W., and Parakkal, P. F. *The Structure and Function of Skin* (3d ed.). New York: Academic, 1974.

Pinkus, H., and Mehregan, A. H. Normal Structure of Skin. In H. Pinkus, *A Guide to Dermatohistopathology* (3d ed.). New York: Appleton-Century-Crofts, 1981.

Chapter 2

Glossary

This glossary introduces the terminology used in dermatopathology. Common pathologic alterations and definitions are listed in the left column. Some diseases in which these alterations can occur are listed on the right.

acantholysis Loss of cohesion between epidermal cells or adnexal keratinocytes owing to loss of intercellular cement substances or faulty formation of intercellular bridges (Fig. 2-1).

Pemphigus
Benign familial pemphigus (Hailey-Hailey disease)
Keratosis follicularis (Darier's disease)
Herpes infections

acanthosis Increased thickness of the epidermis caused by hyperplasia or hypertrophy of the spinous layer.

Psoriasiform hyperplasias
Squamous cell carcinoma
Pseudoepitheliomatous hyperplasia

atrophy Decreased thickness of epidermis and/or dermis.

Lupus erythematosus
Lichen sclerosus et atrophicus
Atrophoderma

ballooning degeneration Epidermal changes characterized by cytoplasmic swelling and vacuolation.

Viral infections (verruca, herpes)
Epidermolytic hyperkeratosis

birefringence Having the power of double refraction. When examined with polarized light, certain materials "light up." In dermatopathology the most commonly encountered birefringent materials are collagen fibers, hair, silica, amyloid, and uric acid crystals (Fig. 2-2).

Amyloidosis

Fig. **2-1.** *Acantholysis from a biopsy of benign familial pemphigus (Hailey-Hailey disease). (×640)*

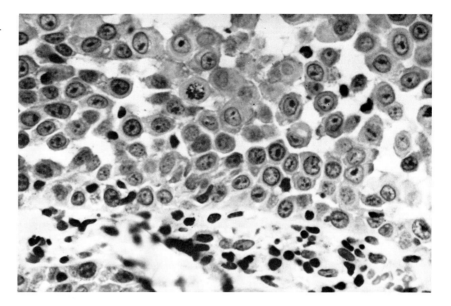

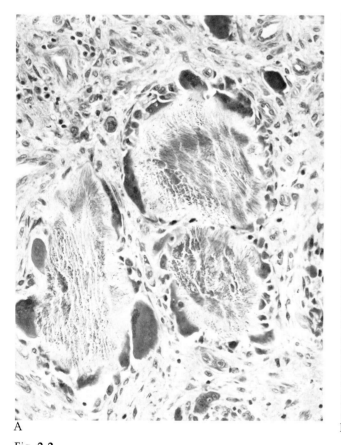

A

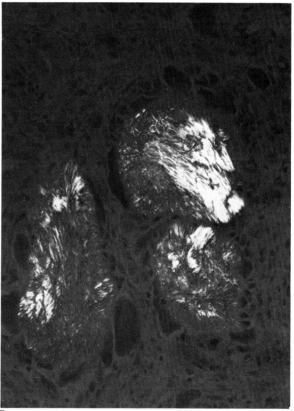

B

Fig. **2-2.**
A. *Giant cells surround sheaves of crystalline urates. (×400)*
B. *Polariscopic examination exhibits birefringence of crystalline material. (×400)*

bulla A blister. The blister cavity and fluid may be located within the epidermis (subcorneal, intraepidermal, suprabasilar) or beneath the epidermis (subepidermal) (Fig. 2-3).

See Chs. 5, 9

Civatte bodies Also called colloid, or hyaline, bodies, Civatte bodies are homogeneous, eosinophilic round structures seen in the epidermis and upper papillary dermis in various diseases. The epidermal bodies are thought to be dyskeratotic, dying, or dead epidermal cells whereas the dermal structures probably represent fragments of altered basement membrane or collagen.

Lichen planus
Lupus erythematosus

colloid bodies *See* Civatte bodies.

corps grains; corps ronds Dyskeratotic, acantholytic basophilic epidermal cells which may be oval (corps grains) or round (corps ronds). The latter usually have perinuclear halos.

Keratosis follicularis (Darier's disease)
Warty dyskeratoma
Transient acantholytic disease

decapitation secretion Term used to describe the proposed mechanism of apocrine secretion whereby the apical portion of the cell is "pinched off" and released into the lumen of the gland (Fig 1-11).

dyskeratosis Abnormal, imperfect, or incomplete keratinization of individual epidermal cells. Histologically dyskeratotic cells usually are intensely eosinophilic and may contain a small, dense basophilic nuclear remnant (Fig. 2-4). Dyskeratosis also refers to densely basophilic cytoplasmic change (as in Darier's disease).

Fig. **2-3.** *Bullous (and vesicular) disorders are classified according to the location of the cleft. (Reprinted with permission from T. H. Kwan and M. C. Mihm. The Skin. In S. L. Robbins and R. S. Cotran (Eds.),* Pathologic Basis of Disease *(2d ed.). Philadelphia: Saunders, 1979.)*

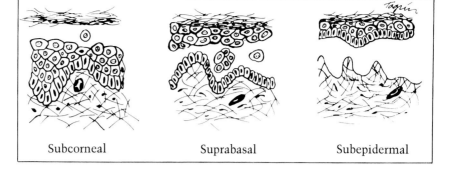

Subcorneal   Suprabasal   Subepidermal

Fig. **2-4.** *Dyskeratotic cells in erythema multiforme. (×400)*

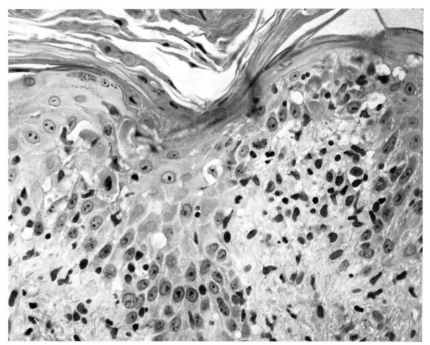

exocytosis A term used in dermatopathology to indicate inflammatory cells and erythrocytes that are "out of place," i.e., in the epidermis instead of the dermis or blood vessels.

Mycosis fungoides
Pityriasis lichenoides et varioliformis acuta
Parapsoriasis en plaques

fibrinoid necrosis of blood vessels Deposition of eosinophilic fibrin in and around vessel walls (Fig. 2-5).

Cutaneous necrotizing vasculitis

foam cell Lipid-laden macrophage with pale vacuolated or "foamy" cytoplasm and a round to oval dark-staining nucleus.

Xanthomas
Juvenile xanthogranuloma

ghost cell (shadow cell) Pale, faintly eosinophilic cell with central unstained area where the nucleus was located (Fig. 2-6).

Pilomatrixoma

giant cell Large, multinucleate cells that may be seen in the epidermis or dermis. *Epidermal multinucleate keratinocytes* usually are seen in a variety of situations; when associated with viral infections such as herpes and measles, characteristic nuclear inclusions and cytopathic effects can be observed. Multinucleate giant cells in the dermis may be derived from *nevocellular nevus cells* or histiocytes. Histiocytic giant cells with nuclei arranged in a horseshoe at the periphery are known as *Langhans-type* giant cells. *Touton-type* histiocytic giant cells characteristically have a ring of nuclei arranged around a central core of cytoplasm; foamy cytoplasm is seen peripheral to the nuclei. *Foreign-body* histiocytic giant cells have nuclei haphazardly scattered throughout the cytoplasm.

Fig. **2-5.** *Fibrinoid necrosis and nuclear dust in cutaneous necrotizing vasculitis. (×400)*

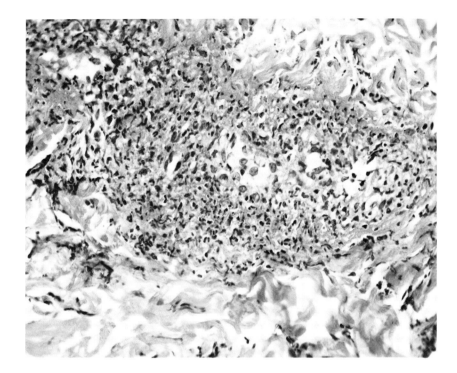

Fig. **2-6.** *Ghost (shadow) cells in pilomatrixoma. (×400)*

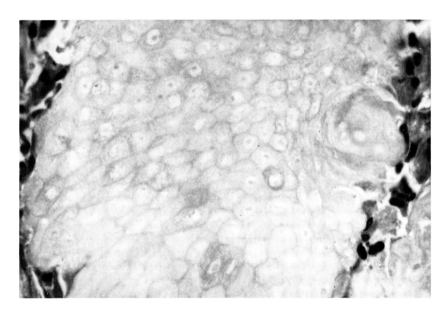

Grenz zone From the German *Granze,* meaning "border." A clear area of uninvolved (usually papillary) dermis between epidermis and dermal inflammatory or neoplastic infiltrate.

Granuloma faciale
Lymphoma cutis
Leukemia cutis

horn cyst Intraepidermal, keratin-filled space resembling a cyst. "Pseudohorn cysts" are formed by obvious epidermal invagination.

Seborrheic keratosis

hyperkeratosis An increase in the thickness of the stratum corneum that is clinically manifested as scale. The thickened stratum corneum may retain its basketweave pattern, may appear delicately layered (stratified, laminated), or may become dense and compact. The term *hyperkeratosis* is used to describe the thickening of the normal anucleate stratum corneum in contradistinction to *parakeratosis,* which describes the thickened stratum corneum with retained keratinocyte nuclei. Parakeratosis, which infers incomplete keratinization, is seen normally in mucous membranes and abnormally in association with numerous inflammatory and neoplastic processes.

Lamellar ichthyosis and ichthyosis vulgaris
Pityriasis rosea
Psoriasis

Langhans giant cell *See* giant cell.

melanophage Histiocyte containing phagocytized melanin.

Postinflammatory hyperpigmentation
Lentigo
Cellular blue nevus
Fixed drug eruption

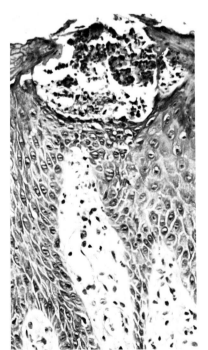

Fig. 2-7. *Munro microabscess in psoriasis. (×256)*

Munro microabscess Neutrophil aggregates within the stratum corneum (Fig. 2-7).

Psoriasis
Seborrheic dermatitis

necrobiosis Refers to altered collagen that loses its normal eosinophilic coloration and fibrillar appearance, becoming slightly bluish, "smudged."

Granuloma annulare
Necrobiosis lipoidica

nuclear dust Nuclear fragments scattered in the dermis, usually around blood vessels (Fig. 2-5).

Vasculitis

papillomatosis Epidermal and papillary dermal proliferation upward in irregular waves or spires (Fig. 2-8).

Seborrheic keratosis, hyperkeratotic type

Pautrier microabscess A collection of three or more atypical mononuclear cells within the epidermis, often surrounded by a clear space, or "halo."

Mycosis fungoides

pigment incontinence Deposition of melanin in the dermis, as either free particles or particles within macrophages.

Lentigo
Postinflammation hyperpigmentation

pleomorphic Usually refers to variation in nuclear size and shape.

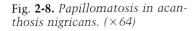

Fig. **2-8.** *Papillomatosis in acanthosis nigricans. (×64)*

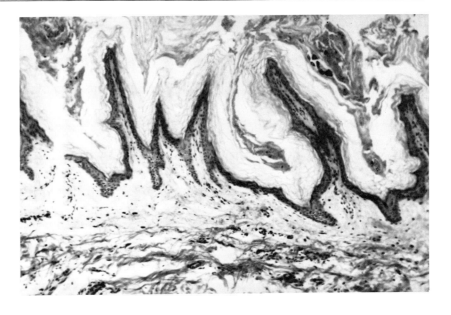

polymorphous With reference to inflammatory infiltrates, this term connotes a mixed infiltrate, e.g., a mixture of lymphocytes, eosinophils, and plasma cells, in contrast to a purely lymphocytic infiltrate.

Mycosis fungoides
Arthropod bite reaction

pseudoepitheliomatous hyperplasia Irregular acanthosis with downward proliferation of the epidermis accompanied by chronic dermal inflammation. The massive degree of proliferation may simulate a well-differentiated squamous cell carcinoma.

Chronic cutaneous ulcers
Granulomatous infections (fungal and mycobacterial)
Pyoderma gangrenosum
Pemphigus vegetans
Iododerma

pustule Fluid-filled space (usually intraepidermal) containing leukocytes and products of inflammation.

Impetigo
Pustular psoriasis
Erythema toxicum neonatorum
Incontinentia pigmenti, first stage

pyknosis Condensation of nuclear chromatin, producing a dense, shrunken-appearing mass.

Usually occurs with cell death

reticular degeneration of epidermis Intracellular edema of epidermal cells with retention of cell walls, producing a reticular, or netlike, appearance (Fig. 2-9).

Viral infections
Epidermolytic hyperkeratosis
Acute eczematous dermatitis

spongiform pustule Collections of neutrophils within the epidermis, often surrounded by clear spaces, or "halos," thus somewhat resembling a sponge.

Psoriasis
Reiter's disease
Geographic tongue
Pustular psoriasis

spongiosis Intercellular edema in the epidermis with separation of keratinocytes, stretching, and rupture of intercellular bridges (Fig. 2-10). Edematous spaces can coalesce, forming spongiotic vesicles.

Acute eczematous dermatitis

Fig. **2-9.** *Reticular degeneration in epidermolytic hyperkeratosis. (×400)*

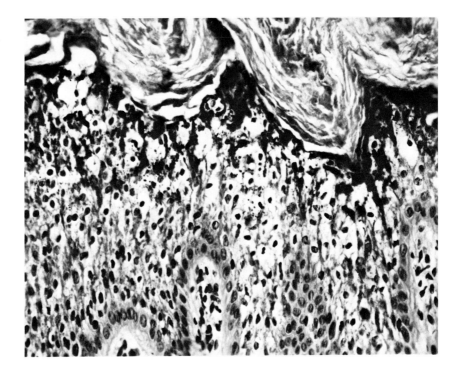

Fig. **2-10.** *Spongiosis and spongiotic vesicles in a biopsy of nummular eczema. (×160)*

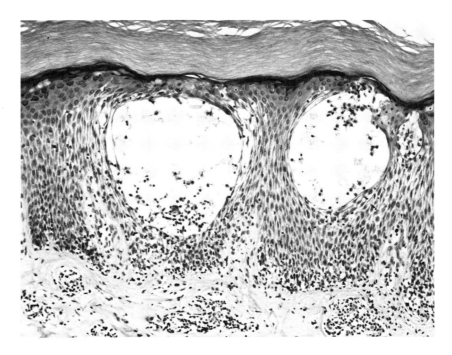

squamotization Replacement of normally cuboidal or columnar, slightly basophilic basal cells by polygonal or flattened eosinophilic keratinocytes (Fig. 2-11).

Lichen planus
Lupus erythematosus
Graft-versus-host reaction

squamous eddies; squamous pearls Concentric layers of squamous cells with increasing keratinization centrally.

Irritated seborrheic keratosis
Squamous cell carcinoma

storiform Refers to the cartwheel pattern that is formed by spindle cells, which appear to emanate from a central anucleate area, recalling the spokes of a wheel. This pattern frequently is seen in fibrous histiocytoma and dermatofibrosarcoma protuberans, but other spindle-cell tumors such as leiomyomas can mimic this pattern.

Fibrous histiocytoma
Dermatofibrosarcoma protuberans

Touton giant cell *See* giant cell.

vesicle Small blister (Fig. 2-3).

See Chs. 5, 9

villus Dermal papilla lined by a row of basal cells, thus resembling "tombstones on a hill" (Fig. 2-12).

Pemphigus
Darier's disease
Warty dyskeratoma

Fig. **2-11.** *Squamotization in lichen planus. (×400)*

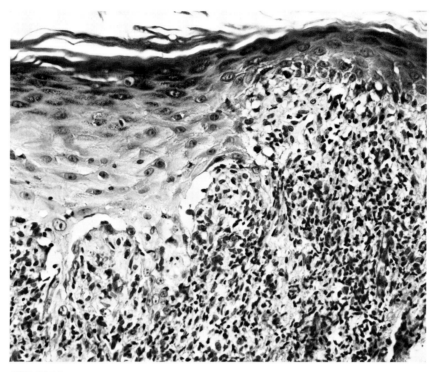

Fig. **2-12.** *Villi in a biopsy of pemphigus vulgaris. (×256)*

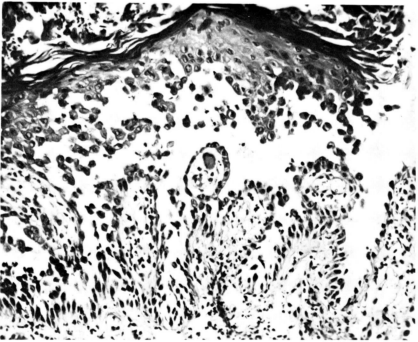

Part **II**

Epidermis

Chapter 3

Hyperkeratosis With or Without Alteration of the Granular Layer

I. Ichthyosis vulgaris
II. Dominant congenital ichthyosiform erythroderma (epidermolytic hyperkeratosis)
III. Recessive congenital ichthyosiform erythroderma (lamellar ichthyosis)
IV. X-linked ichthyosis
V. Acquired ichthyosis
VI. Dermatophytosis

The predominant histologic change demonstrated by the diseases discussed in this chapter is hyperkeratosis, or thickening of the stratum corneum. With the exception of dominant ichthyosiform erythroderma (epidermolytic hyperkeratosis), there is very little alteration in the epidermis or dermis in these diseases; in fact, this change may be subtle and easily overlooked on cursory examination. Many other diseases have hyperkeratosis as a prominent histologic feature, but the hyperkeratosis is associated with other epidermal changes such as hyperplasia, atrophy, and/or dermal inflammation. These diseases are discussed in subsequent chapters.

The Reactive Process and the Disease	Histopathology	Comments
I. Ichthyosis vulgaris	1. Mild to moderate basket-weave or compact **hyperkeratosis** 2. Decreased to absent granular layer (**hypogranulosis**) 3. Flattened rete ridges	*Hypogranulosis* may be seen in: Ichthyosis vulgaris Psoriasis Normal mucous membrane Under parakeratotic scale associated with inflammation
	4. Atrophic to absent sebaceous glands.	Characteristic histologic changes of ichthyosis are best seen in areas of maximal involvement; biopsies obtained from less severely affected areas may be histologically indistinguishable from normal skin
II. Dominant congenital ichthyosiform erythroderma (*epidermolytic hyperkeratosis*) (Fig. 3-1)	1. Marked **compact hyperkeratosis**	Clinical term *epidermolytic hyperkeratosis* is synonymous with dominant congenital ichthyosiform erythroderma; the term also refers to the histologic changes of reticular degeneration and abnormal granule formation seen in other diseases
	2. Prominent granular layer with **reticular degeneration** and abnormal granules (irregular, dark basophilic keratohyaline and eosinophilic trichohyalinelike granules) 3. Intercellular edema of slightly thickened epidermis	Foci of *epidermolytic hyperkeratosis* may be seen in: Normal skin Actinic keratosis Lining of an epidermal cyst Adjacent to or within squamous cell carcinoma Seborrheic keratosis Granuloma annulare Verruca plana Dermatofibroma Systematized linear epidermal nevus

Fig. **3-1.** *Dominant congenital ichthyosiform erythroderma.*
A. *Papillary epidermal hyperplasia with epidermolytic hyperkeratosis.* (×160)
B. Epidermolytic hyperkeratosis *refers to hyperkeratosis and reticular degeneration of keratinocytes with the formation of large, irregularly clumped keratohyaline granules. This histologic pattern occurs in a variety of other conditions besides ichthyosis.* (×400)

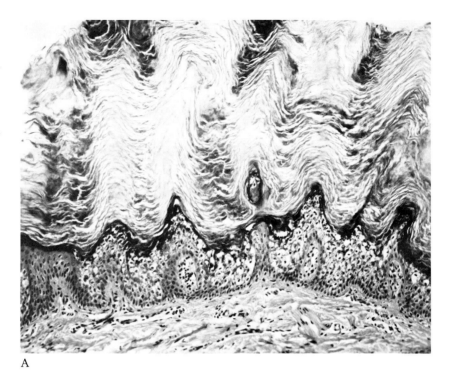

A

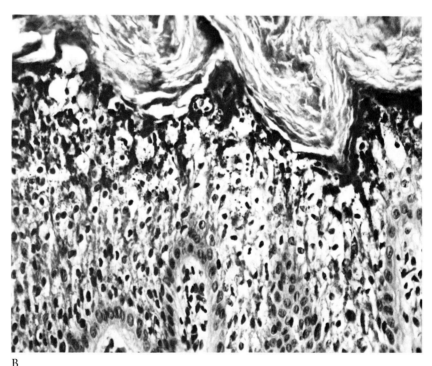

B

III. Recessive congenital ichthyosiform erythroderma (*lamellar ichthyosis*) (Fig. 3-2)

1. Moderate **hyperkeratosis**
2. Focal parakeratosis
3. Normal to increased granular layer

IV. X-linked ichthyosis

1. Moderate compact, laminated, eosinophilic **hyperkeratosis**
2. Parakeratosis
3. Increased granular layer (**hypergranulosis**)
4. Sparse perivenular and periappendageal lymphocytic infiltrate

> *Hypergranulosis* may be seen in any hyperkeratotic lesion but is characteristically seen in:
>
> Epidermolytic hyperkeratosis
> X-linked ichthyosis
> Lichen simplex chronicus
> Epidermal nevus
> Verruca vulgaris
> Lichen planus and its variants

V. Acquired ichthyosis

Histology is identical to that of ichthyosis vulgaris

VI. Dermatophytosis (Fig. 3-3A)

1. Hyphal forms are present in the stratum corneum and sometimes the stratum granulosum
2. Yeast forms may be present; yeast forms alone can be seen as normal commensals
3. Parakeratosis, epidermal hyperplasia, spongiosis, vesiculation, and exocytosis are all variable
4. Perivascular and superficial dermal lymphohistiocytic infiltrates are typical
5. Neutrophilic infiltrates within the epidermis are variable

Special stains (see Appendix) such as PAS highlight organisms

Candidiasis exhibits yeast and pseudohyphal forms (Fig. 3-3B)

Fig. **3-2.** *Recessive congenital ichthyosiform erythroderma (lamellar ichthyosis). The stratum spinosum appears unremarkable, but the stratum corneum exhibits compact hyperkeratosis with platelike scales. Compare this stratum corneum with that of Figure 1-2. (×256)*

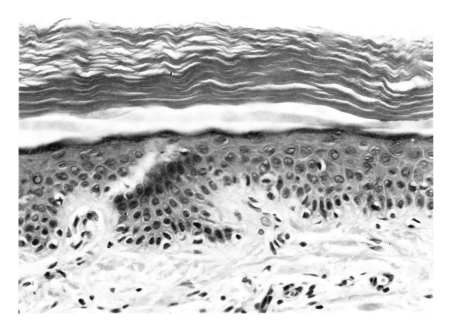

Fig. **3-3.**
A. *Dermatophytosis. PAS stain delineates these septate hyphal forms within the stratum corneum. (×400)*
B. *Candidiasis. Yeast and pseudohyphal forms are present within the stratum corneum and stratum granulosum. (×400)*

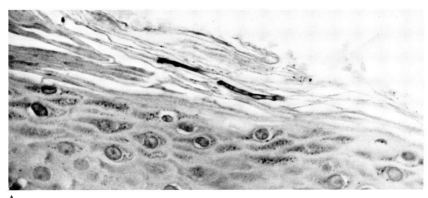

A

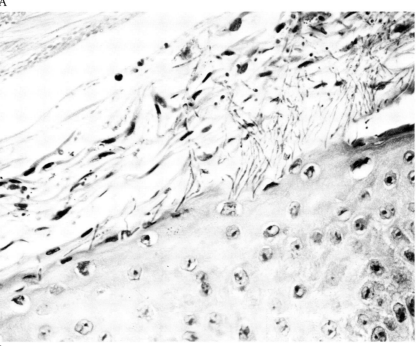

B

Suggested Reading
Ichthyosis

Ackerman, A. B. Histopathologic concept of epidermolytic hyperkeratosis. *Arch. Dermatol.* 102:253, 1970.

Dykes, P. J., and Mark, R. Acquired ichthyosis: Multiple causes for an acquired generalized disturbance in desquamation. *Br. J. Dermatol.* 97:327, 1977.

Feinstein, A., Ackerman, A. B., and Ziprkowski, L. Histology of autosomal dominant ichthyosis vulgaris and X-linked ichthyosis. *Arch. Dermatol.* 101:524, 1970.

Flint, G. L., Flam, M., and Soter, N. A. Acquired ichthyosis: A sign of nonlymphoproliferative malignant disorders. *Arch. Dermatol.* 111:1446, 1975.

Frost, P. Ichthyosiform dermatoses. *J. Invest. Dermatol.* 60:541, 1973.

Goldsmith, L. A. The ichthyoses. *Prog. Med. Genet.* 1:185, 1976.

Marks, R., and Dykes, P. J. *The Ichthyoses.* New York: S.P. Medical and Scientific Books, 1978.

Vandersteen, P. R., and Muller, S. A. Lamellar ichthyosis: An enzyme histochemical light, and electron microscopic study. *Arch. Dermatol.* 106:694, 1972.

Van Scott, E. J., and Yu, R. J. "Ichthyosiform dermatoses" by Frost and Van Scott, August 1966. Commentary: Ichthyosis and keratinization. Concepts in transition. *Arch. Dermatol.* 118:846, 1982.

Dermatophytosis

Rebell, G., and Iaplin, D. *Dermatophytes: Their Recognition and Identification* (rev. ed.). Coral Gables, Fla.: University of Miami Press, 1970.

Stretcher, G. S., and Smith, J. G. Diagnosis and treatment of cutaneous fungus diseases. *D.M.* 1–40, September 1975.

Chapter 4

Psoriasiform Hyperplasia

I. Psoriasiform hyperplasia, psoriatic type
  A. Psoriasis
  B. Chronic eczematous dermatitis
    1. Unclassified or nonspecific
    2. Atopic dermatitis or eczema—chronic lichenified plaque
    3. Allergic contact dermatitis, chronic
    4. Lichen simplex chronicus
    5. Prurigo nodularis
    6. Nummular eczema
  C. Seborrheic dermatitis
  D. Exfoliative dermatitis (erythroderma)
  E. Parapsoriasis en plaques
  F. Pityriasis rubra pilaris
  G. Incontinentia pigmenti, second stage: verrucous lesions
  H. Inflammatory pityriasis rosea
II. Psoriasiform hyperplasia with pustules
  A. Pustular psoriasis including generalized and localized forms, acrodermatitis continua of Hallopeau, and impetigo herpetiformis
  B. Reiter's syndrome
III. Psoriasiform hyperplasia with polymorphous infiltrate
  A. Arthropod bite reaction
  B. Mycosis fungoides
  C. Secondary syphilis

Psoriasiform hyperplasia is a term used to describe epidermal hyperplasia with elongation of the rete ridges. The prototype of psoriasiform hyperplasia is, of course, psoriasis, but it may be seen in chronic eczematous dermatitis, seborrheic dermatitis, exfoliative dermatitis, parapsoriasis en plaques, pityriasis rubra pilaris, incontinentia pigmenti, and inflammatory pityriasis rosea.

Psoriasiform hyperplasia with pustule formation is seen in pustular psoriasis and its variants, acrodermatitis continua, and impetigo herpetiformis as well as Reiter's syndrome.

In contrast to the above diseases, psoriasiform hyperplasia may be accompanied by an intense polymorphous inflammatory infiltrate as in mycosis fungoides, arthropod bite reaction, and secondary syphilis.

The Reactive Process and the Disease	Histopathology	Comments
I. Psoriasiform hyperplasia **A.** Psoriasis (Fig. 4-1)	1. Laminated **hyperkeratosis** 2. Confluent or focal **parakeratosis** 3. Focal **hypogranulosis** 4. Thin suprapapillary plate	The granular layer can be seen in early and treated psoriatic lesions

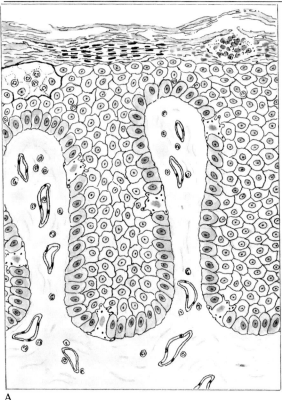

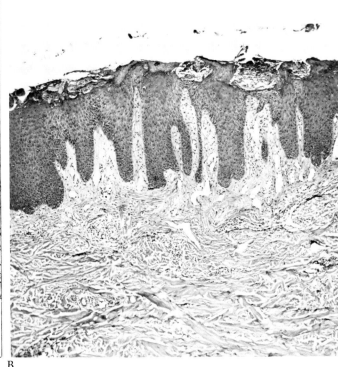

A   B

Fig. **4-1.** *Psoriasis.*
A, B. Psoriasiform hyperplasia, hyperkeratosis, parakeratosis, hypogranulosis, suprapapillary thinning, venular ectasia, spongiform pustules, and Munro microabscesses are characteristic. (B, ×64)

Fig. **4-1** (continued)
   *C. Spongiform pustule.
      (×400) See Figure 3-5,
      pustular psoriasis.*
   *D. A Munro microabscess,
      suprapapillary thinning,
      and venular ectasia.
      (×256.)*

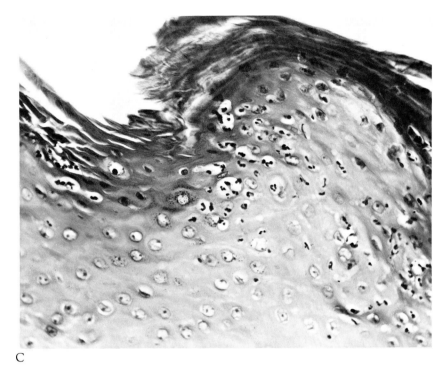

C

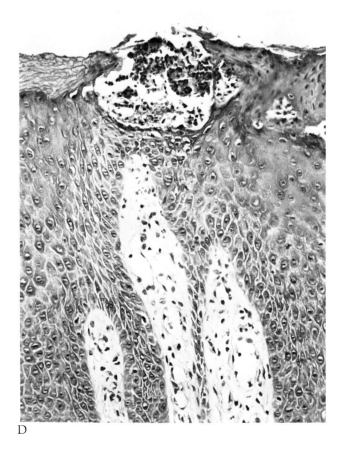

D

5. Relatively regular **psoriasiform hyperplasia** with elongated, club-shaped rete ridges
6. **Spongiform pustule** of Kogoj and/or **Munro microabscess**

In early lesions of psoriasis, epidermal hyperplasia may be minimal

---

Spongiform pustules are present in:

Psoriasis, all types
Subcorneal pustular dermatosis
Reiter's syndrome
Geographic tongue (Fig. 4-2)
Candidiasis
Halogenodermas
Impetigo

---

7. Elongation and edema of dermal papillae
8. Papillary vessel ectasia, proliferation, and tortuosity
9. Sparse perivenular mononuclear cell infiltrate

B. Chronic eczematous dermatitis
   1. Unclassified or nonspecific

1. Hyperkeratosis
2. Focal hypergranulosis
3. Marked **psoriasiform hyperplasia**
4. Slight intercellular edema (spongiosis)
5. Superficial perivascular lymphohistiocytic infiltrate
6. Papillary dermal edema and **fibrosis**
7. Pigment incontinence

Chronic eczematous dermatitis is a general term applied to an end-stage reaction pattern produced by a wide variety of causes

---

Entities exhibiting the histologic pattern of *chronic eczematous dermatitis* include:

Atopic dermatitis
Nummular eczema
Lichen simplex chronicus
Chronic contact dermatitis
Prurigo nodularis
Dermatophytosis
Pityriasis rubra pilaris

---

2. Atopic dermatitis or eczema—chronic lichenified plaque

1. Irregular hyperkeratosis
2. Irregular psoriasiform hyperplasia
3. Slight intercellular edema
4. Occasional lymphocytes invading epidermis
5. Papillary dermal fibrosis
6. Mild to moderate perivascular and intervascular mononuclear cell infiltrate

Fig. **4-2.** *Geographic tongue. Location on the tongue, epidermal hyperplasia, and numerous Munro microabscesses are typical of this disorder. A similar pattern can be seen in psoriasis, candidiasis, and Reiter's disease. (×160.)*

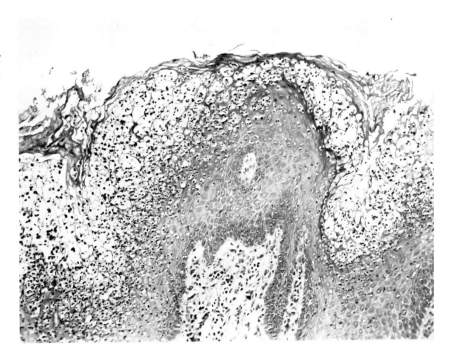

3. Allergic contact dermatitis, chronic

1. Hyperkeratosis
2. Variable psoriasiform hyperplasia
3. Intercellular edema
4. Lymphocytes and **eosinophils** arranged in nodular aggregates about vessels in superficial dermis

Lesions of acute contact dermatitis after several days show epidermal hyperplasia with spongiotic vesicle formation

4. Lichen simplex chronicus (Fig. 4-3)

1. Hyperkeratosis
2. **Hypergranulosis**
3. Psoriasiform hyperplasia with **irregular elongation** of rete ridges
4. Perivascular infiltrate of lymphocytes and eosinophils
5. **Lamellar fibrosis** of papillary dermis
6. Perineural fibrosis

5. Prurigo nodularis

1. **Progressive elongation of rete ridges from edge to center of lesion**
2. Center of lesion may exhibit focal ulceration with fibrin at its base (site of excoriation)
3. **Marked papillary dermal fibrosis and sclerosis**
4. Perineural fibrosis and endoneural hypertrophy
5. Blood vessel proliferation and ectasia
6. Variable superficial dermal infiltrate, often containing numerous eosinophils

Epidermal hyperplasia may simulate pseudoepitheliomatous hyperplasia

6. Nummular eczema

1. Hyperkeratosis
2. Parakeratosis
3. Psoriasiform hyperplasia
4. Spongiosis and intraepidermal vesicle formation

Nummular eczema may resemble acute and chronic contact dermatitis or atopic dermatitis

C. Seborrheic dermatitis

1. Hyperkeratosis
2. Focal parakeratosis
3. Slight to moderate psoriasiform hyperplasia
4. Slight intracellular and intercellular edema (**spongiosis**)
5. Mild perivascular mononuclear cell infiltrate
6. Occasional Munro microabscess

A differentiating point between psoriasis and seborrheic dermatitis is the presence of spongiosis in seborrheic dermatitis

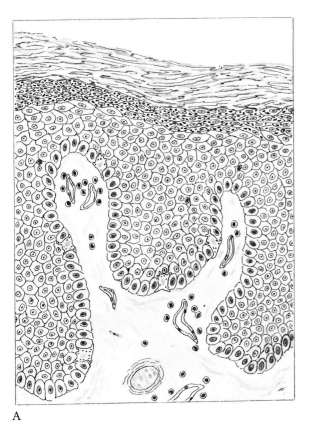

A

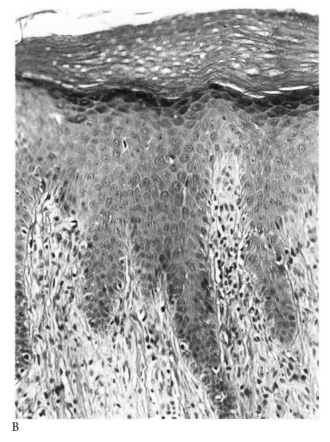

B

Fig. **4-3.** *Lichen simplex chronicus. Irregular psoriasiform hyperplasia, hypergranulosis, a variable degree of perivascular infiltrate, and papillary dermal fibrosis are commonly seen in this disorder. (B, ×256)*

D. Exfoliative dermatitis (erythroderma)

1. Hyperkeratosis
2. Parakeratosis
3. Intercelluar and intracellular edema
4. Psoriasiform hyperplasia
5. Edema of papillary dermis
6. Vascular ectasia
7. Dermal infiltrate of lymphocytes, plasma cells, and occasional eosinophils
8. Exocytosis of mononuclear cells into epidermis

The histology of *exfoliative dermatitis* may vary according to etiology. Various causes include:

Preexisting cutaneous diseases (psoriasis, atopic eczema, mycosis fungoides, lichen planus, seborrheic dermatitis, pemphigus foliaceus, pityriasis rubra pilaris, stasis dermatitis, ichthyosis)

Systemic diseases (leukemia, lymphoma, carcinoma of the lung or rectum, multiple myeloma, Sézary's syndrome)

Drugs [aspirin, arsenic, barbiturates, codeine, diphenylhydantoin (Dilantin), gold, iodine, isoniazid, mephenytoin, mercury, penicillin, quinacrine, quinadine, sulfonamides, trimethadione]

E. Parapsoriasis en plaques (Fig. 4-4)

1. Hyperkeratosis
2. **Mounds of parakeratotic scale** either closely adherent to or separated in toto from the underlying epidermis
3. Normal, hyperplastic, or occasionally atrophic epidermis
4. **Invasion of epidermis by lymphocytes,** ocasionally forming
5. Pautrier-like microabscesses
6. Grenz zone
7. **Bandlike superficial lymphohistiocytic infiltrate** may include eosinophils and plasma cells.

F. Pityriasis rubra pilaris

1. Follicular hyperkeratosis and occasionally "shoulder" parakeratosis
2. Focal parakeratosis
3. Mild psoriasiform hyperplasia
4. Basal vacuolation frequently present
5. Scant lymphohistiocytic perivascular infiltrate

Shoulder parakeratosis describes a column of parakeratotic cells at the edge of the follicular orifice

Pityriasis rubra pilaris may be histologically indistinguishable from chronic eczematous dermatitis

Fig. **4-4.** *Parapsoriasis en plaques. Psoriasiform hyperplasia, focal parakeratosis, exocytosis, intraepidermal mononuclear microabscesses, vacuolation at the dermoepidermal junction, and perivenular lymphohistiocytic infiltrates are present. Parapsoriasis, which is sometimes difficult to define, may exhibit a variety of histologic patterns, ranging from almost normal to the above. Focal parakeratosis is the histologic correlate of the fine, branlike scale observed clinically. (×160)*

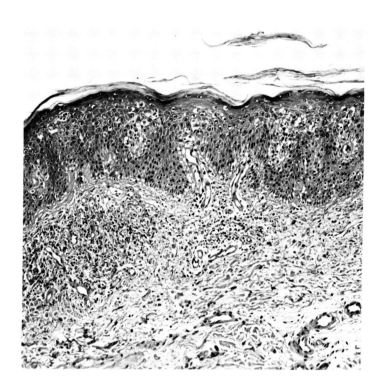

G. Incontinentia pigmenti, second stage: verrucous lesions (see Fig. 4-3)

1. Hyperkeratosis
2. Irregular papillomatosis
3. Marked psoriasiform hyperplasia
4. **Intraepidermal keratinization in whorls**
5. Individual **dyskeratotic cells** scattered throughout the epidermis
6. Mild dermal infiltrate of lymphocytes and histiocytes

H. Inflammatory pityriasis rosea (see Fig. 9-10)

1. Focal mounds of parakeratosis, sometimes called **skipping scale**
2. Occasional scattered dyskeratotic cells in stratum spinosum
3. Variable psoriasiform hyperplasia
4. **Exocytosis** of lymphocytes and erythrocytes
5. Intraepidermal microabscesses containing mononuclear cells
6. **Vacuolation** along the dermal epidermal junction
7. Superficial perivenular lymphohistiocytic infiltrate
8. Extravasation of erythrocytes variable, but may be extensive

See also Ch. 9, II. I; Ch. 11, I.D

II. Psoriasiform hyperplasia with pustules

A. Pustular psoriasis including generalized and localized forms, acrodermatitis continua of Hallopeau, and impetigo herpetiformis (Fig. 4-5)

1. Discrete, large intraepidermal **pustules** filled with many neutrophils and surrounded by spongiform pustules
2. Variable psoriasiform hyperplasia; other changes characteristic of psoriasis may be absent

In localized forms of pustular psoriasis, the pustules tend to be unilocular (for differential diagnosis of spongiform pustule, see Ch. 4, I.A.6)

B. Reiter's syndrome

Similar to pustular psoriasis but hyperkeratosis, parakeratosis, and psoriasiform hyperplasia are more prominent

Fig. **4-5.** *Pustular psoriasis. An intraepidermal pustule with adjacent numerous spongiform pustules on a background of psoriasiform hyperplasia is typical. (×160)*

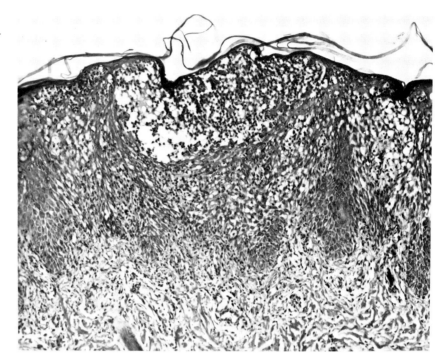

III. Psoriasiform hyperplasia
with polymorphous
infiltrate

A. Arthropod bite reaction
(see Fig. 11-2)

1. **Marked psoriasiform hyper-plasia**
2. An erosion or ulceration may be present
3. Dense, superficial and deep perivascular and/or diffuse infiltrate of lymphocytes, histiocytes, plasma cells, and numerous **eosinophils**
4. Endothelial cell swelling and proliferation
5. Inflammatory infiltrate and endothelial proliferation extend deep into the reticular dermis, even into the subcutaneous fat
6. Lymphoid follicles with germinal centers may be present

See also Ch. 10, IV; Ch. 11, I. F

B. Mycosis fungoides
(Fig. 4-6)

1. Psoriasiform hyperplasia
2. Dermal infiltrate of variable atypical mononuclear cells admixed with eosinophils, neutrophils, and plasma cells. The distribution of the infiltrate may be bandlike, nodular, perivascular, or any combination of the above

Present in the infiltrate are: (1) small, atypical mononuclear cells, 8 to 15 μm in diameter with hyperchromatic convoluted nuclei and minimal cytoplasm; and (2) *larger atypical hyperchromatic mononuclear cells* measuring up to 20 to 25 μm; finding these larger atypical cells is most helpful in establishing the diagnosis of mycosis fungoides

The presence of numerous eosinophils in a dermal infiltrate may be a harbinger of mycosis fungoides

3. **Epidermal invasion by larger atypical cells**

Other diseases with infiltrates that may contain small, *atypical mononuclear cells* include:

Lichen planus
Pityriasis rosea
Chronic contact dermatitis
Basal cell carcinoma
Actinic keratosis
Fixed drug eruption

Fig. **4-6.** *Mycosis fungoides.*
A. *Mycosis fungoides, plaque type. Pautrier's microabscesses and a diffuse dermal infiltrate with numerous atypical lymphocytes are characteristic. (×100)*
B. *Mycosis fungoides, epidermotropic type. An infiltrate of atypical hyperchromatic lymphocytes is present within the lower epidermis. (×400)*
C. *Mycosis fungoides, epidermotropic type. The large cell size and convoluted nuclear outlines of the mycosis cells are easier to appreciate in this Giemsa-stained 1-μm Epon-embedded section from the same patient illustrated in B. (×1008)*

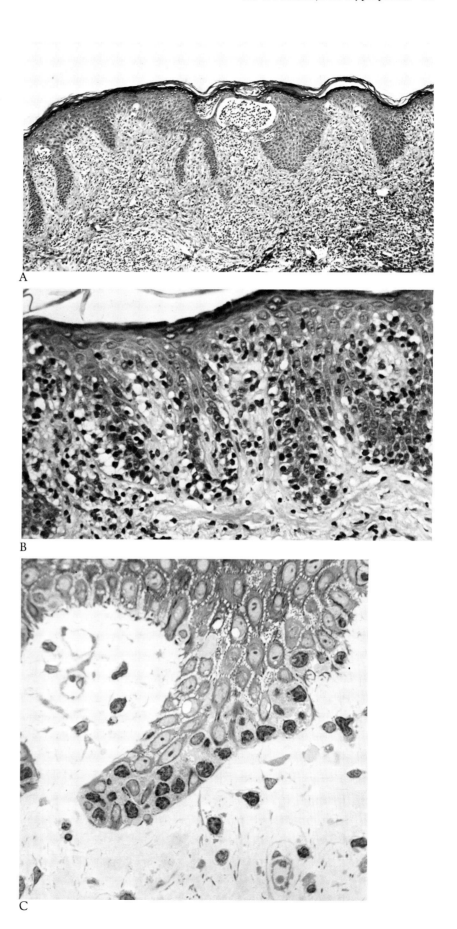

A

B

C

4. **Pautrier microabscess**

Microabscesses similar to those in mycosis fungoides (*Pautrier-like*) may be seen in:

Pityriasis rosea
Dermal contact dermatitis (formaldehyde, nickel)
Parapsoriasis en plaques
Leukemia cutis (acute myelomonocytic leukemia)
Drug eruptions
Pityriasis lichenoides et varioliformis acuta
Poikiloderma vasculare atrophicans

5. Invasion of appendageal epithelium by atypical cells

C. Secondary syphilis (Fig. 4-7)

1. Parakeratosis
2. Psoriasiform hyperplasia
3. Edema and occasional fibrosis of papillary dermis
4. Dermal infiltrate
   a. Bandlike infiltrate of lymphocytes and **plasma cells, often obscuring the dermoepidermal interface**
   b. Superficial and deep perivascular infiltrate of lymphocytes, histiocytes, and **plasma cells**
   c. Epithelioid granulomas admixed with **plasma cells** may be seen
5. **Endothelial cell proliferation and hypertrophy**
6. Pigment incontinence common

Special silver stains (see Appendix) may demonstrate spirochetes within the epidermis or around blood vessels in the upper dermis

Plasma cell infiltrates can be seen in:

Paramucosal surfaces, face and scalp
Secondary syphilis
Mycosis fungoides
Folliculitis
Foreign-body reaction
Rhinoscleroma
Basal cell carcinoma
Actinic keratosis
Syringocystadenoma papilliferum

See also Ch. 10, XIII

Fig. **4-7.** *Secondary syphilis. Psoriasiform hyperplasia with vacuolation at the dermoepidermal junction, exocytosis, perivenular infiltrate of lymphocytes, plasma cells, and endothelial cell swelling are characteristic (A). Sometimes (but not here) the infiltrate contains numerous histiocytes, forming "shoddy granulomas." Plasma cells and endothelial changes (B) usually are considered the hallmark of syphilis, but 25 percent of cases in one series (Abell, Marks, and Wilson-Jones) did not show plasma cells in biopsies. Serologic confirmation should always be obtained. (A, ×160; B, ×640)*

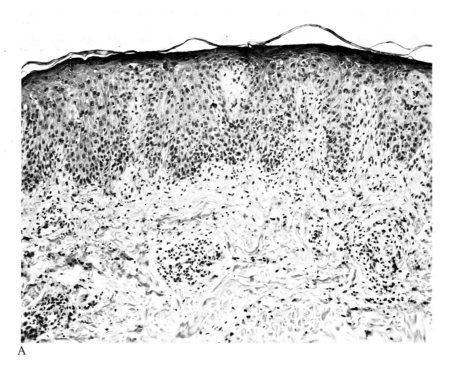

A

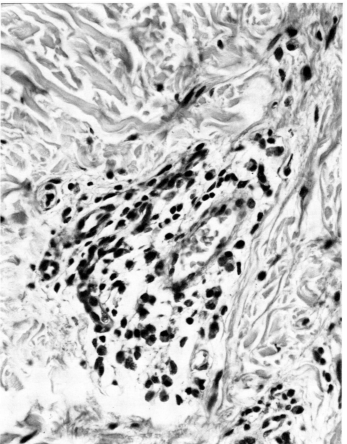

B

Suggested Reading
Psoriasis

Baker, H., and Ryan, T. J. Generalized pustular psoriasis. *Br. J. Dermatol.* 80:771, 1968.

Cox, A. J., and Watson, W. Histological variations in lesions of psoriasis. *Arch. Dermatol.* 106:503, 1972.

Gordon, M., and Johnson, W. C. Histopathology and histochemistry of psoriasis. *Arch. Dermatol.* 95:402, 1967.

Pinkus, H., and Mehregan, A. H. The primary histologic lesion of seborrheic dermatitis and psoriasis. *J. Invest. Dermatol.* 46:109, 1966.

Ragaz, A., and Ackerman, A. B. Evolution, maturation, and regression of lesions of psoriasis. *Am. J. Dermatopathol.* 1:199, 1979.

Soltani, K., and Van Scott, E. J. Patterns and sequence of tissue changes in incipient and evolving lesions of psoriasis. *Arch. Dermatol.* 106:484, 1972.

Eczematous Dermatitis

Blaylock, W. K. Atopic dermatitis: Diagnosis and pathobiology. *J. Allergy Clin. Immunol.* 57:62, 1976.

Doyle, J. A., Connolly, S. M., Hunziker, N., and Winkelmann, R. K. Prurigo nodularis: A reappraisal of the clinical and histologic features. *J. Cutan. Pathol.* 6:392, 1979.

Dvorak, H. F., Mihm, M. C., Jr., Dvorak, A. M., et al. Morphology of delayed type hypersensitivity reactions in man. I. Quantitative description of inflammatory response. *Lab. Invest.* 31:111, 1974.

Hanifin, J. M., and Lobitz, W. C. Newer concepts of atopic dermatitis. *Arch. Dermatol.* 113:663, 1977.

Mihm, M. C., Jr., Soter, N. A., Dvorak, H. F., and Austen, K. F. The structure of normal skin and the morphology of atopic eczema. *J. Invest. Dermatol.* 67:305, 1976.

Norins, A. L. Atopic dermatitis. *Ped. Clin. North Am.* 18:801, 1971.

Shaffer, B., and Beerman, H. Lichen simplex chronicus and its variants. *Arch. Dermatol. Syphilol.* 64:340, 1951.

Seborrheic Dermatitis

Ackerman, A. B. Histopathologic differentiation of eczematous dermatitides from psoriasis and seborrheic dermatitis. *Cutis* 20:619, 1977.

Pinkus, H., and Mehregan, A. H. The primary histologic lesion of seborrheic dermatitis and psoriasis. *J. Invest. Dermatol.* 46:109, 1966.

Exfoliative Dermatitis

Nicolis, G. D., and Helwig, E. B. Exfoliative dermatitis: A clinicopathologic study of 135 cases. *Arch. Dermatol.* 108:788, 1973.

Parapsoriasis

Bonvalet, D., et al. The different forms of parapsoriasis en plaques. A report of 90 cases. *Acta Derm. Venereol. (Stockh.)* 104:18, 1977.

Hu, C. H., and Winkelmann, R. K. Digitate dermatosis. A new look at symmetrical, small plaque parapsoriasis. *Arch. Dermatol.* 107:65, 1973.

Lambert, W. C. Parapsoriasis. In T. B. Fitzpatrick et al. (Eds.), *Dermatology in General Medicine* (2d ed.). New York: McGraw-Hill, 1979.

Samman, P. D. Survey of reticuloses and premycotic eruptions. *Br. J. Dermatol.* 76:1, 1964.

Sanchez, J. F., and Ackerman, A. B. The patch stage of mycosis fungoides. Criteria for histologic diagnosis. *Am. J. Dermatopathol.* 1:5, 1979.

Pityriasis Rubra Pilaris

Brown, J., and Perry, H. O. Pityriasis rubra pilaris. *Arch. Dermatol.* 94:636, 1966.

Lamar, L. M., and Gaethe, G. Pityriasis rubra pilaris. *Arch.Dermatol.* 89:515, 1964.

Incontinentia Pigmenti

Carney, R. G., and Carney, R. G., Jr. Incontinentia pigmenti. *Arch. Dermatol.* 102:157, 1970.

Epstein, S., Vedder, J. S., and Pinkus, H. Bullous variety of incontinentia pigmenti (Bloch-Sulzberger). *Arch. Dermatol. Syphilol.* 65:557, 1952.

Wiklund, D. A., and Weston, W. L. Incontinentia pigmenti. A four-generation study. *Arch. Dermatol.* 116:701, 1980.

Pityriasis rosea Bunch, L. W., and Tilley, J. C. Pityriasis rosea: A histologic and serologic study. *Arch. Dermatol.* 84:79, 1961.
Lipman Cohen, E. Pityriasis rosea. *Br. J. Dermatol.* 79:533, 1967.

Pustular Psoriasis Baker, H., and Ryan, T. J. Generalized pustular psoriasis. *Br. J. Dermatol.* 80:771, 1968.
Kingery, F. A. J., Chinn, H. D., and Saunders, T. S. Generalized pustular psoriasis. *Arch. Dermatol.* 84:912, 1961.

Reiter's Syndrome Perry, H. O., and Mayne, J. G. Psoriasis and Reiter's syndrome. *Arch. Dermatol.* 92:129, 1965.

Mycosis Fungoides Brehmer-Andersson, E. Mycosis fungoides and its relation to Sézary's syndrome, lymphomatoid papulosis, and primary cutaneous Hodgkin's disease. *Acta Derm. Venereol. (Stockh.)* 75:(Suppl. 56):9, 1976.
Degreef, H., Holvoet, C., Van Vloten, W. A., et al. Woringer-Kolopp disease. An epidermotropic variant of mycosis fungoides. *Cancer* 38:2154, 1976.
Jimbow, K., Chiba, M., and Horikoshi, T. Electron microscopic identification of Langerhans cells in the dermal infiltrates of mycosis fungoides. *J. Invest. Dermatol.* 78:102, 1982.
Lutzner, M., Edelson, R., Schein, P., et al. Cutaneous T-cell lymphomas: The Sézary syndrome, mycosis fungoides and related disorders. *Ann. Intern. Med.* 83:534, 1975.
Waldorf, D. S., Ratner, A. C., and Van Scott, E. J. Cells in lesions of mycosis fungoides lymphoma following therapy. Changes in number and type. *Cancer* 21:264, 1968.
Winkelmann, R. K., and Caro, W. A. Current problems in mycosis fungoides and Sézary syndrome. *Annu. Rev. Med.* 28:251, 1977.

Arthropod Bite Reaction Fernandez, N., Torres, A., and Ackerman, A. B. Pathologic findings in human scabies. *Arch. Dermatol.* 113:320, 1977.
Goldman, L., Rockwell, E., and Richfield, D. F., III. Histopathological studies on cutaneous reactions to the bites of various arthropods. *Am. J. Trop. Med. Hyg.* 1:514, 1952.
Horen, W. P. Insect and scorpion sting. *J.A.M.A.* 221:894, 1972.
Larrivee, D. H., Benjamini, E., Feingold, B. F., et al. Histologic studies of guinea pig skin: Different stages of allergic reactivity to flea bites. *Exp. Parasitol.* 15:491, 1964.
Steffen, C. Clinical and histopathologic correlation of midge bites. *Arch. Dermatol.* 117:785, 1981.
Thomson, J., Cochran, T., Cochran, R., and McQueen, A. Histology simulating reticulosis in persistent nodular scabies. *Br. J. Dermatol.* 90:241, 1974.

Secondary Syphilis Abell, E., Marks, R., and Wilson-Jones, E. Secondary syphilis: A clinicopathological review. *Br. J. Dermatol.* 93:53, 1975.
Jeerapaet, P., and Ackerman, A. B. Histologic patterns of secondary syphilis. *Arch. Dermatol.* 107:373, 1973.

Chapter 5

Vesicles and Bullae

I. Intracorneal or subcorneal
   A. Miliaria crystallina
   B. Erythema toxicum neonatorum
   C. Impetigo
   D. Subcorneal pustular dermatosis (Sneddon-Wilkinson)
   E. Pemphigus foliaceus and pemphigus erythematosus
   F. Cutaneous candidiasis
II. Intraepidermal
   A. Epidermolysis bullosa of hands and feet
   B. Friction blisters
   C. Eczematous dermatitis—acute and subacute
   D. Incontinentia pigmenti, first stage: Vesicular lesions
   E. Viral blisters: Herpes simplex, herpes varicella-zoster
   F. Miliaria rubra
   G. Staphylococcal scalded skin syndrome
   H. Dominant congenital ichthyosiform erythroderma (epidermolytic hyperkeratosis)
   I. Bullous dermatosis of diabetes mellitus
   J. Coma bulla (pressure necrosis)
   K. Pustular psoriasis
   L. Erythema multiforme
III. Suprabasilar
   A. Pemphigus vulgaris
   B. Pemphigus vegetans
      1. Early
      2. Late
   C. Benign familial pemphigus (Hailey-Hailey disease)
   D. Keratosis follicularis (Darier's disease)
   E. Transient acantholytic dermatosis (Grover's disease)
   F. Epidermolysis bullosa simplex
IV. Subepidermal vesicles
   A. Bullous pemphigoid
   B. Dermatitis herpetiformis
   C. Epidermolysis bullosa: junctional, dystrophic, and acquired types
   D. Bullous lichen planus
   E. Lichen sclerosus et atrophicus
   F. Lupus erythematosus
   G. Erythema multiforme
   H. Porphyria cutanea tarda
   I. Urticaria pigmentosa
   J. Arthropod bite reaction
   K. Herpes gestationis
   L. Acute graft-versus-host reaction
   M. Toxic epidermal necrolysis
   N. Bullous drug eruptions
   O. Bullous dermatosis of diabetes mellitus
   P. Coma bulla

Vesicles and bullae are best characterized histologically by their location in the skin. This chapter examines those diseases characterized by vesicles that are formed within the stratum corneum and epidermis. Vesicles and bullae that are located beneath the epidermis are discussed in Chapter 9.

The Reactive Process and the Disease	Histopathology	Comments
I. Intracorneal or subcorneal		
A. Miliaria crystallina	Intracorneal or subcorneal vesicles in direct communication with an underlying sweat duct	Multiple sections may be required to demonstrate ductal communication
B. Erythema toxicum neonatorum	Perifollicular subcorneal **pustules** filled with **eosinophils**	
C. Impetigo	1. Subcorneal pustule filled with **neutrophils** and an occasional acantholytic cell	
	2. Spongiosis 3. Neutrophilic exocytosis 4. Moderately intense inflammatory infiltrate (neutrophils, lymphocytes) in the papillary dermis	Special stains may demonstrate bacteria (see Appendix)
D. Subcorneal pustular dermatosis (Sneddon-Wilkinson)	1. Subcorneal pustules containing neutrophils and occasional eosinophils 2. Mild intracellular epidermal edema 3. Spongiform pustules may be present adjacent to subcorneal pustule 4. Slight leukocytic exocytosis 5. Perivascular infiltrate of neutrophils, eosinophils, and mononuclear cells	
E. Pemphigus foliaceus and pemphigus erythematosus	1. **Subcorneal, intragranular, or upper epidermal clefts** 2. **Acantholysis** 3. Dyskeratotic cells in granular cell layer 4. Perivascular infiltrate often with **eosinophils**	
F. Cutaneous candidiasis	Subcorneal pustule filled with neutrophils	Special stains demonstrate organisms within the stratum corneum (see Appendix)

> Differential diagnosis of *subcorneal pustules:*
>
> Impetigo
> Subcorneal pustular dermatosis
> Candidiasis
> Pustular psoriasis
> Geographic tongue

II. Intraepidermal

A. Epidermolysis bullosa of hands and feet (see Fig. 5-9)	1. Degeneration of cells in the upper stratum spinosum 2. Some dyskeratosis	In the several types of epidermolysis bullosa, the blisters form in different regions of the epidermis (see Fig. 5-9)
B. Friction blisters	1. High to mid-intraepidermal cleavage 2. Dermal infiltrate sparse to absent	

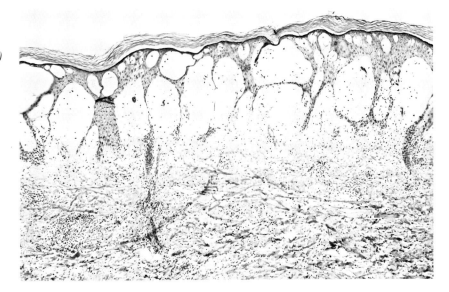

Fig. **5-1.** *Acute eczematous dermatitis. Large intraepidermal vesicles with dermal edema and perivascular inflammation.* (×64)

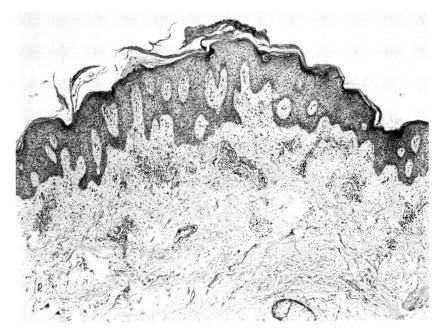

Fig. **5-2.** *Subacute eczematous dermatitis. Irregular psoriasiform hyperplasia with focal hyperkeratosis, parakeratosis, spongiosis, and perivenular inflammation.* (×64)

C. Eczematous dermatitis—acute and subacute (Figs. 5-1, 5-2)

1. Parakeratosis
2. **Spongiosis and vesicles** occurring in lower two-thirds of epidermis
3. Superficial, predominantly perivascular infiltrate of lymphocytes and histiocytes

In acute, subacute, and occasionally chronic eczematous dermatitis, there may be intraepidermal spongiotic vesicles

Spongiosis and retention of the granular layer help differentiate eczema from psoriasis

Spongiotic vesicles may be seen in:

Acute and subacute eczematous dermatitis including atopic, nummular, dyshidrotic, photo-induced, and contact dermatitis
Lichen simplex chronicus
Exfoliative erythroderma
Pityriasis rosea
Pityriasis lichenoides et varioliformis acuta (PLEVA)
Miliaria rubra
Incontinentia pigmenti
Erythema multiforme
Dermatophytosis and candidiasis
Figurate erythemas

D. Incontinentia pigmenti, first stage: Vesicular lesions (Fig. 5-3)

1. Spongiosis
2. Vesicles containing **eosinophils**
3. Eosinophils within epidermis
4. Mild, superficial perivascular and diffuse infiltrate of lymphocytes and eosinophils

Spongiosis with epidermal invasion by eosinophils is seen in:

Pemphigus vulgaris
Allergic contact dermatitis
Urticarial lesions of bullous pemphigoid and herpes gestationis
Incontinentia pigmenti
Erythema toxicum neonatorum

Fig. **5-3.** *Incontinentia pigmenti. Epidermal hyperplasia, intraepidermal eosinophilic microabscesses (center), and melanin-laden macrophages in the upper dermis are hallmarks of this disorder. (×256)*

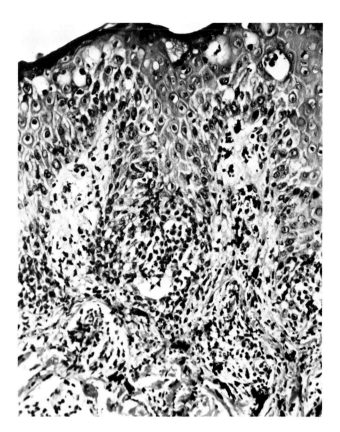

E. Viral blisters: Herpes simplex, herpes varicella-zoster (Fig. 5-4)

1. **Ballooning and reticular degeneration** of epidermis

> Differential diagnosis of *ballooning degeneration:*
>
> Smallpox (variola)
> Vaccinia
> Verruca vulgaris
> Orf
> Picornavirus
> Herpes varicella-zoster
> Herpes simplex

2. **Acantholytic keratinocytes** with homogeneous eosinophilic cytoplasm
3. Large, irregular or **multinucleate keratinocytes**
4. Nuclear margination of chromatin with violet "ground glass" appearance
5. Intranuclear eosinophilic inclusion body surrounded by a faint, clear halo
6. Perivascular infiltrate with mononuclear cells and neutrophils may extend into deep reticular dermis
7. Leukocytoclastic vasculitis with fibrinoid necrosis may be present

Nuclear inclusions may be seen in hair follicles as well as in epidermis

F. Miliaria rubra

1. Intraepidermal spongiotic vesicles in direct communication with a sweat duct
2. Mononuclear cells within vesicles and in subjacent dermis

G. Staphylococcal scalded skin syndrome

1. **Mid-to-upper intraepidermal cleavage**
2. Acantholytic cells
3. **Dermal infiltrate minimal to absent**

H. Dominant congenital ichthyosiform erythroderma (epidermolytic hyperkeratosis) (see Fig. 3-1)

1. Hyperkeratosis
2. Reticular degeneration of granular layer and upper epidermis

See also Ch. 3, I.B

I. Bullous dermatosis of diabetes mellitus

1. Intraepidermal and subepidermal vesicles and bullae
2. Mild superficial perivascular mononuclear cell infiltrate

Fig. **5-4.** *Herpes zoster.*

A. Reticular degeneration with multinucleate giant cells. (×160)

B. Ulcer with acute and chronic inflammation resulting from degeneration and necrosis of epidermis. (×64)

C. Multinucleate cells with ground glass nuclear inclusions are usually found at the edge of the vesicle or ulcer. (×400) Note that herpes zoster and herpes simplex usually cannot be distinguished by histologic features.

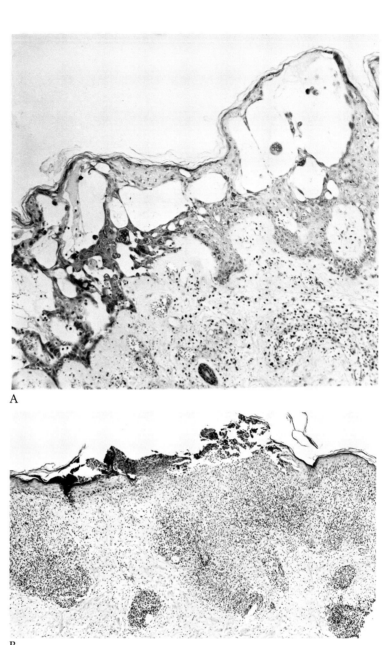

A

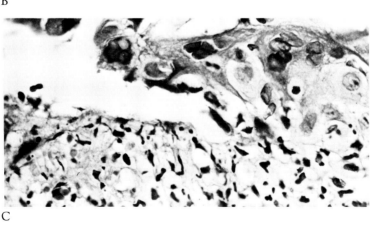

B

C

J. Coma bulla (pressure necrosis) (see Fig. 23-10)

1. Intraepidermal and subepidermal blisters
2. Epidermal necrosis
3. **Eccrine gland necrosis**
4. Variable infiltrate of neutrophils and mononuclear cells in and around necrotic eccrine glands
5. Predominantly neutrophilic infiltrate in and around pilosebaceous structures
6. Dermal hemorrhage
7. Focal areas of necrosis, edema, and acute inflammation in the subcutaneous tissue

See also Ch. 23, I.D.

K. Pustular psoriasis (Fig. 4-5)

See also Ch. 4, II.A

L. Erythema multiforme (see Figs. 9-6 and 9-7)

Intraepidermal vesicles occasionally may occur in erythema multiforme (see also Ch. 5, IV.G; Ch. 9, I.G)

III. Suprabasilar

A. Pemphigus vulgaris (Fig. 5-5)

1. Eosinophils with apparent spongiosis in lower epidermis
2. **Suprabasilar clefts**
3. **Acantholysis**
4. Roof of bulla is composed of intact epidermis
5. Base of bulla composed of basal cell layer on prominent dermal papillae (so-called **villi**)
6. Scant perivascular inflammatory infiltrate composed of lymphocytes, histiocytes, and occasional eosinophils, neutrophils, or plasma cells

Differential diagnosis of *acantholysis* includes:

Pemphigus, all forms
Keratosis follicularis (Darier's disease)
Benign familial pemphigus (Hailey-Hailey disease)
Transient acantholytic dermatosis (Grover's disease)
Actinic keratosis
Viral vesicles
Squamous cell carcinoma
Impetigo
Staphylococcal scalded skin syndrome
Warty dyskeratoma
Subcorneal pustular dermatosis

Suprabasilar acantholysis combined with the loss of intercellular attachments between basal cells gives a "tombstone" appearance to the basal layer

Fig. **5-5.** *Pemphigus vulgaris. Acantholysis with suprabasilar cleft formation is the hallmark of pemphigus vulgaris. The prominent dermal papillae ("villi") also are characteristic. Note the presence of acantholytic cells, i.e., keratinocytes with round shapes resulting from the loss of intercellular connections. (B, ×256)*

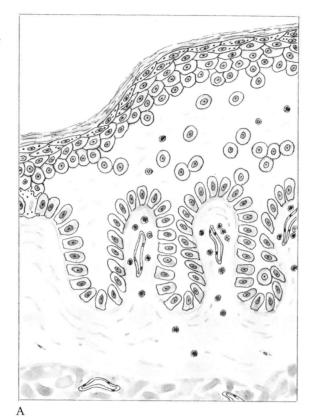

A

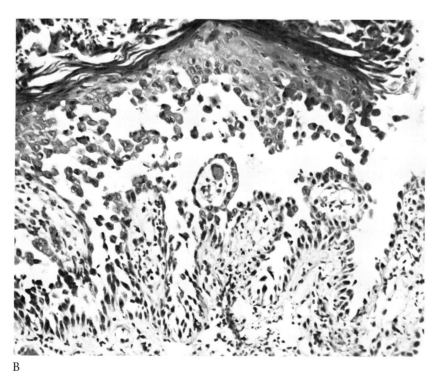

B

B. Pemphigus vegetans

    1. Early

1. **Suprabasilar cleft** formation
2. **Acantholysis**
3. Bullae are filled with eosinophils
4. **Epidermal hyperplasia**
5. Papillary and upper reticular dermal infiltrate composed predominantly of eosinophils

> *Intraepidermal eosinophilic abscesses* may be seen in:
>
> Pemphigus vegetans, rarely foliaceus
> Incontinentia pigmenti
> Bromoderma and iododerma
> Erythema toxicum neonatorum
> Impetigo

    2. Late

1. Epidermal hyperplasia with hyperkeratosis and papillomatosis
2. Acantholysis may be absent at this stage
3. A dense, diffuse infiltrate of eosinophils, lymphocytes, and plasma cells in the papillary and upper reticular dermis

C. Benign familial pemphigus (Hailey-Hailey disease) (Fig. 5-6)

1. Suprabasilar clefts
2. Acantholysis
3. Partial acantholysis throughout the epidermis, giving the appearance of a **dilapidated brick wall**
4. Dyskeratosis, with basal cell shrinkage and alteration in staining of cytoplasm (brightly eosinophilic in color)
5. Elongated papillae may form villi, which protrude into vesicle

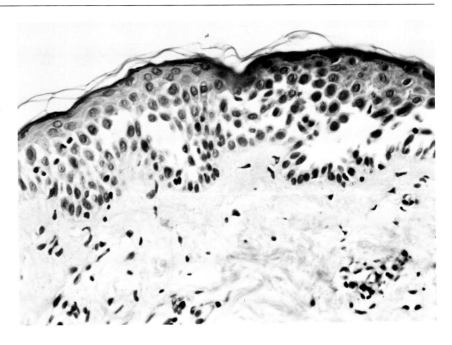

Fig. **5-6.** *Benign familial pemphigus (Hailey-Hailey disease). Acantholysis, which appears incomplete in some areas, results in the "dilapidated brick wall" appearance, a feature that is commonly observed in this disorder. More complete acantholysis, resulting in suprabasal cleft formation, is also present. (×400)*

D. Keratosis follicularis (Darier's disease) (Fig. 5-7)

1. **Hyperkeratosis**
2. Epidermal hyperplasia, even papillary epidermal hyperplasia, and rarely pseudoepitheliomatous hyperplasia have been noted

Fig. **5-7.** *Keratosis follicularis (Darier's disease). Suprabasal cleft formation with corps ronds (cells with apparent perinuclear halos) and corps grains (cells with small, dark oval nuclei resembling millet grains) are typical. (B, ×256)*

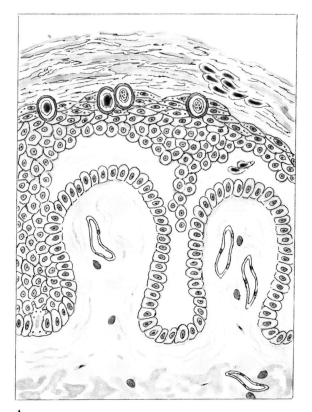

A

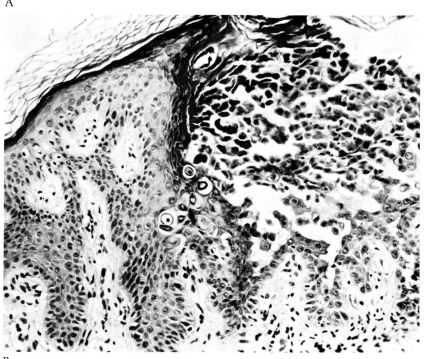

B

3. Acantholytic dyskeratosis resulting in **corps ronds** (granular layer and upper epidermis) and **corps grains** (within cleft and parakeratotic stratum corneum)
4. **Suprabasilar acantholysis** with formation of clefts and lacunae
5. Irregular upward proliferation of papillae with formation of villi
6. Sparse lymphohistiocytic perivascular infiltrate in the upper dermis

E. Transient acantholytic dermatosis (Grover's disease) (Fig. 5-8)

1. Focal suprabasilar clefts and vesicles
2. Occasional corps ronds and corps grains

Transient acantholytic dermatosis (TAD) may also resemble benign familial pemphigus, pemphigus foliaceus, or pemphigus vulgaris; TAD may be differentiated from these diseases by the focal nature of the histologic abnormalities

F. Epidermolysis bullosa simplex (Fig. 5-9)

See Fig. 5-9

Fig. **5-8.** *Transient acantholytic dermatosis (Grover's disease). Dyskeratotic cells, corps ronds, and suprabasal clefts with spongiosis as well as focal parakeratosis and papillary dermal lymphocytic infiltrates are typical. These histologic changes resemble those of a poorly formed Darier's disease. (A, ×160; B, ×160)*

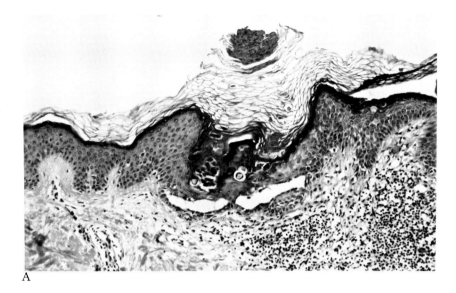

A

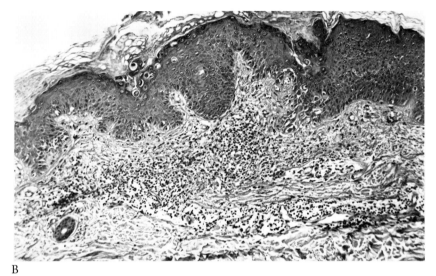

B

IV. Subepidermal vesicles

Most of the entities included in this category are primarily disorders of the papillary dermis and basement membrane zone and are described in Part 3

A. Bullous pemphigoid (see Fig. 9-8)

See Ch. 9, II.A

B. Dermatitis herpetiformis (see Fig. 9-9)

See Ch. 9, II.B

C. Epidermolysis bullosa: junctional, dystrophic, and acquired types (see Fig. 5-9)

D. Bullous lichen planus (see Fig. 9-1)

See also Ch. 9, I.A.1; Ch. 10, I

E. Lichen sclerosus et atrophicus (see Fig. 9-4)

See also Ch. 7, I; Ch. 10, II

F. Lupus erythematosus (see Fig. 9-3)

See also Ch. 7, VI; Ch. 9, I.D, II.D; Ch. 10, III

G. Erythema multiforme (see Figs. 9-6, 9-7)

See also Ch. 5, II.L; Ch. 9, I.G

H. Porphyria cutanea tarda (see Fig. 9-12)

See also Ch. 9, III.A

I. Urticaria pigmentosa (see Figs. 5-10, 16-6)

See also Ch. 16, IV.A

J. Arthropod bite reaction (see Fig. 11-2)

See also Ch. 4, III.A; Ch. 14, I.A.2; Ch. 17, II

K. Herpes gestationis

See also Ch. 9, II.C

L. Acute graft-versus-host reaction (see Fig. 9-5)

See also Ch. 9, I.F

M. Toxic epidermal necrolysis

See also Ch. 9, I.H

N. Bullous drug eruptions

May resemble bullous pemphigoid (see also Ch. 9, II.A, II.G)

O. Bullous dermatosis of diabetes mellitus

See also Ch. 5, II.I

P. Coma bulla (see Fig. 23-10)

See also Ch. 5, II.J

Fig. **5-9.** *Epidermolysis bullosa.*
A. *Epidermolysis bullosa of the hands and feet. Cytolysis and dyskeratosis occur in the mid to upper epidermis.*
B. *Epidermolysis bullosa, junctional (or letalis) type. The vesicle forms at the dermoepidermal junction, and the PAS-positive basement membrane zone is present at the base of the vesicle.*
C. *Epidermolysis bullosa, simplex type. Cleft formation is the result of vacuolation and degeneration of basal cells.*
D. *Epidermolysis bullosa dystrophica (dominant and recessive types) and epidermolysis bullosa acquisita. Vacuolation at the dermoepidermal junction occurs early, but the fully developed vesicle occurs within the superficial papillary dermis.*

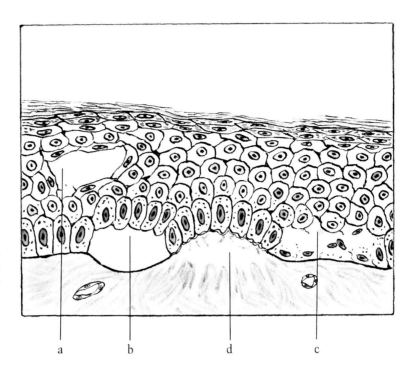

a   b   d   c

Fig. **5-10.** *Mastocytosis, bullous lesion. The extensive dermal mast cell infiltrate is capped by edema and fibrin within a subepidermal bulla. (×160) See also Figure 16-6, urticaria pigmentosa.*

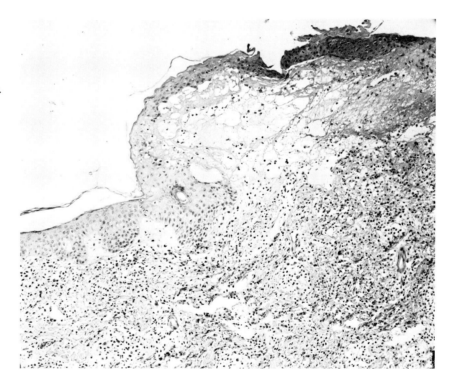

Suggested Reading
Intracorneal or Subcorneal

Miliaria Crystallina
Shelley, W. B., and Horvath, P. N. Experimental miliaria in man. II. Production of sweat retention anidrosis and miliaria crystallina by various kinds of injury. *J. Invest. Dermatol.* 14:9, 1950.

Erythema Toxicum Neonatorum
Freeman, R. G., Spiller, R., and Knox, J. M. Histopathology of erythema toxicum neonatorum. *Arch. Dermatol.* 82:586, 1960.
Luders, D. Histologic observations in erythema toxicum neonatorum. *Pediatrics* 26:219, 1960.

Impetigo
Jordan, W. E., Montes, L. F., and Pittillo, R. F. Microscopic features of pustule formation in experimental impetigo of guinea pig. *J. Cutan. Pathol.* 1:54, 1974.
Peter, G., and Smith, A. L. Group A streptococcal infections of the skin and pharynx. (First of two parts.) *N. Engl. J. Med.* 297:311, 1977.

Subcorneal Pustular Dermatosis
Johnson, S. A. M., and Cripps, D. J. Subcorneal pustular dermatosis in children. *Arch. Dermatol.* 109:73, 1974.
Sneddon, I. B., and Wilkinson, D. S. Subcorneal pustular dermatosis. *Br. J. Dermatol.* 100:61, 1979.
Wilkinson, D. S. Pustular dermatoses. *Br. J. Dermatol.* 81 (Suppl. 3):38, 1969.

Pemphigus Foliaceus
Furtado, T. A. Histopathology of pemphigus foliaceus. *Arch. Dermatol.* 80:66, 1959.
Perry, H. O., and Brunsting, L. A. Pemphigus foliaceus. Further observations. *Arch. Dermatol.* 91:10, 1965.

Intraepidermal

Epidermolysis Bullosa
Bauer, E. A., and Briggaman, R. A. The Mechanobullous Diseases (Epidermolysis Bullosa). In T. B. Fitzpatrick et al. (Eds.), *Dermatology in General Medicine* (2d ed.). New York: McGraw-Hill, 1979.
Briggaman, R. A., and Wheeler, C. E., Jr. Epidermolysis bullosa dystrophica-recessive: A possible role of anchoring fibrils in the pathogenesis. *J. Invest. Dermatol.* 65:203, 1975.
Haneke, E., and Anton-Lamprecht, I. Ultrastructure of blister formation in epidermolysis bullosa hereditaria: V. Epidermolysis bullosa simplex localisata type Weber-Cockayne. *J. Invest. Dermatol.* 78:219, 1982.
Lowe, L. B., Jr. Hereditary epidermolysis bullosa. *Arch. Dermatol.* 95:587, 1967.
Pearson, R. W., Potter, B., and Strauss, F. Epidermolysis bullosa hereditaria letalis: Clinical and histological manifestations and course of the disease. *Arch. Dermatol.* 109:349, 1974.
Roenigk, H. H., Jr., Ryan, J. G., and Bergfeld, W. F. Epidermolysis bullosa acquisita. *Arch. Dermatol.* 103:1, 1971.
Yaoita, H., Briggaman, R. A., Lawley, T. J., et al. Epidermolysis bullosa acquisita: Ultrastructural and immunological studies. *J. Invest. Dermatol.* 76:288, 1981.

Friction Blisters
Braun-Falco, O. The Pathology of Blister Formation. In A. W. Kopf and R. Andrade (Eds.), *The Year Book of Dermatology.* Chicago: Year Book, 1969.
Sulzberger, M. B., Cortese, T. A., Fishman, L., and Wiley, H. S. Studies on blisters produced by friction. *J. Invest. Dermatol.* 47:456, 1966.

Eczematous Dermatitis
Blaylock, W. K. Atopic dermatitis: Diagnosis and pathobiology. *J. Allergy Clin. Immunol.* 57:62, 1976.
Doyle, J. A., Connolly, S. M., Hunziker, N., and Winkelmann, R. K. Prurigo nodularis: A reappraisal of the clinical and histologic features. *J. Cutan. Pathol.* 6:392, 1979.

Dvorak, H. F., et al. Morphology of delayed type hypersensitivity reactions in man. I. Quantitative description of inflammatory response. *Lab. Invest.* 31:111, 1974.

Hanifin, J. M., and Lobitz, W. C. Newer concepts of atopic dermatitis. *Arch. Dermatol.* 113:663, 1977.

Mihm, M. C., Jr., Soter, N. A., Dvorak, H. F., and Austen, K. F. The structure of normal skin and the morphology of atopic eczema. *J. Invest. Dermatol.* 67:305, 1976.

Norins, A. L. Atopic dermatitis. *Ped. Clin. North Am.* 18:801, 1971.

Shaffer, B., and Beerman, H. Lichen simplex chronicus and its variants. *Arch. Dermatol. Syphilol.* 64:340, 1951.

Incontinentia Pigmenti

Carney, R. G., and Carney, R. G., Jr. Incontinentia pigmenti. *Arch. Dermatol.* 102:157, 1970.

Epstein, S., Vedder, J. S., and Pinkus, H. Bullous variety of incontinentia pigmenti (Bloch-Sulzberger). *Arch. Dermatol. Syphilol.* 65:557, 1952.

Wiklund, D. A., and Weston, W. L. Incontinentia pigmenti. A four-generation study. *Arch. Dermatol.* 116:701, 1980.

Viral Blisters

Kaplan, A. S. *The Herpesviruses.* New York: Academic, 1973.

McSorley, J., Shapiro, L., Brownstein, M. H., and Hsu, K. C. Herpes simplex and varicella-zoster: Comparative histopathology of 77 cases. *Int. J. Dermatol.* 13:69, 1974.

Miliaria Rubra

Shelley, W. B., and Horvath, P. N. Experimental miliaria in man. *J. Invest. Dermatol.* 14:193, 1950.

Staphylococcal Scalded Skin Syndrome

Elias, P. M., Fritsch, P., and Epstein, E. H., Jr. Staphylococcal scalded skin syndrome: Clinical features, pathogenesis, and recent microbiological and biochemical developments. *Arch. Dermatol.* 113:207, 1977.

Lyell, A. Toxic epidermal necrolysis (the scalded skin syndrome): A reappraisal. *Br. J. Dermatol.* 100:69, 1979.

Bullous Dermatosis of Diabetes Mellitus

Allen, G. E., and Hadden, D. R. Bullous lesions of the skin in diabetes (bullosis diabeticorum). *Br. J. Dermatol.* 82:216, 1970.

Bernstein, J. E., Medenica, M., Soltani, K., and Griem, S. F. Bullous eruption of diabetes mellitus. *Arch. Dermatol.* 115:324, 1979.

Cantrell, A. R., and Martz, W. Idiopathic bullae in diabetics. Bullous diabeticorum. *Arch. Dermatol.* 96:42, 1967.

Coma Bulla

Arndt, K. A., Mihm, M. C., Jr., and Parrish, J. A. Bullae: A cutaneous sign of a variety of neurologic diseases. *J. Invest. Dermatol.* 60:312, 1973.

Suprabasilar

Pemphigus Vulgaris

Emmerson, R. W., and Wilson-Jones, E. Eosinophilic spongiosis in pemphigus: A report of an unusual histological change in pemphigus. *Arch. Dermatol.* 97:252, 1968.

Lever, W. F. *Pemphigus and Pemphigoid.* Springfield, Ill.: Thomas, 1965.

Pemphigus Vegetans

Director, W. Pemphigus vegetans: A clinicopathological correlation. *Arch. Dermatol. Syphilol.* 66:343, 1952.

Guerra-Rodrigo, F., and Morais-Cardoso, J. P. Pemphigus vegetans. *Arch. Dermatol.* 104:412, 1971.

Benign Familial Pemphigus

Gottlieb, S. K., and Lutzner, M. A. Hailey-Hailey disease—An electron microscopic study. *J. Invest. Dermatol.* 54:368, 1970.

Michel, B. "Familial benign chronic pemphigus" by Hailey and Hailey, April 1939. Commentary: Hailey-Hailey disease, familial benign chronic pemphigus. *Arch. Dermatol.* 118:774, 1982.

Palmer, D. D., and Perry, H. O. Benign familial chronic pemphigus. *Arch. Dermatol.* 86:493, 1962.

Keratosis Follicularis (Darier's Disease)

Baden, H. P. Darier-White Disease (Keratosis Follicularis) and Miscellaneous Hyperkeratotic Disorders. In T. B. Fitzpatrick et al. (Eds.), *Dermatology in General Medicine* (2d ed.). New York: McGraw-Hill, 1979.

Getzler, N. A., and Flint, A. Keratosis follicularis: A study of one family. *Arch. Dermatol.* 93:545, 1966.

Gottlieb, S. K., and Lutzner, M. A. Darier's disease: An electron microscopic study. *Arch. Dermatol.* 107:225, 1973.

Transient Acantholytic Dermatosis

Ackerman, A. B. Focal acantholytic dyskeratosis. *Arch. Dermatol.* 106:702, 1972.

Chalet, M., Grover, R., and Ackerman, A. B. Transient acantholytic dermatosis. A reevaluation. *Arch. Dermatol.* 113:431, 1977.

Grover, R. W. Transient acantholytic dermatosis. *Arch. Dermatol.* 101:426, 1970.

Heaphy, M. R., Tucker, S. B., and Winkelmann, R. K. Benign papular acantholytic dermatosis. *Arch. Dermatol.* 112:814, 1976.

General

Beutner, E. H., Chorzelski, T. P., and Bean, S. F. (Eds). *Immunopathology of the Skin* (2d ed.). New York: Wiley, 1979.

Lever, W. F. *Pemphigus and Pemphigoid.* Springfield, Ill.: Thomas, 1965.

Pearson, R. W. Advances in the Diagnosis and Treatment of Blistering Diseases: A Selective Review. In F. D. Malkinson and R. W. Pearson (Eds.), *Year Book of Dermatology.* Chicago: Year Book, 1977.

Chapter 6

Neoplastic Patterns of the Epidermis

I. Benign hyperplastic disorders
  A. Seborrheic keratosis
    1. Hyperkeratotic
    2. Acanthotic
    3. Adenoidal
    4. Irritated (inverted follicular)
  B. Linear epidermal nevus
  C. Verruca vulgaris and verruca plantaris
  D. Condyloma acuminatum
  E. Verruca plana
  F. Molluscum contagiosum
  G. Fibroepithelial polyp
  H. Warty dyskeratoma
  I. Clear cell acanthoma (Degos' tumor)
II. Hyperplastic disorders, unclassified
  A. Keratoacanthoma
  B. Pseudoepitheliomatous hyperplasia
III. Atypical keratinocytic proliferation
  A. Actinic keratosis
    1. Hypertrophic
    2. Atrophic
    3. Acantholytic
    4. Lichenoid
IV. Malignancy
  A. Squamous cell carcinoma
    1. In situ
      a. Bowen's disease
      b. Erythroplasia of Queyrat
      c. Intraepidermal epithelioma of Jadassohn
    2. Invasive
  B. Basal cell carcinoma
    1. Superficial (multifocal)
    2. Sclerosing (morphealike)
    3. Metatypical (basosquamous carcinoma)
  C. Fibroepithelioma of Pinkus
  D. Extramammary Paget's disease; Paget's disease of the breast

The Reactive Process and the Disease	Histopathology	Comments
I. Benign hyperplastic disorders		
A. Seborrheic keratosis (Fig. 6-1)		
1. Hyperkeratotic (Fig. 6-2)	1. Marked laminated hyperkeratosis 2. Papillary epidermal hyperplasia (papillomatosis) 3. Proliferation of basaloid cells 4. Horn cysts may or may not be present	*Papillary epidermal hyperplasia (papillomatosis)* often seen in: Seborrheic keratosis Actinic keratosis Epidermal nevus Verruca vulgaris Acanthosis nigricans (Fig. 6-3) Acrokeratosis verruciformis (Hopf) Fibroepithelial polyp Seborrheic keratoses are usually elevated above the normal skin surface

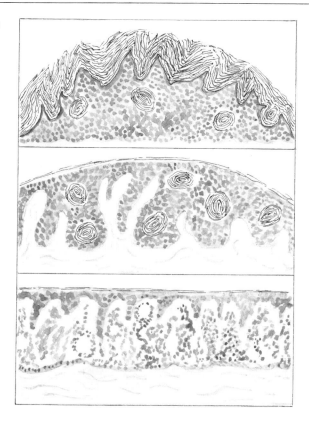

Fig. **6-1.** *Seborrheic keratosis. The histologic patterns illustrated here include the hyperkeratotic* (top), *acanthotic* (middle), *and adenoidal* (lower) *types.*

Fig. **6-2.** *Seborrheic keratosis, hyperkeratotic pattern. Epidermal nevi may also exhibit this histology. (×160) (Reprinted with permission from T. H. Kwan and M. C. Mihm. The Skin. In S. L. Robbins and R. S. Cotran (Eds.),* Pathologic Basis of Disease *(2d ed.). Philadelphia: Saunders, 1979.)*

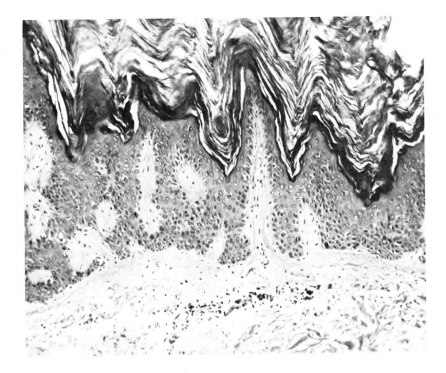

Fig. **6-3.** *Acanthosis nigricans. Papillomatosis with minimal acanthosis and hyperkeratosis are typical. (×64)*

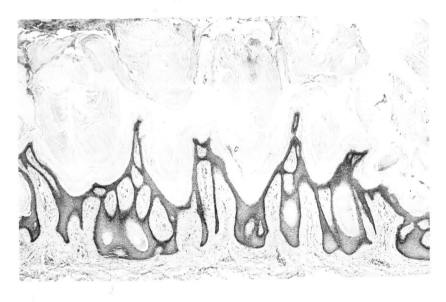

2. Acanthotic
(Fig. 6-4)

1. Hyperkeratosis
2. Sheets of basaloid cells
3. Keratin-filled horn cysts and pseudohorn cysts

3. Adenoidal (Fig. 6-4)

1. Hyperkeratosis
2. Lacelike strands of basaloid cells
3. Horn cysts may be absent

4. Irritated (inverted follicular) (Fig. 6-5)

1. Hyperkeratosis
2. Basaloid proliferation of cells, often arising from a hair follicle
3. Squamous eddies or pearls (concentric layers of squamous cells with increasing keratinization toward the center)

Squamous eddies may be seen in:

Seborrheic keratosis
Actinic keratosis
Squamous cell carcinoma
Warty dyskeratoma
Keratoacanthoma

B. Linear epidermal nevus

1. Hyperkeratosis
2. Focal parakeratosis
3. Papillomatosis

Fig. **6-4.** *Seborrheic keratosis. A mixture of adenoidal and acanthotic patterns is present. (× 100)*

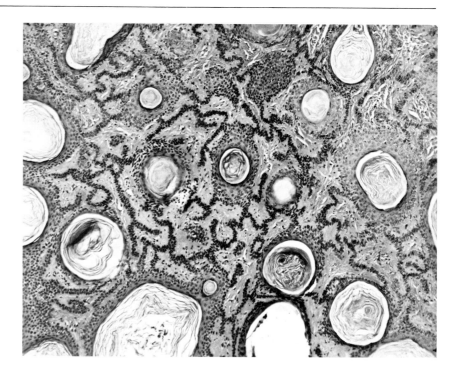

Fig. **6-5.** *Irritated seborrheic keratosis.*
A. *Papillary epidermal hyperplasia with areas of squamous change, squamous eddies, and chronic inflammation are typical. (×47)*
B. *Squamous eddies. (×400)*

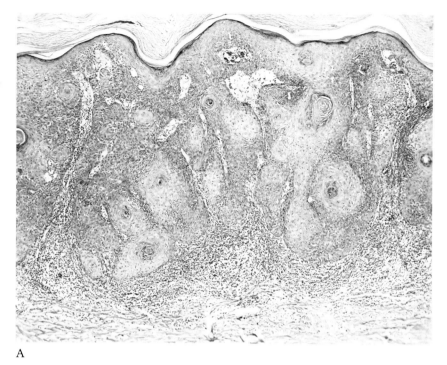

A

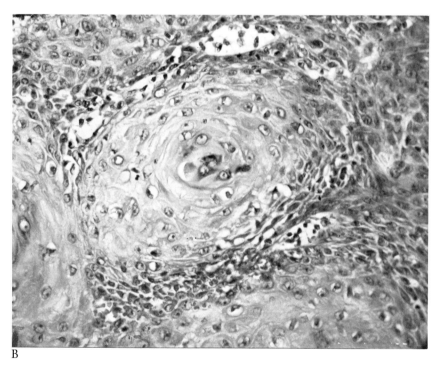

B

C. Verruca vulgaris and verruca plantaris (Fig. 6-6A,B,D)

1. Marked hyperkeratosis
2. Marked focal **parakeratosis** over papillary projections
3. Papillomatosis
4. Elongated hyperplastic rete ridges curving inward toward the center of the lesion
5. Large, vacuolated keratinocytes **(ballooning degeneration)** with deeply **basophilic inclusion bodies** replacing the nucleus located in the granular and upper spinous layers
6. Intranuclear, irregularly shaped eosinophilic bodies within clear spaces
7. **Large keratohyaline granules** in vacuolated (infected) and nonvacuolated (noninfected) cells
8. **Dilated, elongated vessels in papillary dermis**

Ballooning degeneration is a term used to describe the cytoplasmic swelling and vacuolation in keratinocytes that occurs in some viral infections (see also Ch. 5, II.E)

D. Condyloma acuminatum (Fig. 6-6 C)

1. Diffuse **parakeratosis**
2. Filiform papillary epidermal hyperplasia with thickening and elongation of the rete ridges
3. **Perinuclear vacuolation**
4. Eccentrically located, hyperchromatic irregularly shaped nuclei
5. Edematous dermis with dilated capillaries and moderately dense mononuclear cell infiltrate

Lesions usually occur on mucosal surfaces; pseudoepitheliomatous hyperplasia occurs rarely (giant condylomata of Buschke and Lowenstein)

E. Verruca plana

1. Basketweave hyperkeratosis
2. Epidermal hyperplasia
3. Numerous vacuolated cells in the upper third of the epidermis—so-called **bird's-eye cells**
4. Nucleus has dense chromatin and prominent nucleolus

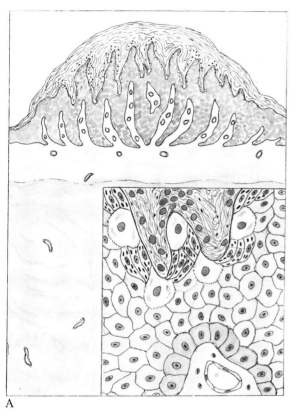

A

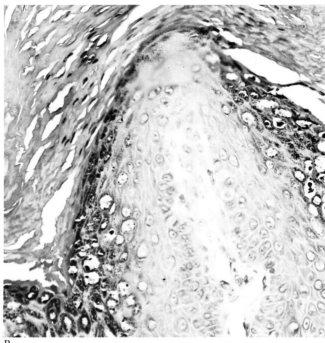

B

Fig. **6-6.** *Verruca vulgaris, condyloma acuminatum, and verruca plantaris. Epidermal hyperplasia, papillomatosis, hyperkeratosis, parakeratosis, densely basophilic nuclear inclusions, and disturbed keratohyaline granule formation are seen in varying degrees in lesions caused by the wart virus(es).*
A. Verruca vulgaris. Inset: nuclear inclusions, large keratohyaline granules, and ballooning cytoplasmic changes.
B. Verruca vulgaris. Photomicrograph for comparison. (approximately ×400)
C. Condyloma acuminatum.
D. Verruca plantaris.

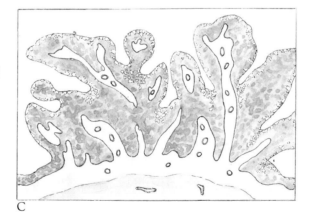

C

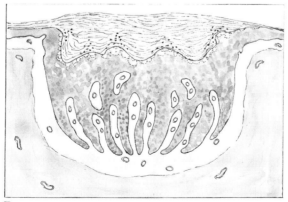

D

F. Molluscum con-
   tagiosum (Fig. 6-7)

1. Epithelial hyperplasia extending downward in a lobulated
   fashion to form a cup-shaped
   lesion
2. Hyperkeratosis
3. **"Molluscum bodies"**

Molluscum bodies are homogeneous, eosinophilic intracytoplasmic inclusions that en-
large to compress and flatten
the nucleus; these molluscum
bodies become basophilic at
the level of granular layer

G. Fibroepithelial polyp

1. Hyperkeratosis
2. Papillomatosis
3. Variable epidermal hyperplasia
4. Dermal connective-tissue
   stalk composed of loose collagen fibers and capillaries

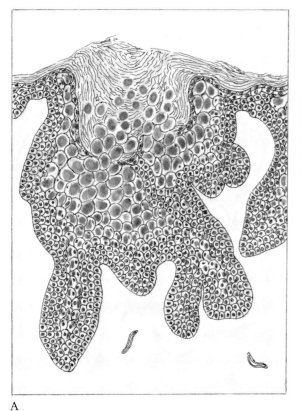

A

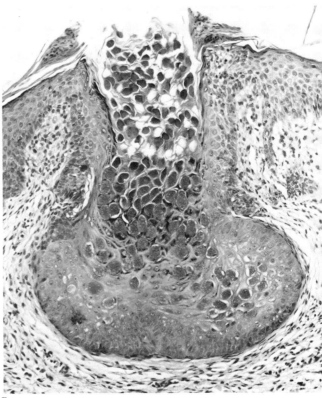

B

Fig. **6-7.** *Molluscum contagiosum.
Hyperplasia and invagination of
the epidermis with the characteristic eosinophilic cytoplasmic inclusions are diagnostic. (B, ×256)*

H. Warty dyskeratoma (Fig. 6-8)

1. Central cup-shaped invagination filled with hyperkeratotic and parakeratotic debris
2. Acantholytic and dyskeratotic cells at base of the lesion
3. Prominent papillary projections, called **villi**, are lined by basal cells

The histology of warty dyskeratoma may be identical to that of keratosis follicularis (Darier's disease)

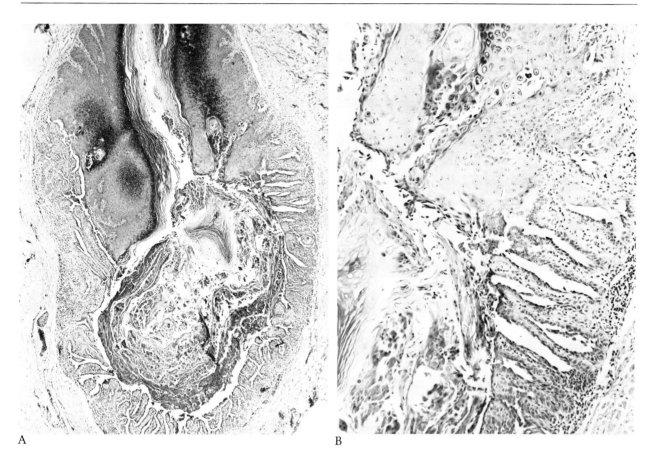

A   B

Fig. **6-8.** *Warty dyskeratoma.*
A. An epidermal invagination filled with keratinaceous material exhibits suprabasal cleft formation and villous papillary epidermal hyperplasia. (×37)
B. This higher magnification exhibits corps ronds and papillomatosis. (×100)

I. Clear cell acanthoma (Degos' tumor)

1. Parakeratosis
2. Sharply demarcated area of epidermal hyperplasia with elongated, intertwined rete ridges
3. **Large, pale or "clear" keratinocytes**
4. Slight spongiosis
5. Neutrophilic invasion of epidermis and formation of neutrophilic microabscesses
6. Prominent vascular dilation
7. Dermal mononuclear cell infiltrate in dermis

Clear cells contain abundant glycogen, which is PAS-positive and diastase-labile

II. Hyperplastic disorders, unclassified

A. Keratoacanthoma (Fig. 6-9)

1. **Cup-shaped** invagination of epidermis with keratin-filled central crater and lateral "lip-like" extensions over the sides of the crater
2. Peripheral small cuboid cells surround **large cells with pale, eosinophilic "glassy" cytoplasm**
3. Intraepidermal neutrophilic abscesses containing collagen, elastic fibers, and occasional dyskeratotic cell
4. Predominantly mononuclear cell infiltrate beneath proliferating epidermis

Differential diagnosis:
  Squamous cell carcinoma
  Inverted follicular keratosis
  Molluscum contagiosum
  Hypertrophic actinic keratosis
  Pseudoepitheliomatous hyperplasia
  Prurigo nodularis

Unilocular intraepidermal neutrophilic abscesses with marked epidermal hyperplasia may be seen in:

Clear cell acanthoma
Keratoacanthoma
Deep fungal infection
Pilonidal tract
Iododerma
Bromoderma

B. Pseudoepitheliomatous hyperplasia

1. Variable hyperkeratosis and parakeratosis
2. Extensive epidermal hyperplasia
3. Elongated rete ridges
4. Normal maturation from basal layer to stratum corneum
5. Mitoses occasionally present

Pseudoepitheliomatous hyperplasia is observed:
  At the edge of chronic ulcers and sinus tracts
  In association with chronic infectious processes (deep fungal and mycobacterial infections, tertiary syphilis, and granuloma inguinale)

Overlying granular cell tumors
Extensive epidermal proliferation with dysplasia and atypia favors a diagnosis of squamous cell carcinoma

Fig. **6-9.** *Keratoacanthoma. The overall cup shape and well-demarcated borders (A), the orderly architecture of basaloid cells surrounding nests of "glassy" squamous cells (B), and lack of significant cytologic atypism allow one to diagnose keratoacanthoma with certainty. (A, ×9; B, ×400)*

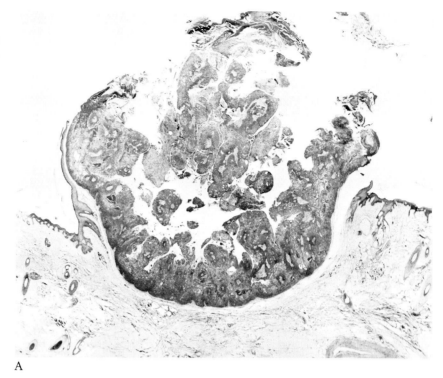

A

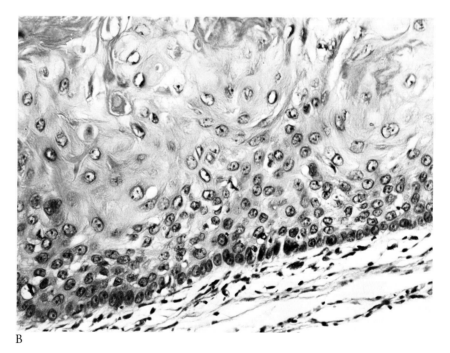

B

III. Atypical keratinocytic proliferation

A. Actinic keratosis (Fig. 6-10)

1. Pronounced hyperkeratosis
2. Focal parakeratosis
3. Epidermal atrophy alternating with hyperplasia
4. **Pleomorphism** of large, irregular hyperchromatic nuclei in the lower layers of the epidermis
5. **Loss of cellular polarity,** especially in lower epidermis, with teardroplike proliferation of cells in basal layer (these changes may be seen in all actinic keratoses)

Solar elastotic changes as well as a mononuclear cell infiltrate are frequently found beneath an actinic keratosis

1. Hypertrophic

Changes described above with emphasis on hyperkeratosis and acanthosis

2. Atrophic

Changes described above with emphasis on epidermal atrophy

It is not necessary to subclassify actinic keratoses for clinical reasons, but subtypes present distinctive histologic patterns and so are mentioned here

Actinic keratoses may exhibit marked hyperpigmentation of keratinocytes; these lesions are sometimes called *pigmented* actinic keratosis

3. Acantholytic

1. Pronounced hyperkeratosis
2. Focal parakeratosis
3. Suprabasilar clefts with acantholysis
4. Cellular atypia in basal cell layer

4. Lichenoid (see Fig. 10-2)

1. Hyperkeratosis
2. Focal parakeratosis
3. Epidermal hyperplasia
4. Dyskeratosis often present
5. Mild atypicality of cells in basal layer
6. Dense, bandlike mononuclear cell infiltrate in the upper dermis

Lichenoid actinic keratosis may be similar histologically to lichen planus (see also Ch. 9, I.A)

Fig. **6-10.** *Actinic keratosis. The hallmark of this disorder is proliferation of atypical keratinocytes associated with solar elastosis. Parakeratosis and chronic inflammation frequently are present. In actinic keratosis, the atypical keratinocytes are* not *transepidermal, unlike squamous cell carcinoma in situ in which the atypical keratinocytes are present at all levels of the epidermis. (A, ×100; B, ×256)*

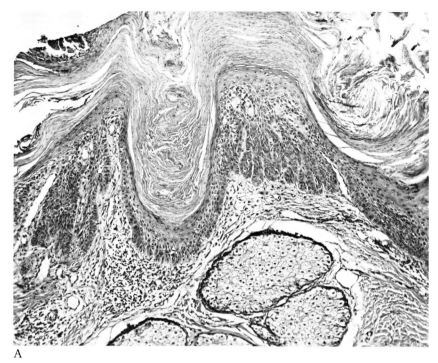

A

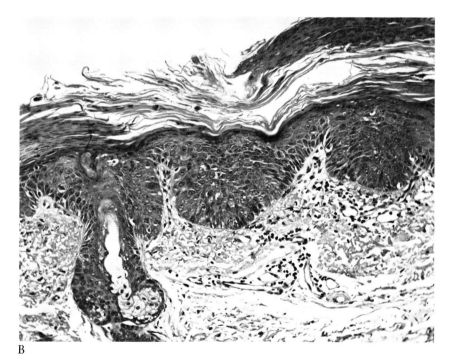

B

Fig. **6-11.** *Squamous cell carcinoma in situ.*

A. Transepidermal cytologic atypia is diagnostic. Note the sharp demarcation between atypical and hyperplastic epidermis (right). *(×64)*

B. Dyskeratosis, atypical mitotic figures, hyperkeratosis, and chronic inflammation in the dermis are frequently observed. (×400)

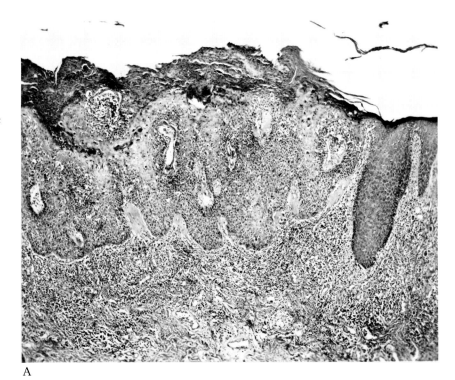

A

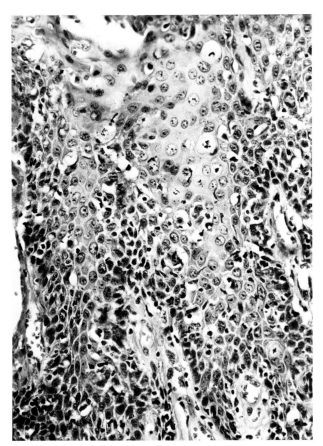

B

IV. Malignancy

    A. Squamous cell carcinoma

        1. In situ (Fig. 6-11)

a. Bowen's disease	1. Marked parakeratosis 2. Acanthosis common, but atrophy occasionally seen 3. **Loss of normal polarity** 4. Atypia and pleomorphism of keratinocytes with frequent mitoses extending **throughout the entire epidermis** 5. Multinucleated epidermal cells 6. Dyskeratosis 7. Apparently normal basal cells on a PAS-positive basement membrane, which delineates a sharp border between epidermis and dermis

b. Erythroplasia of Queyrat

This term refers to carcinoma in situ located on the glans penis or the vulva

c. Intraepidermal epithelioma of Jadassohn (Fig. 6-12)

    1. Hyperkeratosis
    2. Variable papillomatosis and epidermal hyperplasia
    3. **Discrete nests of atypical keratinocytes within the epidermis**
    4. Individual atypical cells may be pigmented, pale, acantholytic, dyskeratotic, or multinucleated
    5. Intact basal cell layer and basement membrane

> Tumors *apparently* arising within and confined to the epidermis include:
>
> Squamous cell carcinoma
> Basal cell carcinoma
> Malignant melanoma
> Paget's disease
> Eccrine poroma
> Hidradenoma
> Clear cell acanthoma

Fig. **6-12.** *Intraepidermal epithelioma, actinic keratosis type. The nests of cells exhibit intercellular bridges (indicating keratinocytic origin) and a moderate degree of cytologic atypia. (×160)*

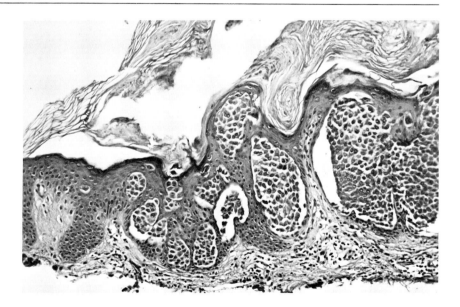

2. Invasive (Fig. 6-13)

1. Irregular masses of atypical (pleomorphic, dysplastic) cells with variable keratinization proliferating downward and **invading the dermis**
2. Squamous pearls
3. Marked inflammatory dermal infiltrate composed predominantly of mononuclear cells

Atypism is minimal to absent in well-differentiated squamous cell carcinoma.

Occasionally cells may be predominantly spindle-shaped (Fig. 6-14)

Morbidity and mortality are said to be greater in squamous cell carcinoma arising from non–sun-exposed skin

Fig. **6-13.** *Invasive squamous cell carcinoma. Irregular tongues of moderately well-differentiated squamous cell carcinoma invade the dermis, apparently arising from the epidermis. A lymphocytic infiltrate surrounds some tumor nests at left. (×64).*

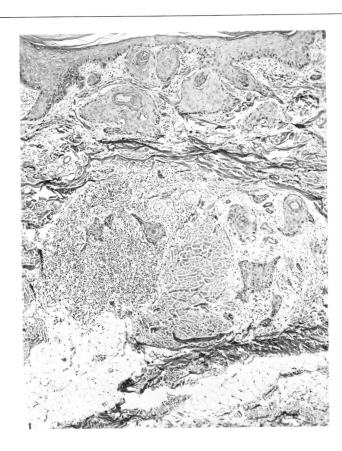

Fig. **6-14.** *Pseudosarcomatous (spindle cell) squamous cell carcinoma. The differential diagnosis of this spindle cell tumor (A) includes atypical fibroxanthoma, malignant fibrous histiocytoma, and spindle cell or desmoplastic melanoma. Squamous cell carcinoma can be diagnosed if origin from epidermal keratinocytes is observed, if areas of squamous differentiation such as bridges and squamous pearls are present, or by immunoperoxidase stains for keratin (B) in the appropriate clinical setting. (A, B, ×400) (Immunoperoxidase preparation courtesy of Geraldine Pinkus, M.D.)*

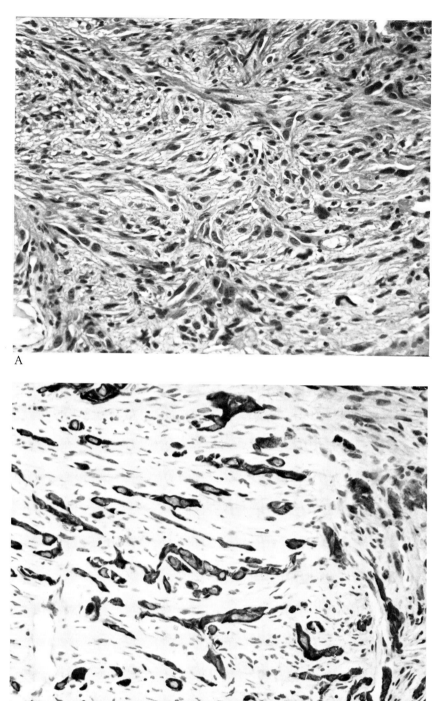

A

B

B. Basal cell carcinoma (Fig. 6-15A,B)

1. Organoid proliferation of **undifferentiated basaloid cells** with a relatively uniform round to oval hyperchromatic nucleus without nucleoli, surrounded by scanty cytoplasm
2. Intercellular bridges are decreased to absent as viewed with the light microscope
3. **Peripheral palisading** of basaloid cells
4. Tumor often surrounded by a fibrous and inflammatory stroma
5. **Separation (retraction) artifact** between tumor cells and stroma is frequently observed
6. Tumor lobules frequently connect to overlying epidermis or adjacent hair follicles

The histologic appearance of basal cell carcinoma varies considerably with regard to the presence or absence of surface ulceration, adnexal involvement, pigmentation, keratinization, acid mucopolysaccharide (mucin) deposition, or cystic spaces. Consequently descriptive adjectives such as *ulceronodular, cystic, pigmented*, and so forth are often used in diagnosing basal cell carcinoma. For practical, prognostic, and therapeutic purposes, however, it is most important to qualify the diagnosis in three instances:
Superficial or multifocal basal cell carcinoma
Sclerosing or morphea-like basal cell carcinoma
Metatypical basal cell or basosquamous carcinoma

1. Superficial (multifocal) (Fig. 6-15C)

1. Small **buds** of deeply basophilic cells extend from the epidermis into superficial dermis
2. Separation artifact may be prominent

Superficial and sclerosing basal cell carcinomas may have microscopic extension far beyond clinically apparent borders

Fig. **6-15.** *Basal cell carcinoma.*
A. Solid and pseudocystic pat-
*   terns. (×64)*
B. Pseudocystic and pseudoglan-
*   dular patterns. (×100)*
C. Superficial type. (×100)

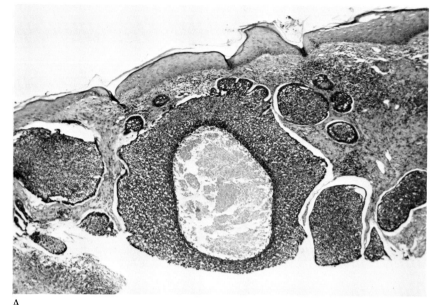

A

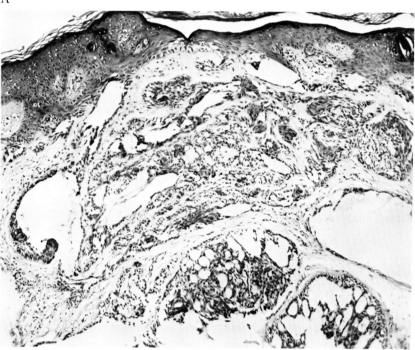

B

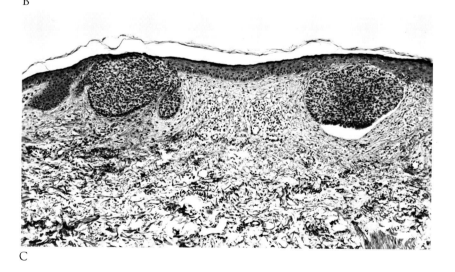

C

Fig. **6-15** *(continued)*
D. *Sclerosing type. (×400)*
E. *Metatypical or basosquamous
    type. (×256)*

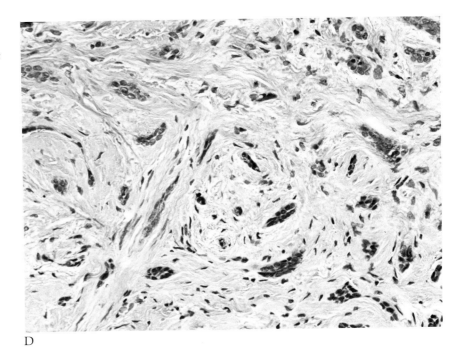

D

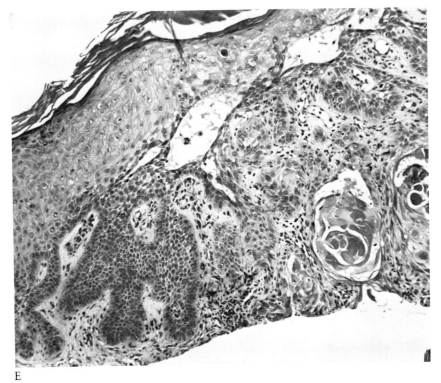

E

2. Sclerosing (morphealike) (Fig. 6-15D)

1. Small, often **linear and branching** aggregates of tumor cells embedded in a **fibrotic dermis**

2. Overlying epidermal attachment may be minimal to absent

Fibrous stroma may be the predominant feature since the total number of tumor cells present in sclerosing basal cell carcinoma may be quite small

Differential diagnosis: Metastatic carcinoma, especially adenocarcinoma of the breast (helpful distinguishing feature: metastatic carcinoma grows in nonbranching lines)

3. Metatypical (basosquamous carcinoma) (Fig. 6-15E)

1. Variable hyperkeratosis
2. Basaloid tumor cells resembling a typical basal cell carcinoma
3. Foci of cells with squamous differentiation resembling squamous cell carcinoma (metatypical region)
4. Areas of typical basal cell carcinoma may merge into a metatypical region

Metatypical basal cell carcinomas may be quite locally aggressive and may even metastasize

C. Fibroepithelioma of Pinkus (Fig. 6-16)

1. Narrow anastomosing strands of basaloid cells extend from epidermis deep into dermis
2. Fibrotic stroma surrounds tumor

Some controversy exists over whether this tumor is a variant of basal cell carcinoma or seborrheic keratosis

Fig. **6-16.** *Fibroepithelioma of Pinkus. Basaloid cells within a fibrous stroma extend in an anastomosing trabecular pattern deep into the dermis.* (×46)

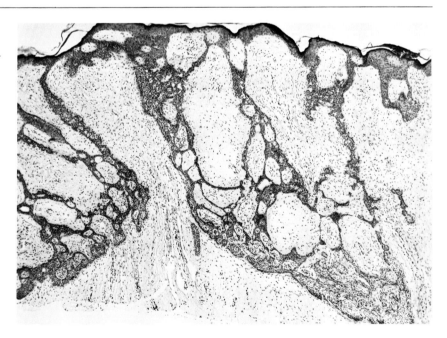

D. Extramammary Paget's disease; Paget's disease of the breast (Fig. 6-17)

1. Epidermal hyperplasia is frequent
2. Epidermal infiltration by single cells or groups of cells
3. **Paget's cells** are variably pleomorphic, with pale, often vacuolated cytoplasm, large nuclei, and no intercellular bridges
4. Tumor cells may be disposed along basement membrane zone or throughout epidermis
5. In the lower epidermis, tumor cells often compress or flatten the underlying basal cells

Paget's cells are PAS positive, diastase-resistant, and stain with alcian blue at pH 2.5

Differential diagnosis:
Malignant melanoma
Carcinoma in situ (Bowen's disease)

Compression of the basal cells is a finding that helps differentiate Paget's disease from malignant melanoma

Fig. **6-17.** *Paget's disease. Large cells with clear to granular cytoplasm and hyperchromatic nuclei pepper the epidermis. Note the superficial resemblance to intraepidermal malignant melanoma. (×640)*

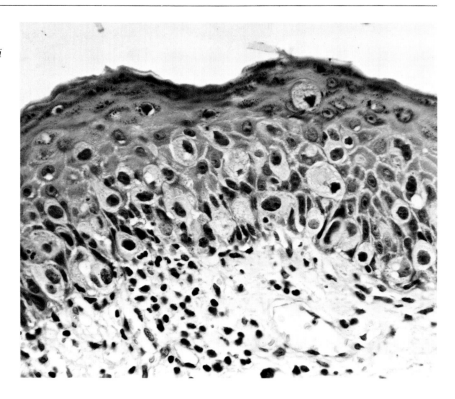

Suggested Reading
Seborrheic Keratosis

Bedi, T. R. Familial congenital multiple seborrheic verrucae. *Arch. Dermatol.* 113:1441, 1977.

Berman, A., and Winkelmann, R. K. Seborrheic keratoses: Appearance in course of exfoliative erythroderma and regression associated with histologic mononuclear cell infiltration. *Arch. Dermatol.* 118:615, 1982.

Braun-Falco, O., and Kint, A. Zur histogenese der verruca seborrhoica. I. Mittelung. *Arch. Klin. Exp. Dermatol.* 216:615, 1963.

Mevorah, B., and Mishima, Y. Cellular response of seborrheic keratosis following croton oil irritation and surgical trauma. *Dermatologica* 131:452, 1965.

Sanderson, K. V. The structure of seborrhoeic keratoses. *Br. J. Dermatol.* 80:588, 1968.

Sperry, K., and Wall, J. Adenocarcinoma of the stomach with eruptive seborrheic keratoses: The sign of Leser-Trelat. *Cancer* 45:2434, 1980.

Linear Epidermal Nevus

Altman, J., and Mehregan, A. H. Inflammatory linear verrucose epidermal nevus. *Arch. Dermatol.* 104:385, 1971

Dupre, A., and Christol, B. Inflammatory linear verrucose epidermal nevus. A pathologic study. *Arch. Dermatol.* 113:767, 1977.

Solomon, L. M., Fretzin, D. F., and Dewald, R. L. The epidermal nevus syndrome. *Arch. Dermatol.* 97:273, 1968.

Molluscum Contagiosum

Lutzner, M. A. Molluscum contagiosum, verruca and zoster viruses: Electron microscopic studies in the skin. *Arch. Dermatol.* 87:436, 1963.

Warty Dyskeratoma

Szymanski, F. J. Warty dyskeratoma: A benign cutaneous tumor resembling Darier's disease microscopically. *Arch. Dermatol.* 75:567, 1957.

Clear Cell Acanthoma

Brownstein, M., Fernando, S., and Shapiro, L. Clear cell acanthoma: Clinicopathologic analysis of 37 new cases. *Am. J. Clin. Pathol.* 59:306, 1973.

Trau, H., Fisher, B. K. and Schewach-Millet, M. Multiple clear cell acanthomas. *Arch. Dermatol.* 116:433, 1980.

Keratoacanthoma

Fathizadeh, A., Medenica, M. M., Soltani, K., et al. Aggressive keratoacanthoma and internal malignant neoplasm. *Arch. Dermatol.* 118:112, 1982.

Fisher, E. R., McCoy, M. M., and Wechsler, H. L. Analysis of histopathologic and electron microscopic determinants of keratoacanthoma and squamous cell carcinoma. *Cancer* 29:1387, 1972.

Ghadially, F. N., Barton, B. W., and Kerridge, D. F. The etiology of keratoacanthoma. *Cancer* 16:603, 1963.

King, D. F., and Barr, R. J. Intraepithelial elastic fibers and intracytoplasmic glycogen: Diagnostic aids in differentiating keratoacanthoma from squamous cell carcinoma. *J. Cutan. Pathol.* 7:140, 1980.

Reed, R. J. Keratoacanthoma: Entity or syndrome? *Bull. Tulane Univ. Med. Fac.* 26:117, 1967.

Takaki, Y., Masutani, M., and Kawada, A. Electron microscopic study of keratoacanthoma. *Acta Derm. Venereol.* 51:21, 1971.

Weedon, D., and Barnett, L. Keratoacanthoma centrifugum marginatum. *Arch. Dermatol.* 111:1024, 1975.

Actinic Keratosis

Ackerman, A. B., and Reed, R. J. Epidermolytic variant of solar keratosis. *Arch. Dermatol.* 107:104, 1973.

Pinkus, H. Keratosis senilis. *Am. J. Clin. Pathol.* 29:193, 1958.

Pinkus, H. Actinic Keratosis—Actinic Skin. In R. Andrade et al. (Eds.), *Cancer of the Skin.* Philadelphia: Saunders, 1976.

Shapiro, L., and Ackerman, A. Solitary lichen planus-like keratosis. *Dermatologica* 132:386, 1966.

Squamous Cell Carcinoma

Johnson, W. C., and Helwig, E. B. Adenoid squamous cell carcinoma (adenoacanthoma): A clinicopathologic study of 155 patients. *Cancer* 19:1639, 1966.

Lichtiger, B., Mackay, B., and Tessmer, C. F. Spindle-cell variant of squamous carcinoma. *Cancer* 26:1311, 1970.

Lund, H. Z. Squamous Cell Carcinoma. In *Tumors of the Skin. Atlas of Tumor Pathology.* Sec. 1, Fasc. 2. Washington: Armed Forces Institute of Pathology, 1957. P. 235.

Schlegel, R., Banks-Schlegel, S., McLeod, J. A., and Pinkus, G. S. Immunoperoxidase localization of keratin in human neoplasms. *Am. J. Pathol.* 101:41, 1980.

Stern, R. S., Thibodeau, L. A., Kleinerman, R. A., et al. Risk of cutaneous carcinoma in patients treated with oral methoxsalen photochemotherapy for psoriasis. *N. Engl. J. Med.* 300:809, 1979.

Bowen's Disease

Berger, B. W., and Hori, Y. Multicentric Bowen's disease of the genitalia: Spontaneous regression of lesions. *Arch. Dermatol.* 114:1698, 1978.

Bowen, J. Precancerous dermatoses. *J. Cutan. Dis.* 30:241, 1912.

Graham, J. H., and Helwig, E. B. Bowen's disease and its relationship to systemic cancer. *Arch. Dermatol.* 80:133, 1959.

Graham, J. H., and Helwig. E. B. Erythroplasia of Queyrat: A clinicopathologic and histochemical study. *Cancer* 32:1396, 1973.

McGovern, V. J. Bowen's disease. *Aus. J. Dermatol.* 8:48, 1965.

Rickert, R. R., Brodkin, R. H., and Hutter, R. V. Bowen's disease. *CA* 27:160, 1977.

Taylor, D. R., Jr., and South, D. A. Bowenoid papulosis: A review. *Cutis* 27:92, 1981.

Ulbright, T. M., Stehman, F. B., Roth, L. M., et al. Bowenoid dysplasia of the vulva. *Cancer* 50:2910, 1982.

Wade, T. R., Kopf, A. W., and Ackerman, A. B. Bowenoid papulosis of the penis. *Cancer* 42:1890, 1978.

Basal Cell Epithelioma

Caro, M. R., and Howell, J. B. Morphea-like epithelioma. *Arch. Dermatol. Syphilol.* 65:53, 1951.

Costanza, M. E., Dayal, Y., Binder, S., and Nathanson, L. Metastatic basal cell carcinoma. *Cancer* 34:230, 1974.

Farmer, E. R., and Helwig, E. B. Metastatic basal cell carcinoma: A clinicopathologic study of seventeen cases. *Cancer* 46:748–757, 1980.

Freeman, R. G., and Winkelmann, R. K. Basal cell tumor with eccrine differentiation (eccrine epithelioma). *Arch. Dermatol.* 100:234, 1969.

General

Gelfant, S. A new concept of tissue and tumor cell proliferation. *Cancer Res.* 37:3845, 1977.

Graham, J. H., and Helwig, E. B. Premalignant Cutaneous and Mucocutaneous Diseases. In J. H. Graham, W. C. Johnson, and E. B. Helwig (Eds.), *Dermal Pathology.* Hagerstown, Md.: Harper & Row, 1972.

Kopf, A. W., Bart, R. S., and Andrade, R. *Atlas of Tumors of the Skin.* Philadelphia: Saunders, 1978.

Lever, W. F. Pathology of common skin tumors. *J. Surg. Oncol.* 3:235, 1971.

Chapter 7

Atrophic Processes of the Epidermis

The Reactive Process and the Disease	Histopathology	Comments
I. Lichen sclerosus et atrophicus (Fig. 9-4)		
A. Early	1. Variable hyperkeratosis 2. Epidermal atrophy	

> *Epidermal atrophy* may be a prominent feature in:
>
> Atrophic actinic keratosis
> Atrophic lichen planus
> Scleroderma
> Lentigo maligna
> Chronic graft-versus-host reaction
> Aged or actinically damaged skin
> Following chronic use of topical corticosteroid preparations
> Acrodermatitis chronica atrophicans
> Radiodermatitis
> Necrobiosis lipoidica
> Lupus erythematosus
> Dermatomyositis
> Epidermis overlying tumors

The Reactive Process and the Disease	Histopathology	Comments
	3. Vacuolation of dermoepidermal junction	See also Ch. 9, I.E
	4. Markedly edematous and **homogenized, broadened papillary dermis**	Subepidermal hemorrhagic bulla occasionally present
	5. Vascular ectasia	
	6. Bandlike mononuclear cell infiltrate beneath the edematous papillary dermis extending about and between venules and into the upper reticular dermis	See also Ch. 9, I.E; Ch. 10, II
B. Late	1. Marked hyperkeratosis 2. **Follicular plugging** 3. Marked epidermal **atrophy** alternating with epidermal hyperplasia	
	4. **Vacuolation** along the dermoepidermal interface	See also Ch. 9, I.E
	5. **Squamotization** of basal cell layer	

	6. **Homogenization of papillary dermis** with **sclerosis** of collagen	Differential diagnosis:
		  Morphea
		  Lupus erythematosus
		  Chronic radiodermatitis

	7. Patchy mononuclear cell infiltrate chronic in upper dermis	

II. Parapsoriasis	Parapsoriasis variegata and parapsoriasis en plaques (Fig. 4-4) at times may exhibit variable atrophy of the epidermis	See also Ch. 4, I.E; Ch. 10, VIII
III. Porokeratosis (Fig. 7-1)	1. **Coronoid lamella:** A column of parakeratotic stratum corneum arising within a keratin-filled invagination of epidermis 2. **Absence of granular layer at the base of the coronoid lamella;** cells may be vacuolated or dyskeratotic 3. Epidermis overlying the central portion of the lesion may be normal, atrophic, or even hyperplastic 4. Mild lymphohistiocytic perivascular infiltrate in dermis	These changes often are less well formed in disseminated superficial actinic porokeratosis
IV. Acrodermatitis chronica atrophicans		
A. Inflammatory phase	1. Hyperkeratosis 2. Parakeratosis 3. Epidermal atrophy with spongiosis 4. Grenz zone	

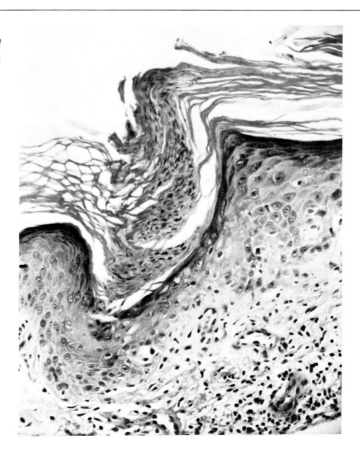

Fig. **7**-1. *Porokeratosis. The column of parakeratotic cells, called the* coronoid lamella, *rests within an epidermal invagination and overlies an area of hypogranulosis and dyskeratosis. Epidermal atrophy is typical. (×256)*

5. Patchy lymphohistiocytic infiltrate around and between vessels throughout edematous dermis and subcutaneous fat

6. Atrophic sebaceous glands and hair follicles; eccrine glands preserved

B. Atrophic phase

1. Profound **atrophy of epidermis, dermis, and subcutaneous fat**

2. Inflammatory infiltrate scant to absent

See also Ch. 10, VII; Ch. 18, X

V. Poikiloderma vasculare atrophicans (Fig. 7-2)

1. Hyperkeratosis
2. Focal parakeratosis
3. **Epidermal atrophy** with flattening of rete ridges
4. Dyskeratosis

> *Poikiloderma* may be:
>
> Congenital
> Idiopathic
> Associated with dermatomyositis
> Associated with mycosis fungoides

5. **Vacuolation** along dermoepidermal interface

See also Ch. 9, II.F

6. **Bandlike lymphohistiocytic dermal infiltrate**

See also Ch. 10, IX

7. Vascular ectasia
8. Pigment incontinence may be prominent

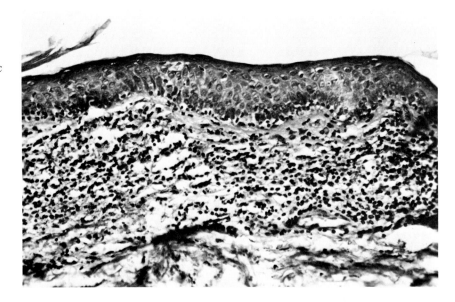

Fig. **7-2.** *Poikiloderma. Thinning of the epidermis, vacuolation of the dermoepidermal junction, lymphocytes lined up in the basal layer, and bandlike chronic inflammation of the dermis are characteristic. Severe atypism of lymphocytes is seen in mycosis fungoides–associated poikiloderma vasculare atrophicans. (×256)*

VI. Lupus erythematosus (see Fig. 9-3)

1. Hyperkeratosis
2. Follicular plugging
3. Epidermal atrophy
4. Squamotization of basal cell layer
5. Thickened basement membrane zone

Direct immunofluorescence studies are often helpful in diagnosis

Demonstration of thickened basement membrane with PAS stain is helpful in diagnosis of lupus erythematosus

See Ch. 9, I.D, II.D

6. **Vacuolation** along dermal epidermal junction both **above and below basement membrane zone**
7. Edema of papillary dermis
8. Vascular ectasia
9. **Lymphohistiocytic dermal infiltrate** may be:
   a. Bandlike, occasionally obscuring the dermal interface
   b. Patchy and disposed about vessels and appendages in reticular dermis, occasionally extending into subcutaneous fat
10. Pigment incontinence common
11. Increased deposition of acid mucopolysaccharide in reticular dermis

Based on histology alone, it is not possible to differentiate cutaneous (discoid) lupus erythematosus from systemic lupus erythematosus

See also Ch. 10, III

See also Ch. 14, I.B.1; Ch. 22, I.G

Fig. **7-3.** *Kyrle's disease.*
A. *An epidermal invagination is plugged by parakeratotic and basophilic material. Note the attenuation of the epidermis at the base of the plug. (×256)*
B. *Where the plug contacts the dermis, neutrophils and altered collagen bundles can be observed. (×256)*

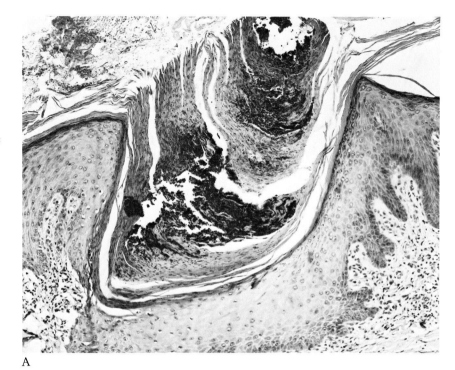

A

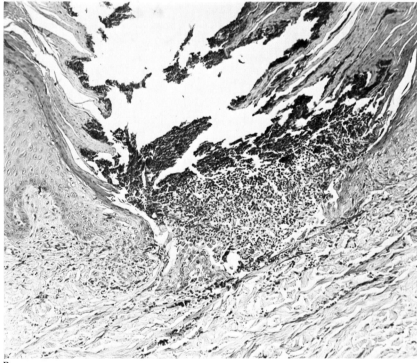

B

VII. Kyrle's disease (Fig. 7-3)

1. Epidermal invagination filled with keratin plug and basophilic debris
2. Focal atrophy of epidermal wall at base of invagination associated with loss of granular layer
3. Keratin plug at times in direct contact with dermis
4. Mononuclear cell infiltrate in dermis

Kyrle's disease is classified with other *perforating disorders* of the skin:

Perforating folliculitis
Reactive perforating collagenosis (Fig. 7-4)
Elastosis perforans serpiginosa
Perforating granuloma annulare

Fig. **7-4.** *Perforating collagenosis. At the base of an invagination similar to that of Fig. 7-3, collagen fibers appear to traverse the epidermis. (×400)*

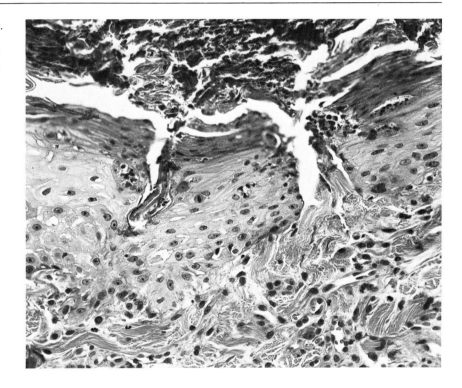

Suggested Reading
Lichen Sclerosus et Atrophicus

Bergfeld, W. F., and Lesowitz, S. A. Lichen sclerosus et atrophicus. *Arch. Dermatol.* 101:247, 1970.
Steigleder, G. K., and Raab, W. P. Lichen sclerosus et atrophicus. *Arch. Dermatol.* 84:219, 1961.

Parapsoriasis

Bonvalet, D. The different forms of parapsoriasis en plaques. A report of 90 cases. *Acta Derm. Venereol. (Stockh.)* 104:18, 1977.
Hu, C. H., and Winklemann, R. K. Digitate dermatosis. A new look at symmetrical, small plaque parapsoriasis. *Arch. Dermatol.* 107:65, 1973.
Lambert, W. C. Parapsoriasis. In T. B. Fitzpatrick et al. (Eds.), *Dermatology in General Medicine* (2nd ed.). New York: McGraw-Hill, 1979.
Samman, P. D. The natural history of parapsoriasis en plaques (chronic superficial dermatitis) and prereticulotic poikiloderma. *Br. J. Dermatol.* 87:405, 1972.
Sanchez, J. F., and Ackerman, A. B. The patch stage of mycosis fungoides. Criteria for histologic diagnosis. *Am. J. Dermatopathol.* 1:5, 1979.

Porokeratosis

Mikhail, G. R., and Wertheimer, F. W. Clinical variants of porokeratosis (Mibelli). *Arch. Dermatol.* 98:124, 1968.
Reed, R. J., and Leone, P. Porokeratosis—A mutant clonal keratosis of the epidermis. I. Histogenesis. *Arch. Dermatol.* 101:340, 1970.

Acrodermatitis Chronica Atrophicans

Burgdorf, W. H. C., Worret, W. I., and Schultka, O. Acrodermatitis chronica atrophicans. *Int. J. Dermatol.* 18:595, 1979.
Montgomery, H., and Sullivan, R. R. Acrodermatitis atrophicans chronica. *Arch. Dermatol. Syphilol.* 51:32, 1945.

Poikiloderma Vasculare Atrophicans

Watsky, M. S., and Lynfield, Y. L. Poikiloderma vasculare atrophicans. *Cutis* 17:938, 1976.
Wolf, D. J., and Selmanowitz, V. J. Poikiloderma vasculare atrophicans. *Cancer* 25:682, 1970.

Lupus Erythematosus

Biesecker, G., Lavin, L., Ziskind, M., and Koffler, D. Cutaneous localization of the membrane attack complex in discoid and systemic lupus erythematosus. *N. Engl. J. Med.* 306:264, 1982.
Brown, M. M., and Yount, W. J. Skin immunopathology in systemic lupus erythematosus. *J.A.M.A.* 243:38, 1980.
Clark, W. H., Reed, R. J., and Mihm, M. C., Jr. Lupus erythematosus: Histopathology of cutaneous lesions. *Hum. Pathol.* 4:157, 1973.
Dubois, E. L. *Lupus Erythematosus: A Review of the Current Status of Discoid and Systemic Lupus Erythematosus and Their Variants* (2d ed.). Los Angeles: University of Southern California Press, 1974.
McCreight, W. G., and Montgomery, H. Cutaneous changes in lupus erythematosus. *Arch. Dermatol. Syphilol.* 61:1, 1950.
Provost, T. T., Zone, J. J., Synkowski, D., et al. Unusual cutaneous manifestations of systemic lupus erythematosus. I. Urticaria-like lesions. Correlation with clinical and serological abnormalities. *J. Invest. Dermatol.* 75:495, 1980.
Prunieras, M., and Montgomery, H. Histopathology of cutaneous lesions in systemic lupus erythematosus. *Arch. Dermatol.* 74:177, 1956.
Prystowsky, S. D., and Gilliam, J. N. Discoid lupus erythematosus as part of a larger disease spectrum. *Arch. Dermatol.* 111:1448, 1975.
Synkowski, D. R., Reichlin, M., and Provost, T. T. Serum autoantibodies in systemic lupus erythematosus and correlation with cutaneous features. *J. Rheumatol.* 9:380, 1982.
Tuffanelli, D. L., Kay, D., and Fukuyama, K. Dermal-epidermal junction in lupus erythematosus. *Arch. Dermatol.* 99:652, 1969.
Winkelmann, R. K. Spectrum of lupus erythematosus. *J. Cutan. Pathol.* 6:457, 1979.

Kyrle's Disease

Carter, V. H., and Constantine, V. S. Kyrle's disease. I. Clinical findings in five cases and review of literature. *Arch. Dermatol.* 97:624, 1968.

Constantine, V. S., and Carter, V. H. Kyrle's disease. II. Histopathologic findings in five cases and review of the literature. *Arch. Dermatol.* 97:633, 1968.

Hood, A. F., Hardegen, G. L., Zarate, A. R., et al. Kyrle's disease in patients with chronic renal failure. *Arch. Dermatol.* 118:85, 1982.

Squier, C. A., Eady, R. A., and Hopps, R. M. The permeability of epidermis lacking normal membrane-coating granules: An ultrastructural tracer study of Kyrle-Flegel disease. *J. Invest. Dermatol.* 70:361, 1978.

Chapter 8

Disorders of the Melanocyte

I. Hypermelanosis
   A. Circumscribed
      1. Ephelis (freckle)
      2. Café-au-lait spot
      3. Postinflammatory hyperpigmentation
      4. Melasma
   B. Diffuse
II. Hyperplasia
   A. Lentigo simplex
   B. Lentigo senilis
III. Neoplasia
   A. Benign
      1. Nevocellular nevus
         a. Junctional nevus
         b. Compound nevus
         c. Dermal nevus
         d. Congenital pigmented nevus
         e. Halo nevus
      2. Blue nevus
         a. Common
         b. Cellular
      3. Mongolian spot
      4. Spindle and epithelioid cell nevus (compound nevus of Spitz)
   B. Premalignant
      1. Lentigo maligna
   C. Malignant melanoma
      1. Lentigo maligna melanoma
      2. Superficial spreading melanoma
      3. Acral lentiginous melanoma
      4. Nodular melanoma
IV. Hypomelanosis
   A. Circumscribed
      1. Vitiligo and piebaldism
      2. Halo nevus
      3. Postinflammatory hypopigmentation
   B. Generalized
      1. Albinism, oculocutaneous
      2. Vitiligo
      3. Chédiak-Higashi syndrome

The Reactive Process and the Disease	Histopathology	Comments
I. Hypermelanosis		
A. Circumscribed		
1. Ephelis (freckle) (Fig. 8-1)	Increased melanin in basal cell layer; normal number of melanocytes	
2. Café-au-lait spot	Increased melanin in basal cell layer; probably increased number of melanocytes	Solitary café-au-lait spots are seen in the general population, but when multiple they may be associated with neurofibromatosis or Albright's syndrome
3. Postinflammatory hyperpigmentation	1. Increased melanin in basal cell layer; occasional increased number of melanocytes 2. Free and/or phagocytized melanin in dermis	Postinflammatory hyperpigmentation is seen in association with or following disorders that involve the dermoepidermal junction, such as lichen planus, lupus erythematosus, and drug eruptions
4. Melasma	1. Increased melanin in basal cell layer 2. Free and/or phagocytized melanin in dermis	

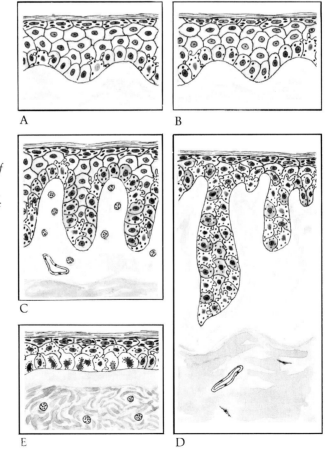

Fig. **8-1.** *Some disorders of intraepidermal melanocytes.*
A. *Normal: one melanocyte for every four to nine basal cells is usual.*
B. *Freckle: increased pigmentation of basal cells but normal or increased numbers of melanocytes are seen.*
C. *Lentigo simplex: increased pigmentation of basal cells with increased numbers of melanocytes and elongation of rete ridges is typical.*
D. *Lentigo senilis: similar to lentigo simplex but elongation of rete ridges is pronounced.*
E. *Lentigo maligna: increased numbers of atypical melanocytes on a background of sun-damaged skin with epidermal atrophy and solar elastosis.*

B. Diffuse

1. Increased melanin in basal cell layer; apparently normal number of melanocytes
2. Free and/or phagocytized melanin in dermis

Diffuse hypermelanosis may be seen in a wide variety of diseases including:

Addison's disease
Argyria
Hemochromatosis
Porphyria cutanea tarda
Arsenic intoxication
Busulfan administration
Progressive systemic sclerosis
Chronic hepatic insufficiency
Whipple's disease
Malignant melanoma
Radiation exposure
Ultraviolet light exposure

II. Hyperplasia

A. Lentigo simplex (Fig. 8-2)

1. **Elongation of rete ridges**
2. **Increased number of melanocytes**
3. **Increased melanin** in melanocytes, basal cells, and keratinocytes
4. Occasionally, small nests of nevus cells at the dermoepidermal junction
5. Melanophages in upper dermis
6. Occasionally, mild superficial mononuclear cell infiltrate

These histologic features also may be observed in:
Nevus spilus
Multiple lentigines syndrome
Peutz-Jeghers syndrome
Becker's nevus

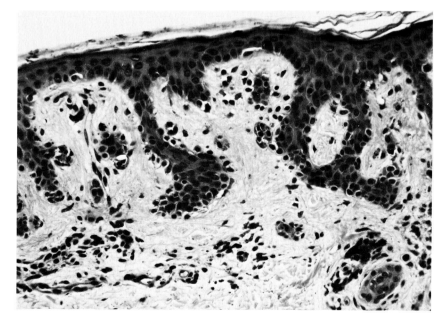

Fig. 8-2. *Lentigo. Melanocytic hyperplasia, hyperpigmented elongated rete ridges, and dermal melanophages are characteristic. (×400)*

B. Lentigo senilis

1. **Elongated, club-shaped rete ridges**
2. Increased number of melanocytes
3. Increased melanin in basal cells
4. Melanophages in upper dermis

A pigmented actinic keratosis may show proliferative "buds" and hyperpigmentation, somewhat resembling a lentigo. See also Ch. 6,III.A

III. Neoplasia

   A. Benign

      1. Nevocellular nevus

These lesions are composed of polygonal nevus cells (which are melanocytic cells of neuroectodermal origin) and are subclassified into junctional, compound, and dermal types

In contrast, collections of *dendritic* melanocytes in the dermis are characteristic of blue nevi

        a. Junctional nevus

1. **Nests of nevus cells within the lower part of the epidermis**
2. Nevus cell characteristics:

    Shape: cuboidal, oval, or spindle
    Cytoplasm: gray, often distinctly outlined
    Nucleus: large, round to oval
    Nucleolus: small
    Melanin: when present, disposed in variably large clumps

        b. Compound nevus (Fig. 8-3)

Intraepidermal and dermal nevus cells; stromal proliferation often observed

Fig. **8-3.** *Compound nevus. Nests of nevus cells are present within both the epidermis and dermis. (B, ×160)*

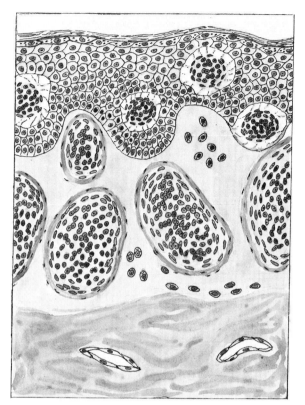

A

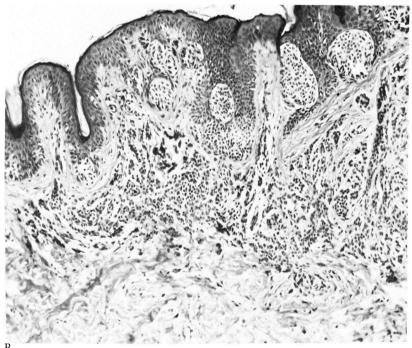

B

c. Dermal nevus	1. **Nests and cords of nevus cells in dermis**	Lower dermal portions of nevi sometimes exhibit a neuroid appearance with an increased number of mast cells; these changes are referred to as *neurotization* (Fig. 8-4)
	2. Nevus cell characteristics vary according to location within the dermis:	
	Upper dermis	
	Shape: cuboidal or oval	
	Cytoplasm: distinctly outlined, homogeneous	
	Nucleus: large, round or oval, pale or vesicular	
	Melanin: when present, finely granular	
	Lower dermis	
	Shape: elongate or spindle	
	Cytoplasm: pale blue-gray, homogeneous without distinct cellular outline	
	Nucleus: spindle-shaped	
	Melanin: usually absent; melanin may be present in adjacent melanophages	
d. Congenital pigmented nevus	The lesions may have the pattern of any nevocellular nevus but usually exhibit nevus cells in:	
	1. Middle to **lower dermis** and subcutis	
	2. Appendages and/or nerves	
	3. Single-cell array between collagen bundles	

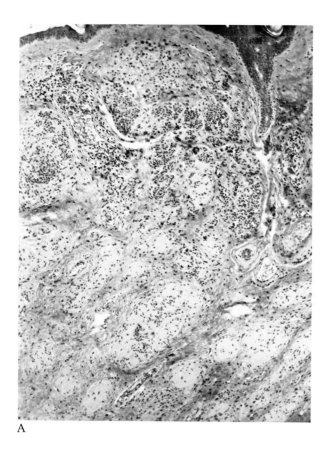

A

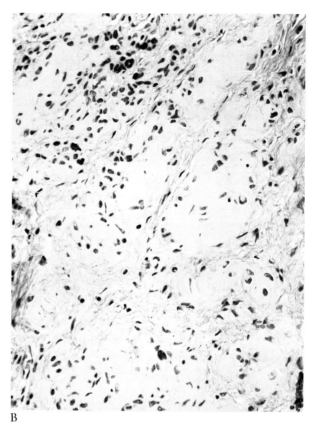

B

Fig. **8-4.** *Neurotized nevus.*
A. *Dermal nevus with neurotiza-*
   tion of deeper areas. (×100)
B. *At higher magnification a few*
   nevocellular nevus cells are
   evident in the upper central
   area, and neurotized nevus
   cells with copious lightly
   eosinophilic fibrillar cytoplasm
   are present elsewhere. (×400)

e. Halo nevus
(Figs. 8-5, 8-9)

1. **Absence of melanocytes within the depigmented halo**
2. **Nevus cells associated with an intense infiltrate of lymphocytes and histiocytes**
3. Nuclei of nevus cells frequently large with prominent nucleoli
4. Dermal fibrosis may be prominent

Dermal fibrosis may be associated with the inflammatory infiltrate; older lesions may exhibit fibrosis without inflammation

2. Blue nevus
a. Common
(Fig. 8-6)

1. Epidermis normal
2. Elongated, slender **dendritic melanocytes** are filled with fine melanin granules and are irregularly dispersed throughout the reticular dermis
3. **Melanophages** filled with coarse melanin granules
4. Dermal fibrosis

Dermal melanocytes in blue nevi similar to but more numerous than those seen in Mongolian spot

Differential diagnosis:
Mongolian spot
Nevus of Ota
Nevus of Ito
Tattoo

Fig. **8-5.** *Halo nevus. At the right and lower portions of the field, nevus cells are admixed with lymphocytes and histiocytes. Nevus cells without much inflammation are present in the upper portions of the micrograph. Older lesions of halo nevus may exhibit less inflammation and more fibrosis. (×400)*

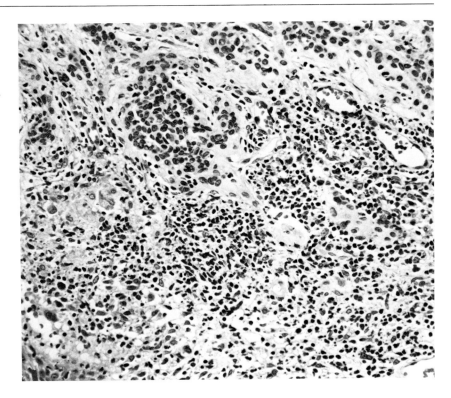

Fig. **8-6.** *Blue nevus.*
A. *The low-power impression is that of numerous pigmented cells in the dermis. Inset: At higher power two populations can be distinguished—dendritic melanocytes with rather delicate pigment (blue nevus cells) and numerous polygonal melanophages with abundant coarse cytoplasmic pigment.*
B. *Micrograph for comparison with A. Fibrosis, here delicate, frequently accompanies blue nevi. (×100)*

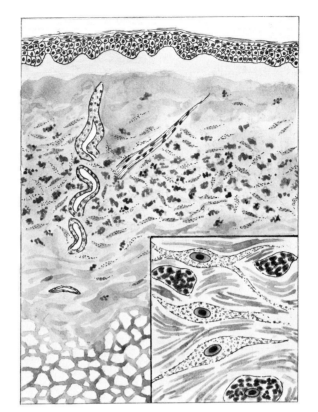

A

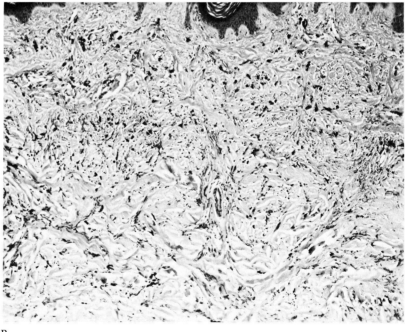

B

b. Cellular (Fig. 8-7)

Biphasic pattern with:

1. Zones of **pigmented dendritic melanocytes** and melanophages
2. Intersecting bundles of aggregated, large, **spindle-shaped and epithelioid cells** with ovoid nuclei, and abundant pale cytoplasm, containing **little or no melanin**

Differential diagnosis:
  Malignant melanoma
  Fibrosarcoma
  Dermatofibroma
  Leiomyoma
  Neurofibroma
  Dermatofibrosarcoma protuberans

3. Spindle-shaped cells may exhibit cytologic atypism
4. Mitoses may be numerous but not atypical

Spindle-shaped cells may give a neuroid or sarcomatous appearance

3. Mongolian spot

1. Ribbonlike, wavy dendritic cells containing evenly dispersed melanin granules are located in the dermis and lie parallel to the surface
2. Melanophages absent

Differential diagnosis:
  Blue nevus
  Nevus of Ota
  Nevus of Ito
  Tattoo

Nevus of Ota displays similar histology, but the distribution of the melanocytes tends to be more superficial

Fig. **8-7.** *Cellular blue nevus.*
A. *Proliferation of dendritic and spindle-type melanocytes with numerous melanophages fills the dermis. The biphasic pattern of bundles of spindle cells alternating with aggregates of dendritic melanocytes is characteristic of cellular blue nevus. (×29)*
B. *This higher magnification illustrates a spindle cell population organized in nests (*lower half of field*), dendritic melanocytes scattered between collagen bundles (*upper half of field*), and numerous heavily pigmented melanophages. (×256).*

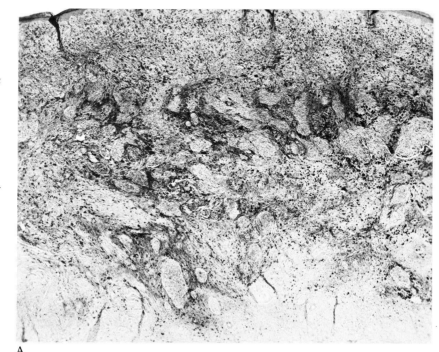

A

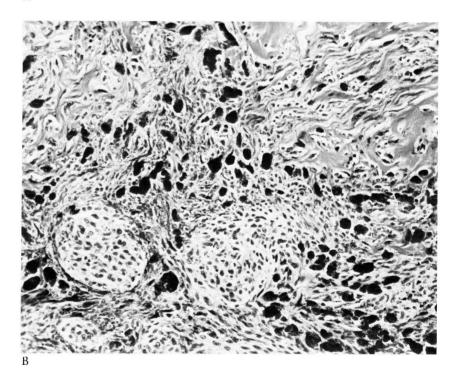

B

4. Spindle and epithelioid cell nevus (compound nevus of Spitz) (Fig. 8-8)

1. Nevus cells extend downward from the dermoepidermal junction, in irregular ("raining down") strands
2. Compound pattern most common, but purely junctional or dermal proliferation may occur
3. Cell types
   a. **Spindle-shaped:** characteristically arranged in whorls; rarely multinucleated
   b. **Epithelioid:** large, polygonal, well-demarcated cells with pale, variably staining cytoplasm
4. Chromatin finely disposed around the nuclear membrane; cytoplasm often "wispy" and usually not pigmented
5. Edema of upper dermis with ectatic capillary venules
6. Melanin may be found in small amounts, usually in macrophages
7. Mitotic figures may be present
8. Nevus cells at lower border infiltrate between collagen bundles
9. Bandlike chronic inflammatory infiltrate occasionally present

Differential diagnosis: malignant melanoma

Tumor cells may be predominantly spindle-shaped, epithelioid, or a mixture of both

Epithelioid cells may possess bizarre nuclei with large nucleoli; nevoid giant cells sometimes present

Staining of the cytoplasm varies from pale blue or mauve to bright pink

The halo phenomenon may occur in spindle and epithelioid cell nevi (Fig. 8-9) and melanoma as it does in nevocellular nevi

Fig. **8-8.** *Spindle cell nevus.*
A. *Plump spindle cells with variable amounts of amphophilic cytoplasm and melanin pigment are organized into nests at the dermoepidermal junction and into fasicles within the dermis.* Inset: *Nucleoli may appear very prominent.*
B. *Photomicrograph for comparison. Numerous junctional nests here are composed of spindle cells. A mitotic figure is present in the center of the field. (×400)*

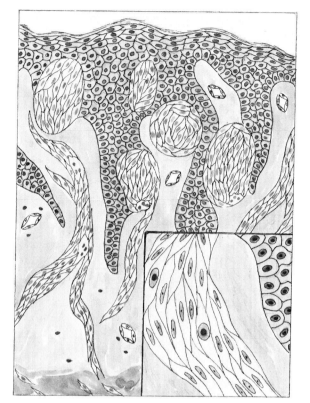

A

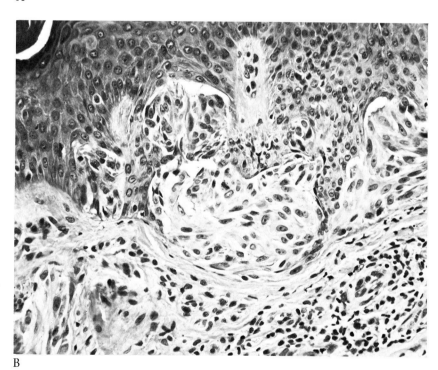

B

B. Premalignant
    1. Lentigo maligna
       (see Fig. 8-1E)

1. **Epidermal atrophy**
2. **Increased number of intraepidermal pleomorphic melanocytes** with variable hyperchromatism, vacuolated cytoplasm, and melanin granules
3. Melanocytes haphazardly dispersed along dermoepidermal junction with (a) occasional extension into the upper epidermis and (b) **downward extension into hair follicles and eccrine ducts**
4. **Solar elastosis** of upper dermis
5. Bandlike mononuclear cell infiltrate may be present
6. Melanophages

Fig. **8-9.** *Halo spindle cell nevus.*
A. Note the typical pattern of spindle cell nevus (compare with Fig. 8-8). (×100)
B. Superimposed upon this nevus is an inflammatory process composed of numerous lymphocytes in close association with nevus cells. (×400)

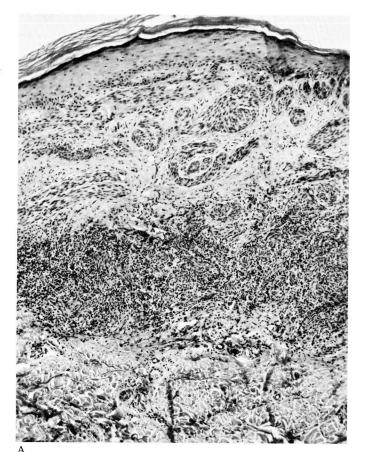

A

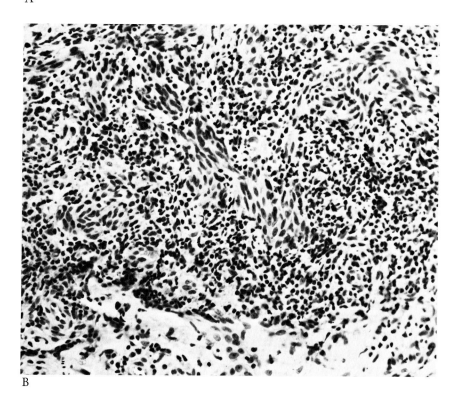

B

C. Malignant melanoma

1. Lentigo maligna melanoma (Fig. 8-10)

1. Histologic features of **lentigo maligna with dermal invasion by atypical, often spindle-shaped melanocytes**

Histologic features of atypical melanocytes include:
1. Increased nuclear-cytoplasmic ratio

Fig. **8-10.** *Lentigo maligna melanoma.*
A. *Nests of tumor cells are most prominent at the dermoepidermal junction of both the epidermis and the hair follicles. Prominent solar elastosis and epidermal atrophy accompany this tumor frequently. (×100)*
B. *Tumor cells invade the dermis accompanied by an underlying lymphocytic infiltrate. (×400)*

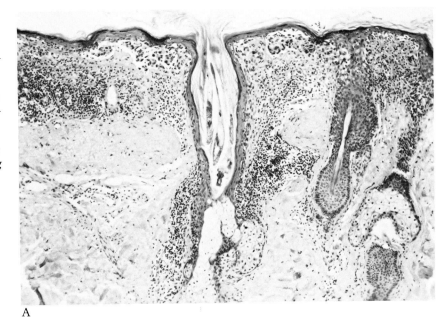

A

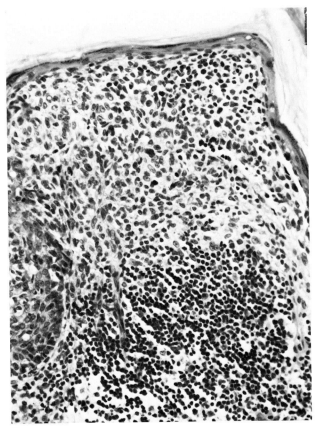

B

2. Mitoses frequent
3. Fibrosis and mononuclear cell infiltrate often associated with invading tumor cells

2. Nuclear pleomorphism and hyperchromatism
3. Occasional atypical mitotic figures (asymmetric, tripolar)

2. Superficial spreading melanoma (Fig. 8-11)

1. **Invasion of dermis** by malignant, commonly epithelioid melanocytes

Fig. **8-11.** *Malignant melanoma, superficial spreading type.*
A. Horizontal and vertical growth phases are evident at lower magnification. (×100)
B. Fibrosis and chronic inflammation within the dermis are frequently associated with tumor cells. (×256)

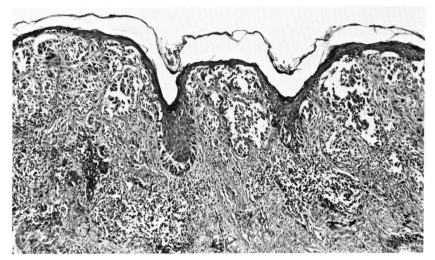

A

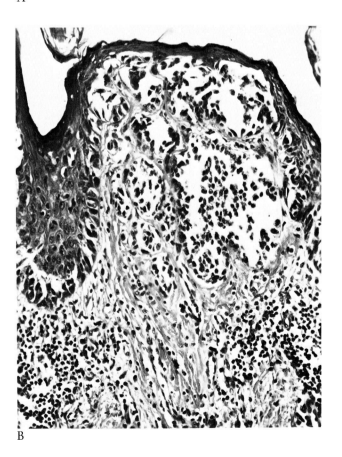

B

2. Marked pleomorphism with variable but often marked mitoses
3. Individual cells exhibit irregular chromatin clumping around nuclear membrane; nucleoli often prominent
4. Dusty pink-tan cytoplasm owing to intracellular melanin granules
5. Epidermis adjacent to invasive areas often exhibits a **pagetoid (single-cell) spread** of large atypical melanocytes

In superficial spreading melanoma and acral lentiginous melanoma, malignant intraepidermal cells extend more than three rete ridges from the areas of dermal invasion

3. Acral lentiginous melanoma

1. **Marked lentiginous hyperplasia of epidermis**
2. **Dermal invasion** by variably shaped pleomorphic malignant melanocytes
3. Epidermis adjacent to areas of invasion exhibits large, **heavily pigmented melanocytes with prominent dendrites** and large, round nuclei with prominent nucleoli
4. Stromal fibrosis with mononuclear cell infiltrate
5. Invasion of nerves by tumor cells may be present

Lentiginous hyperplasia connotes elongation of the rete ridges with hyperpigmentation and increased numbers of melanocytes

4. Nodular melanoma (Fig. 8-12)

1. Pleomorphic malignant melanocytes invade dermis with **little or no lateral intraepidermal component**
2. Nuclei exhibit irregular clumping of chromatin
3. Nucleoli large and sometimes multiple
4. Numerous atypical mitoses often present

In nodular melanoma, lateral spread (atypical melanocytic cells within the epidermis) is usually confined to three or fewer rete ridges

Tumor cells at the base of the lesion often (but not always) appear to *"push,"* or compress the collagen, rather than infiltrate between collagen bundles; the presence of a "pushing border" may be helpful in distinguishing between malignant melanoma and spindle and epithelioid cell nevus

Each melanoma must be (1) *measured* by a micrometer from the top of the granular cell layer to the base of the tumor (excluding periappendageal involvement) and (2) *categorized by the level of invasion:*

   I. Intraepidermal tumor
  II. Invasion into papillary dermis
 III. Tumor fills papillary dermis and extends to, but does not invade, reticular dermis
 IV. Invasion into reticular dermis
  V. Invasion into subcutaneous fat

Fig. **8-12.** *Malignant melanoma, nodular type.*

A. *Lack of lateral spread within the epidermis and nodular downward growth characterize this tumor. (×24)*

B. *Cytologic features of this tumor can vary widely. Large vesicular nuclei with prominent nucleoli and amphophilic cytoplasm with dusty pigment are illustrated here. (×400)*

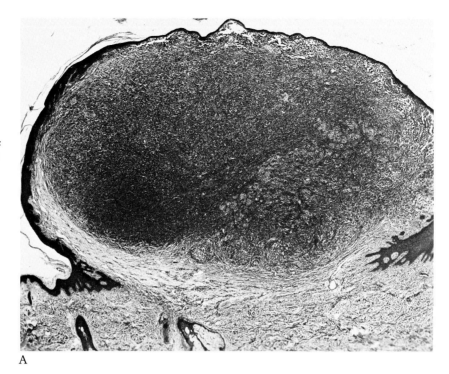

A

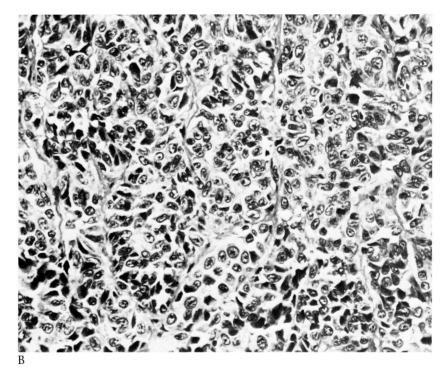

B

IV. Hypomelanosis

A. Circumscribed

1. Vitiligo and piebaldism	Absence of melanocytes	Melanocyte populations are difficult to define on H&E stained sections; electron microscopy will define cells with melanosomes (the ultrastructural hallmark of the melanocyte); DOPA-oxidase preparations define enzymatic functional activity in these cells
2. Halo nevus	Melanocytes are absent in areas of hypopigmentation	
3. Postinflammatory hypopigmentation	Decreased melanin in basal cells but melanocytes are present	

B. Generalized

1. Albinism, oculocutaneous	Absence of melanin in basal cells; melanocytes present
2. Vitiligo	Absence of melanocytes
3. Chédiak-Higashi syndrome	Irregularly shaped, large melanin granules in basal cells, upper dermis, and within melanophages

Suggested Reading
Hypermelanosis and Hypomelanosis

Jimbow, K., Fitzpatrick, T. B., Szabo, T., et al. Congenital circumscribed hypomelanosis: A characterization based on electron microscopic study of tuberous sclerosis, nevus depigmentosus, and piebaldism. *J. Invest. Dermatol.* 64:50, 1975.

Miller, R. A. Psoralens and UV-A–induced stellate hyperpigmented freckling. *Arch. Dermatol.* 118:619, 1982.

Mishima, Y. Histopathology of functional pigmentary disorders. *Cutis* 21:225, 1978.

Morris, T. J., Johnson, W. G., and Silvers, D. N. Giant pigment granules in biopsy specimens from café au lait spots in neurofibromatosis. *Arch. Dermatol.* 118:385, 1982.

Mosher, D. B., Fitzpatrick, T. B., and Ortonne, J. P. Abnormalities of Pigmentation. In T. B. Fitzpatrick et al. (Eds.) *Dermatology in General Medicine* (2d ed.). New York: McGraw-Hill, 1979.

Nevocellular Nevus

Bhawan, J. Melanocytic nevi. A review. *J. Cutan. Pathol.* 6:153, 1979.

Clark, W. H., Reimer, R. R., Greene, M., et al. Origin of familial malignant melanomas from heritable melanocytic lesions, "the B-K mole syndrome." *Arch. Dermatol.* 114:732, 1978.

Elder, D. E., Goldman, L. I., Goldman, S. C., et al. Dysplastic nevus syndrome: A phenotypic association of sporadic cutaneous melanoma. *Cancer* 46:1787, 1980.

Shaffer, B. Pigmented nevi. *Arch. Dermatol.* 72:120, 1955.

Congenital Nevus

Hendrickson, M. R., and Ross, J. C. Neoplasms arising in congenital giant nevi: Morphologic study of seven cases and a review of the literature. *Am. J. Surg. Pathol.* 5:109, 1981.

Mark, G. J., Mihm, M. C., and Liteplo, M. G. Congenital melanocytic nevi of the small and garment type. Clinical, histologic and ultrastructural studies. *Hum. Pathol.* 4:395, 1973.

Halo Nevus

Wayte, D. M., and Helwig, E. B. Halo nevi. *Cancer* 22:69, 1968.

Blue Nevus

Dorsey, C. S., and Montgomery, H. Blue nevus and its distinction from Mongolian spot and the nevus of Ota. *J. Invest. Dermatol.* 22:225, 1954.

Leopold, J. G., and Richards, D. B. Cellular blue naevi. *J. Pathol. Bact.* 94:247, 1967.

Rodriguez, H. A., and Ackerman, L. V. Cellular blue nevus. *Cancer* 21:393, 1968.

Spindle and Epithelioid Cell Nevus

McWhorter, H. E., and Woolner, L. B. Treatment of juvenile melanomas and malignant melanomas in children. *J.A.M.A.* 156:695, 1954.

Paniago-Pereira, C., Maize, J. C., and Ackerman, A. B. Nevus of large spindle and/or epithelioid cells (Spitz's nevus). *Arch. Dermatol.* 114:1811, 1978.

Reed, R. J., Ichinose, H., Clark, W. H., Jr., and Mihm, M. C., Jr. Common and uncommon melanocytic nevi and borderline melanomas. *Semin. Oncol.* 2:119, 1975.

Malignant Melanoma

Balch, C., Murad, T. M., Soong, S.-J., et al. A multifactorial analysis of melanoma: Prognostic histopathological features comparing Clark's and Breslow's staging methods. *Ann. Surg.* 188:732, 1978.

Day, C. L., Mihm, M. C., Sober, A. J., et al. Narrower margins for clinical stage I malignant melanoma. *N. Engl. J. Med.* 306:479, 1982.

Feibleman, C. E., Stoll, H., and Maize, J. C. Melanomas of the palm, sole and nailbed; a clinicopathologic study. *Cancer* 46:2492, 1980.

Gromet, M. A., Epstein, W. L., and Blois, M. S. The regressing thin malignant melanoma, a distinctive lesion with metastatic potential. *Cancer* 42:2282, 1978.

Kopf, A. W., Bart, R. S., Rodriguez-Sains, R. S., et al. *Malignant Melanoma.* New York, Masson, 1979.

McGovern, V. J., Shaw, H. M., Milton, G. W., et al. Prognostic significance of the histological features of malignant melanoma. *Histopathology* 3:385, 1979.

Sober, A. J., Fitzpatrick, T. B., and Mihm, M. C. Primary melanoma of the skin: Recognition and management. *J. Am. Acad. Dermatol.* 2:179, 1980.

Part III

Basement Membrane Zone, Papillary Dermis, and Superficial Venular Plexus

Chapter 9

Vacuolation of the Basement Membrane Zone

I. With inflammation and squamotization
   A. Lichen planus
      1. Bullous lichen planus
      2. Mucosal lichen planus
      3. Hypertrophic lichen planus
      4. Atrophic lichen planus
   B. Lichen planus–like drug eruption
   C. Lichenoid keratosis
   D. Lupus erythematosus
   E. Lichen sclerosus et atrophicus, older lesions
   F. Graft-versus-host reaction (GVHR)
   G. Erythema multiforme (EM), epidermal type (recurrent, Hebra type)
   H. Toxic epidermal necrolysis (TEN)
   I. Fixed drug eruption
II. With inflammation but without squamotization
   A. Bullous pemphigoid
   B. Dermatitis herpetiformis
   C. Herpes gestationis
   D. Lupus erythematosus
   E. Dermatomyositis
   F. Poikiloderma vasculare atrophicans (idiopathic)
   G. Bullous drug eruption
   H. Morbilliform viral exanthem
   I. Inflammatory pityriasis rosea
   J. Pityriasis lichenoides et varioliformis acuta (PLEVA, Mucha-Habermann disease)
   K. Light eruptions including photoallergic reaction and polymorphous light eruption
   L. Secondary syphilis
III. Without inflammation
   A. Porphyria cutanea tarda
   B. Epidermolysis bullosa dystrophica and acquisita
   C. Acute radiodermatitis

Many inflammatory and vesiculobullous cutaneous diseases are characterized histologically by the presence of vacuoles along the dermoepidermal junction. These vacuoles may be located above the basement membrane, below the basement membrane, or, as in lupus erythematosus, both above and below. Coalescence of the vacuoles may result in subepidermal cleft formation or clinical blisters. Vacuolation along the dermoepidermal junction may or may not be accompanied by inflammation. Diseases with inflammation may be subdivided further into those with or without squamotization of the basal layer, a situation in which the normally cuboidal or columnar basal cells are replaced by polygonal or even flattened keratinocytes (see Fig. 2-11).

The Reactive Process and the Disease	Histopathology	Comments
I. With inflammation and squamotization		
A. Lichen planus (Fig. 9-1)	1. Hyperkeratosis 2. **Hypergranulosis** 3. Irregular hyperplasia of epidermis with characteristic **sawtooth** changes of the rete ridges 4. Homogeneous, eosinophilic hyaline bodies (**Civatte bodies**) in the epidermis and papillary dermis 5. Squamotization of basal cell layer	Parakeratosis more commonly observed in lichenoid drug eruptions, hypertrophic lichen planus, and mucosal lichen planus *Lichenoid infiltrates and Civatte bodies* may be seen in many disorders, including: Lichen planus Lichen planopilaris Graft-versus-host reaction Lupus erythematosus Poikiloderma vasculare atrophicans Lichen planus–like drug eruption Actinic keratosis Lichenoid keratosis Halo nevus Spindle and epithelioid cell nevus
	6. **Vacuolation of basal cell layer** 7. **Bandlike infiltrate** of lymphocytes, histiocytes, and macrophages which may obscure the dermoepidermal interface 8. Variable number of melanophages	Vacuoles may coalesce to form subepidermal clefts (Max-Joseph spaces) The presence of eosinophils raises the question of lichen planus–like drug eruption Melanophages are often associated with inflammation in the area of the dermoepidermal junction

Fig. **9-1.** *Lichen planus. Typical features include irregular acanthosis ("sawtoothing"), hyperkeratosis, hypergranulosis, a lymphocytic infiltrate that "hugs" the basal layer, vacuolation at the dermoepidermal junction, Civatte bodies (A, anucleate pink bodies near the dermoepidermal junction), and a squamotized basal layer (see also Fig. 2-11). (×100)*

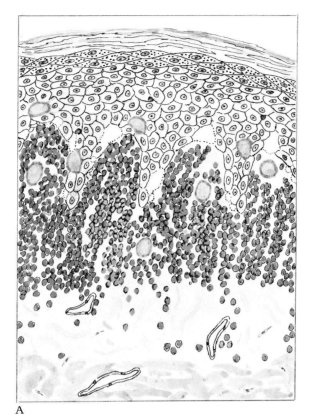

A

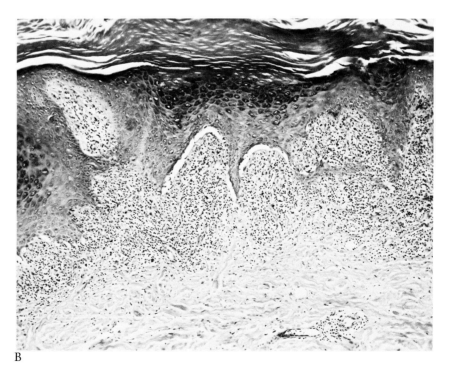

B

All the following are characterized by **squamotization, vacuolation,** and **bandlike infiltrate**

1. Bullous lichen planus

1. **Subepidermal bulla** with marked squamotization of basal cells in roof of bulla
2. Sawtooth papillae may protrude into base of bulla

2. Mucosal lichen planus (Fig. 9-1)

1. **Hypergranulosis**
2. Squamotization and bandlike infiltrate

The presence of keratohyaline granules in most mucosal epithelium represents hypergranulosis since the granular cell layer is normally absent

3. Hypertrophic lichen planus

1. Hyperkeratosis and parakeratosis
2. Marked hypergranulosis
3. **Marked epidermal hyperplasia**
4. Hyperplastic papillary dermis often contains melanophages
5. Mononuclear cell infiltrate focally along dermoepidermal junction and around superficial venules

When no bandlike infiltrate is present, consider lichen simplex chronicus or prurigo nodularis

4. Atrophic lichen planus

1. Epidermal **atrophy**
2. Vacuolation of dermoepidermal junction

Atrophic lichen planus may be difficult to distinguish from lupus erythematosus or lichenoid (actinic) keratosis

B. Lichen planus–like drug eruption

1. Variable hyperkeratosis
2. Parakeratosis common
3. Hypergranulosis often less prominent than lichen planus
4. Variable number of Civatte bodies
5. Vacuolation and squamotization of basal layer may be focal
6. Hyperplastic epidermis with sawtooth rete pattern
7. Dermal infiltrate contains **eosinophils, plasma cells,** and rare neutrophils in addition to lymphocytes and histiocytes
8. Infiltrate extends more prominently about superficial venules and about mid-dermal small vessels than along dermoepidermal junction

Lichen planus and some lichen planus–like drug eruptions may be virtually indistinguishable

Reported causes of *lichen planus–like drug eruptions* include:

Heavy metals: gold, mercury
Arsenicals
Iodides
Quinine
Antibiotics: tetracycline, streptomycin
Para-amino salicylic acid
Phenothiazines
Color-film developer, topically applied
Diuretics: chlorothiazide, hydrochlorothiazide
Antimetabolites: methotrexate

C. Lichenoid keratosis (Fig. 9-2)

1. Hyperkeratosis
2. Focal parakeratosis
3. Dyskeratosis
4. Focal atypia of epidermal cells may be present
5. Variable vacuolation of basal layer
6. Bandlike infiltrate with melanin-laden macrophages irregularly distributed in papillary dermis

The concept of lichenoid keratosis is somewhat confusing, but the term is usually used to describe an erythematous lesion on sun-exposed skin that histologically resembles lichen planus (see *lichenoid actinic keratosis*, Ch. 6, III.A.4)

Fig. **9-2.** *Lichenoid keratosis. A lymphohistiocytic infiltrate "hugs" the dermoepidermal junction. The overlying epidermis appears acanthotic but lacks the distinctive features of lichen planus such as hypergranulosis and sawtoothing. (×256)*

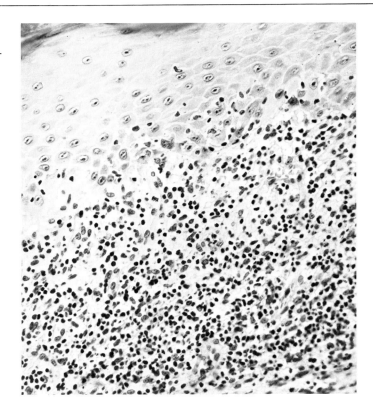

D. Lupus erythematosus (Fig. 9-3)

1. Hyperkeratosis
2. **Follicular keratin plugs**
3. Epidermal atrophy
4. Squamotization of basal cell layer
5. Variable thickening of basement membrane zone
6. Vacuolation along dermoepidermal junction above and below basement membrane
7. Variable edema of papillary dermis
8. Dilated or ectatic vessels

PAS stain confirms thickening of basement membrane zone

See also Ch. 7, VI; Ch. 10, III; Ch. 14, I.B.1

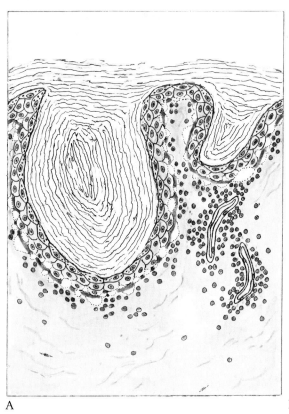

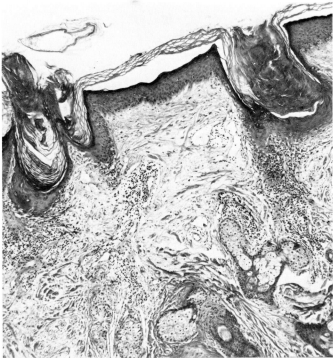

A   B

Fig. **9-3.** *Lupus erythematosus. A, B. Follicular plugging, epidermal atrophy, a predominantly lymphocytic infiltrate dispersed about appendages and vessels, vacuolation, and thickening of the basement membrane zone characterize the usually discoid lesions. (B, ×100)*

C, D. *Similar changes but with edema, vascular ectasia, and sometimes smudged fibrinoid material about vessels are more typical of the lesions of systemic lupus erythematosus. A clear-cut distinction, however, between discoid and systemic erythematosus cannot be made on the basis of routine histopathology. (C, ×256; D, ×400)*

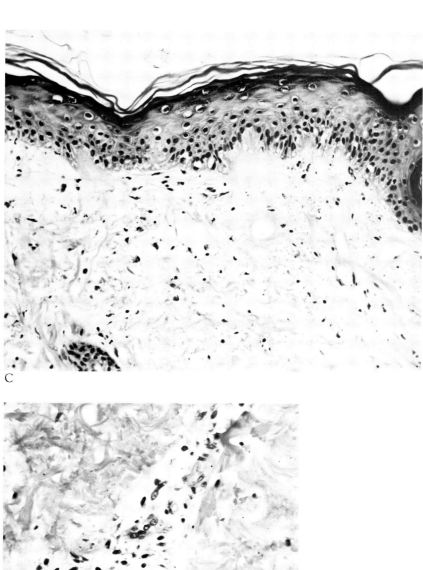

C

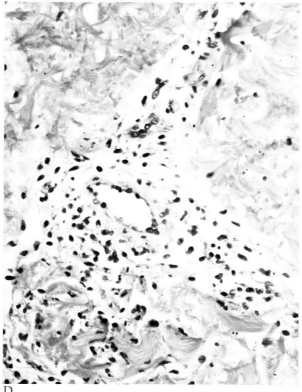

D

9. Bandlike or patchy perivenular lymphohistiocytic dermal infiltrate rarely may obscure the dermoepidermal interface
10. Focal dermal hemorrhage may be present, especially in early lesions
11. **Perivascular and periappendageal lymphohistiocytic infiltrate** in reticular dermis occasionally extends into subcutaneous fat
12. **Infiltrate extends into appendageal epithelium with vacuolation of basal cells**
13. Mucin (hyaluronic acid) deposition in the reticular dermis

Thirty-five percent of patients with systemic lupus erythematosus exhibit lesions clinically and histologically indistinguishable from discoid lupus erythematosus; therefore, it is unwise to attempt to diagnose the type of lupus (systemic or discoid) on the basis of histologic features; the results of direct immunofluorescence and serologic studies may be helpful

Mucin deposition may be so extensive as to resemble myxedema
Histologically it is often difficult to differentiate the lesions of dermatomyositis from acute lupus erythematosus

E. Lichen sclerosus et atrophicus (older lesions) (Fig. 9-4)

1. Marked vacuolation at dermoepidermal junction
2. Focal squamotization
3. **Edematous, homogeneous hyalinized papillary dermis**
4. Sparse, bandlike, lymphohistiocytic infiltrate may be present beneath hyalinized zone

See also Ch. 7, I; Ch. 10, II

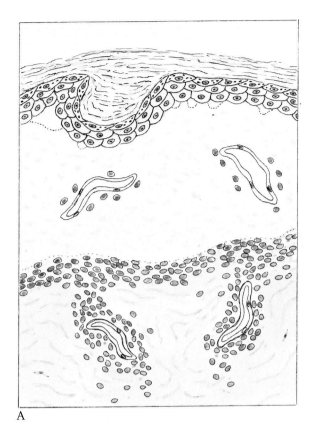

A

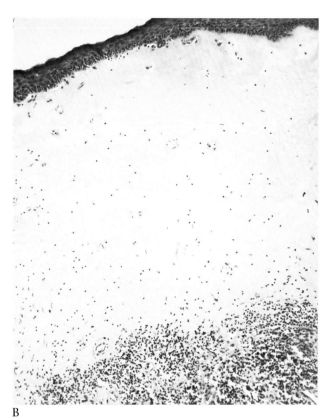

B

Fig. 9-4. *Lichen sclerosus et atrophicus. Vacuolation at the dermoepidermal interface (A, C), homogenization of the upper dermis, and an underlying bandlike lymphocytic infiltrate are the hallmarks of this disorder. Follicular plugging (A) and epidermal atrophy frequently accompany the features described above. (B, ×160; C, ×160)*

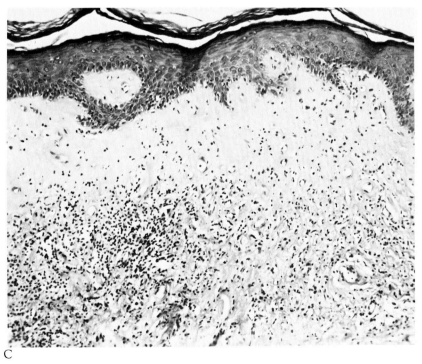

C

F. Graft-versus-host reaction (GVHR) (Fig. 9-5)

1. Hyperkeratosis
2. **Epidermal thinning** with **loss of polarity** of epidermal cells
3. **Dyskeratotic epidermal cells** in clear lacunae occasionally surrounded by lymphocytes
4. **Vacuolation** at dermoepidermal junction
5. Mild perivenular infiltrate with extension into epidermis
6. Melanin incontinence
7. Sclerosis of papillary and reticular dermis with appendageal entrapment in subacute and chronic lesions
8. Subepidermal bullae and ulceration occasionally observed

Early lesions may be confused with erythema multiforme; the prominent disarray of epidermal cells and sparse infiltrate in GVHR helps differentiate the entities

Late (chronic GVHR) lesions can be misdiagnosed as scleroderma if epidermal changes are overlooked

G. Erythema multiforme (EM), epidermal type (recurrent, Hebra type) (Figs. 9-6, 9-7) (see Ch. 11, I.B, for drug-induced erythema multiforme)

1. Focal dyskeratosis
2. Focal intercellular edema
3. Vacuolation of basal cell layer with lymphocytes along the dermoepidermal junction
4. Subepidermal bulla formation may occur
5. Perivenular lymphohistiocytic and rarely eosinophilic infiltrate
6. Endothelial cell hypertrophy of affected cutaneous vessels
7. Melanin incontinence may be present

Numerous dyskeratotic cells may be observed in drug-induced erythema multiforme and the lichenoid phase of pityriasis lichenoides et varioliformis acuta

The histopathology of fixed drug eruption may be indistinguishable from erythema multiforme

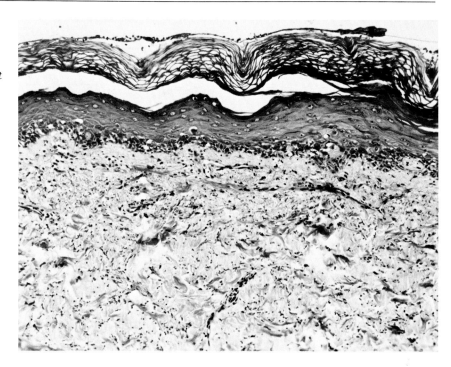

Fig. **9-5.** *Acute graft-versus-host reaction. Numerous dyskeratotic cells, a lymphocytic infiltrate closely applied to the lower stratum Malpighii, vacuolation at the dermoepidermal junction, and irregular, disturbed epidermal maturation are illustrated. (×160)*

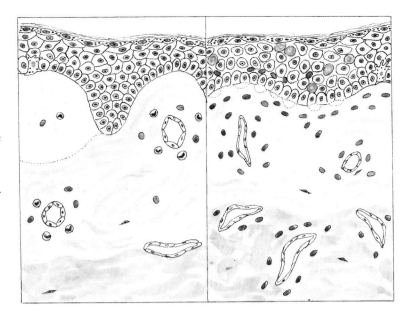

Fig. **9-6.** *Comparison of the noninflammatory and inflammatory types of erythema multiforme.* Left: *Subepidermal cleft formation with edema of the papillary dermis and sparse mononuclear infiltrates is typical of the noninflammatory type of erythema multiforme, of which toxic epidermal necrolysis can be considered an example.* Right: *Dyskeratosis and spongiosis within the epidermis, vacuolation at the dermoepidermal interface, and lymphocytes lined up at the same location and around venules are characteristic of an early lesion of erythema multiforme, inflammatory type.*

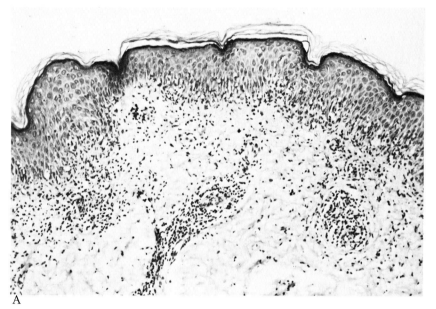

Fig. **9-7.** *Erythema multiforme, inflammatory type. Dermoepidermal junction changes include vacuolation and lymphocytic infiltration. The infiltrate is also disposed about superficial vessels and focally within the epidermis. Spongiosis and dyskeratosis are typical.*
A. *An early lesion with minimal dyskeratosis.* (×160)
B. *A later lesion with numerous dyskeratotic cells and separation at the dermoepidermal junction.* (×160)

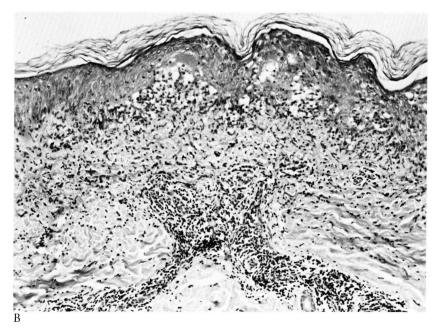

H. Toxic epidermal necrolysis (TEN) (Fig. 9-6)

1. **Full-thickness epidermal necrosis with subepidermal bullae**
2. Vacuolation along dermoepidermal junction adjacent to necrotic epidermis
3. Dermal infiltrate may be sparse

Full-thickness epidermal necrosis may occasionally be observed in erythema multiforme; some observers consider TEN to be a type of noninflammatory EM

I. Fixed drug eruption

1. Focal hyperkeratosis
2. Intercellular edema
3. Focal dyskeratosis most prominent along the basal layer
4. Exocytosis of lymphocytes into lower epidermal region
5. **Vacuolation along the dermoepidermal junction**
6. Lymphohistiocytic infiltrate along dermoepidermal junction may be bandlike
7. Perivenular lymphohistiocytic infiltrate about superficial and deep vessels
8. **Melanin incontinence**

In late stages epidermal changes are minimal, but vacuolation persists associated with numerous melanophages and sometimes a slight inflammatory infiltrate

Differential diagnosis:
Erythema multiforme
Lichenoid drug eruption
Graft-versus-host reaction

II. With inflammation but without squamotization

A. Bullous pemphigoid (Fig. 9-8)

1. **Subepidermal bulla** with roof composed of relatively normal epidermis
2. Vacuolation along the dermoepidermal junction adjacent to bulla
3. Eosinophils may migrate into the epidermis in early lesions
4. Bullous edematous papillae protrude into blister cavity

> *Epidermal invasion by eosinophils* may be seen in:
>
> Bullous pemphigoid
> Pemphigus vulgaris
> Insect bite reaction
> Allergic contact dermatitis
> Incontinentia pigmenti

5. Scattered superficial and deep dermal infiltrate of **eosinophils and lymphocytes** with some aggregation about venules

The number of eosinophils varies; when present in great numbers, they may extend through the dermis and into subcutaneous fat; immunofluorescence studies are usually diagnostic

Fig. **9-8.** *Bullous pemphigoid.*
A. Noninflammatory type. Sub-epidermal cleft formation with small numbers of lymphocytes and eosinophils is characteristic. (×160)
B, C. Inflammatory type. Sub-epidermal cleft formation with numerous eosinophils and lymphocytes within the bulla and dermis is characteristic. (C, ×256)

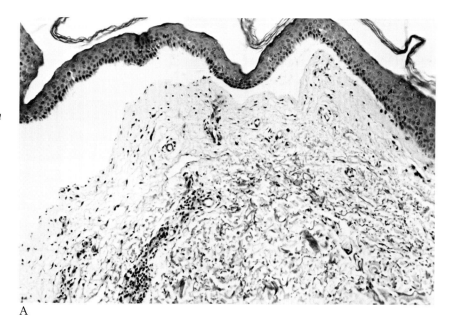

A

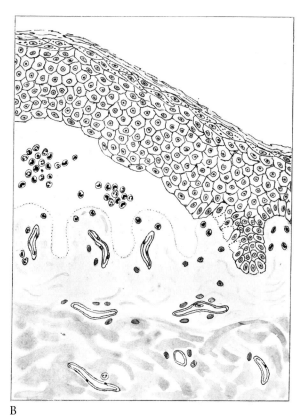

B

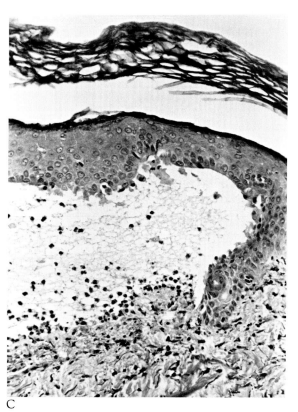

C

B. Dermatitis herpetiformis (Fig. 9-9)	1. Accumulation of neutrophils and basophilic debris below the basement membrane zone 2. Subsequent accumulation of **neutrophils in papillary microabscesses** 3. Separation at the basement membrane zone above microabscesses to form subepidermal clefts 4. Eosinophils appear in the papillary dermis and bulla cavity as lesion evolves 5. Necrosis of epidermis in roof of bulla is *not* seen until late 6. Perivenular infiltrate of lymphocytes and polymorphonuclear leukocytes	Although the presence of papillary neutrophilic abscesses is more typical of dermatitis herpetiformis, this finding is occasionally observed in bullous pemphigoid and bullous lupus erythematosus; immunofluorescence studies are helpful in differentiating these disorders
C. Herpes gestationis	Changes may resemble bullous pemphigoid	Immunofluorescence findings similar to bullous pemphigoid
D. Lupus erythematosus (Fig. 9-3)	Basal vacuoles may coalesce to form subepidermal clefts	See also I.D; Ch. 7, VI; Ch. 10, III

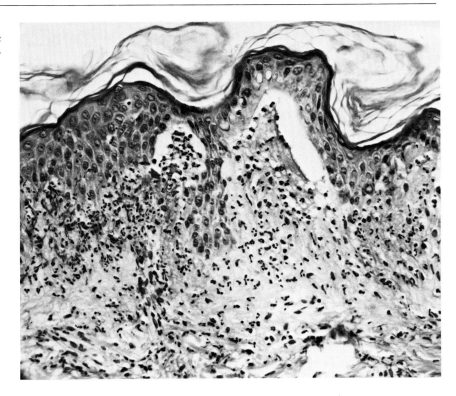

Fig. **9-9.** *Dermatitis herpetiformis. Neutrophilic microabscesses and fibrin are present within dermal papillae. Vacuolation and early cleft formation are evident at right and centrally. (×400)*

E. Dermatomyositis

1. Normal to atrophic epidermis
2. Marked dermal edema with deposition of acid mucopoly-saccharides
3. Scanty lymphohistiocytic infiltrate present about venules in superficial dermis
4. Older lesions may have extensive dermal calcification, especially in children

Edematous, erythematous lesions may be indistinguishable histologically from lupus erythematosus

Older lesions clinically and histologically may resemble poikiloderma (see also Ch. 7, V; Ch. 9, II.F; Ch. 10, IX)

F. Poikiloderma vasculare atrophicans (idiopathic) (see Fig. 7-2)

1. Hyperkeratosis
2. Focal parakeratosis
3. Epidermal atrophy
4. Dyskeratosis in lower epidermal cells
5. Vacuolation at the dermoepidermal interface
6. Bandlike lymphohistiocytic dermal infiltrate with exocytosis
7. Dilated dermal capillaries common

Pautrier-like microabscesses of normal lymphocytes may be observed

See also Ch. 7, V; Ch. 10, IX

G. Bullous drug eruption

1. Vacuolation along dermoepidermal junction
2. **Subepidermal bullae**
3. Edema of papillary dermis
4. Variable perivascular lymphohistiocytic and **eosinophilic infiltrate** in superficial and deep dermis

Differential diagnosis:
    Bullous pemphigoid
    Epidermolysis bullosa acquisita
    Erythema multiforme

See also Ch. 11, I.E

H. Morbilliform viral exanthem

1. Focal dyskeratosis
2. Multinucleated giant cells may be present depending on the causative agent
3. Vacuolation along dermoepidermal junction
4. Focal, scant lymphohistiocytic perivenular infiltrate
5. Focal extravasation of erythrocytes may be present

I. Inflammatory pity-riasis rosea (Fig. 9-10)

1. **Focal "mounds" or "caps" of parakeratosis**
2. **Focal dyskeratosis**
3. Intercellular edema (spongiosis)
4. Exocytosis of lymphocytes into epidermis
5. Pautrier-like microabscesses often present containing normal-appearing mononuclear cells
6. Variable psoriasiform hyperplasia
7. **Vacuolation** along dermoepidermal junction
8. Superficial perivascular lymphohistiocytic infiltrate
9. Extravasation of erythrocytes variable but may be extensive

Differential diagnosis:
Pityriasis lichenoides et varioliformis acuta
Subacute eczematous dermatitis

See also Ch. 4, I.H; Ch. 11, I.D

J. Pityriasis lichenoides et varioliformis acuta (PLEVA, Mucha-Habermann disease) (Fig. 9-11)

1. Focal parakeratosis
2. Accumulation of fibrin and nuclear debris in stratum corneum, forming a crust (older lesions)
3. **Dyskeratosis** often extensive
4. Exocytosis of lymphocytes into epidermis, occasionally forming Pautrier-like microabscesses that contain normal-appearing mononuclear cells
5. **Focal vacuolation** along dermoepidermal junction
6. Perivascular lymphocytic infiltrate with **endothelial cell hypertrophy often resulting in luminal obliteration**
7. Variable **extravasation of erythrocytes** into papillary dermis and epidermis

See also Ch. 11, III.F; Ch. 14, I.B.5

These vascular changes have been called *lymphocytic vasculitis*

K. Light eruptions including photoallergic reaction and polymorphous light eruption (see Fig. 4-2)

See also Ch. 14, I.A.4 and I.B.2

An uncommon persistent light eruption known as *actinic reticuloid* may exhibit atypical mononuclear cells in the dermis and epidermis

L. Secondary syphilis (see Fig. 4-7)

See also Ch. 4, III.C; Ch. 10, XIII

Fig. **9-10.** *Inflammatory pityriasis rosea. Focal parakeratosis, spongiosis, vacuolization at the dermoepidermal junction, edema, and hemorrhage in the papillary dermis with mostly perivascular lymphohistiocytic infiltrates are typical but not diagnostic for this disorder. (×256)*

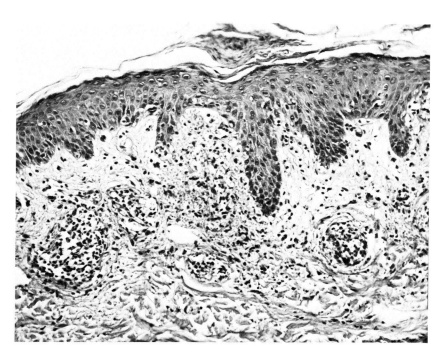

Fig. **9-11.** *Pityriasis lichenoides et varioliformis acuta (Mucha-Habermann disease). Dyskeratosis, extravasation of erythrocytes and leukocytes into the epidermis and dermis, vacuolization and inflammation at the dermoepidermal junction, and "lymphocytic vasculitis" (vessel lumens appear compromised because of endothelial cell swelling and lymphoid infiltrates) are characteristic. (×400)*

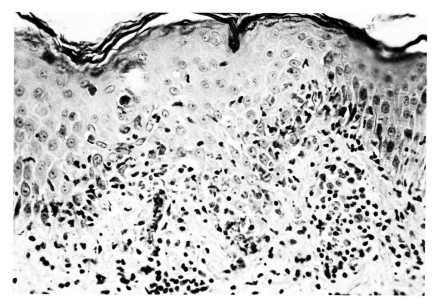

Fig. **9-12.** *Porphyria cutanea tarda.*
A. *Subepidermal cleft formation with "festooning." The latter refers to the remarkably well-preserved shape of dermal papillae. (×160)*
B. *PAS-positive material encircles superficial capillary-venules. (×640)*

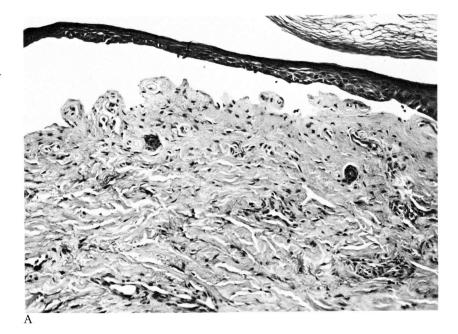

A

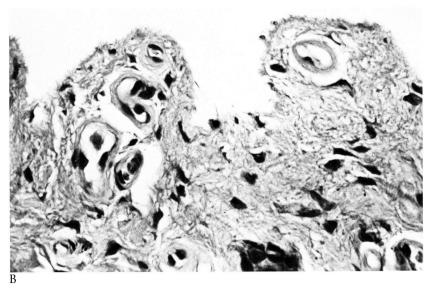

B

III. Without inflammation

A. Porphyria cutanea tarda (Fig. 9-12)

1. **Subepidermal bulla** with intact epidermal roof
2. Dermal papillae protrude irregularly into bulla cavity, giving a ragged appearance to the base of the blister ("festooning")
3. **PAS-positive, diastase-resistant hyaline material deposited around dermal capillaries** in some lesions

B. Epidermolysis bullosa dystrophica and acquisita (see Fig. 5-9)

Subepidermal bulla

C. Acute radiodermatitis

1. Focal dyskeratosis
2. Epidermal necrosis may be present
3. Vacuolation along the dermoepidermal junction
4. Subepidermal bulla formation occasionally observed
5. Edema of papillary and upper reticular dermis
6. Variable pyknosis of fibroblasts and histiocytes
7. Vacuolation of endothelial cells

See also Ch. 18, I

Suggested Reading

Lichen Planus

Altman, J., and Perry, H. O. The variations and course of lichen planus. *Arch. Dermatol.* 84:179, 1961.

Black, M. M. St. John's Hospital Dermatological Society: Symposium on lichen planus. *Clin. Exp. Dermatol.* 2:303, 1977.

Ellis, F. A. Histopathology of lichen planus based on analysis of one hundred biopsy specimens. *J. Invest. Dermatol.* 48:143, 1967.

Ragaz, A., and Ackerman A. B. Evolution, maturation and regression of lesions of lichen planus: New observations and correlations of clinical and histologic findings. *Am. J. Dermatopathol.* 3:5, 1981.

Shklar, G. Erosive and bullous oral lesions of lichen planus. *Arch. Dermatol.* 97:411, 1968.

Lichen Planus–Like (Lichenoid) Drug Eruption

Fry, L. Skin disease from colour developers. *Br. J. Dermatol.* 77:456, 1965.

Penneys, N. S., Ackerman, A. B., and Gottlieb, N. L. Gold dermatitis: A clinical and histopathological study. *Arch. Dermatol.* 109:372, 1974.

Winer, L. H., and Leeb, A. J. Lichenoid eruptions: A histopathological study. *Arch. Dermatol. Syphilol.* 70:274, 1954.

Lichenoid Keratosis

Berman, A., Herszenson, S., and Winkelmann, R.K. The involuting lichenoid plaque. *Arch. Dermatol.* 118:93, 1982.

Goette, I. K. Benign lichenoid keratosis. *Arch. Dermatol.* 116:780, 1980.

Shapiro, L., and Ackerman, A. B. Solitary lichen planus–like keratosis. *Dermatologica* 132:386, 1966.

Lupus Erythematosus

Biesecker, G., Lavin, L., Ziskind, M., and Koffler, D. Cutaneous localization of the membrane attack complex in discoid and systemic lupus erythematosus. *N. Engl. J. Med.* 306:264, 1982.

Brown, M. M., and Yount, W. J. Skin immunopathology in systemic lupus erythematosus. *J.A.M.A.* 243:38, 1980.

Clark, W. H., Reed, R. J., and Mihm, M. C., Jr. Lupus erythematosus: Histopathology of cutaneous lesions. *Hum. Pathol.* 4:157, 1973.

Dubois, E. L. *Lupus Erythematosus: A Review of the Current Status of Discoid and Systemic Lupus Erythematosus and Their Variants* (2nd ed.). Los Angeles: University of Southern California Press, 1974.

McCreight, W. G., and Montgomery, H. Cutaneous changes in lupus erythematosus. *Arch. Dermatol. Syphilol.* 61:1, 1950.

Provost, T. T., Zone, J. J., Synkowski, D., et al. Unusual cutaneous manifestations of systemic lupus erythematosus: I. Urticaria-like lesions. Correlations with clinical and serological abnormalities. *J. Invest. Dermatol.* 75:495, 1980.

Prunieras, M., and Montogomery, H. Histopathology of cutaneous lesions in systemic lupus erythematosus. *Arch. Dermatol.* 74:177, 1956.

Prystowsky, S. D., and Gilliam, J. N. Discoid lupus erythematosus as part of a larger disease spectrum. *Arch. Dermatol.* 111:1448, 1975.

Synkowski, D. R., Reichlin, M., and Provost, T. T. Serum autoantibodies in systemic lupus erythematosus and correlation with cutaneous features. *J. Rheumatol.* 9:380, 1982.

Tuffanelli, D. L., Kay, D., and Fukuyama, K. Dermal-epidermal junction in lupus erythematosus. *Arch. Dermatol.* 99:652, 1969.

Winkelmann, R. K. Spectrum of lupus erythematosus. *J. Cutan. Pathol.* 6:457, 1979.

Lichen Sclerosus et Atrophicus

Bergfeld, W. F., and Lesowitz, S. A. Lichen sclerosus et atrophicus. *Arch. Dermatol.* 101:247, 1970.

Steigleder, G. K., and Raab, W. P. Lichen sclerosus et atrophicus. *Arch. Dermatol.* 84:219, 1961.

Graft-versus-Host Reaction

Hood, A. F., Soter, N. A., Rappeport, J., and Gigli, I. Graft-versus-host reaction: Cutaneous manifestations following bone marrow transplantation. *Arch. Dermatol.* 113:1087, 1977.

Lerner, K. G. Histopathology of graft-versus-host reaction (GVHR) in human recipients of marrow from HLA-matched sibling donors. *Transplant Proc.* 6:367, 1974.

Erythema Multiforme

Ackerman, A. B., Penneys, N. S., and Clark, W. H., Jr. Erythema multiforme exudativum: Distinctive pathological process. *Br. J. Dermatol.* 84:554, 1971.

Bedi, T. R., and Pinkus, H. Histopathological spectrum of erythema multiforme. *Br. J. Dermatol.* 95:243, 1976.

O'Loughlin, S., Schroeter, A. L., and Jordon, R. E. Chronic urticaria-like lesions in systemic lupus erthematosus. A review of 12 cases. *Arch. Dermatol.* 114:879, 1978.

Orfanos, C. E., Schaumburg-Lever, G., and Lever, W. F. Dermal and epidermal types of erythema multiforme. *Arch. Dermatol.* 109:682, 1974.

Toxic Epidermal Necrolysis

Lyell, A. Toxic epidermal necrolysis (the scalded skin syndrome): A reappraisal. *Br. J. Dermatol.* 100:69, 1979.

Bullous Pemphigoid

Bean, S. F., Michel, B., Furey, N., et al. Vesicular pemphigoid. *Arch. Dermatol.* 112:1402, 1976.

Eng, A. M., and Moncada, B. Bullous pemphigoid and dermatitis herpetiformis. *Arch. Dermatol.* 110:51, 1974.

Lever, W. F. *Pemphigus and Pemphigoid.* Springfield, Ill.: Thomas, 1965.

Pearson, R. W. Advances in the Diagnosis and Treatment of Blistering Diseases: A Selective Review. In F. D. Malkinson and R. W. Pearson (Eds.), *Year Book of Dermatology.* Chicago: Year Book, 1977.

Dermatitis Herpetiformis

Connor, B. L., Marks, R., and Wilson-Jones, E. Dermatitis herpetiformis: Histological discriminants. *Trans. St. Johns Hosp. Dermatol. Soc.* 58:191, 1972.

Fry, L., and Seah, P. P. Dermatitis herpetiformis: An evaluation of diagnostic criteria. *Br. J. Dermatol.* 90:137, 1974.

Katz, S. I., and Strober, W. The pathogenesis of dermatitis herpetiformis. *J. Invest. Dermatol.* 70:63, 1978.

Seah, P. P., and Fry, L. Immunoglobulins in the skin in dermatitis herpetiformis and their relevance in diagnosis. *Br. J. Dermatol.* 92:157, 1975.

Herpes Gestationis

Carruthers, J. A., Black, M. M., and Ramnarain, N. Immunopathological studies in herpes gestationis. *Br. J. Dermatol.* 96:35, 1977.

Hertz, K. C., Katz, S. I., Maize, J., and Ackerman, A. B. Herpes gestationis: A clinicopathologic study. *Arch. Dermatol.* 112:1543, 1976.

Schaumburg-Lever, G., Saffold, O. E., Orfanos, C. E., and Lever, W. F. Herpes gestationis: Histology and ultrastructure. *Arch. Dermatol.* 107:888, 1973.

Dermatomyositis

Janis, J. F., and Winkelmann, R. K. Histopathology of the skin in dermatomyositis: A histopathologic study of 55 cases. *Arch. Dermatol.* 97:640, 1968.

Porphyria

Cormane, R. H., Szabo, E., and Hoo, T. T. Histopathology of the skin in acquired and hereditary porphyria cutanea tarda. *Br. J. Dermatol.* 85:531, 1972.

Epstein, J. H., Tuffanelli, D. L., and Epstein, W. L. Cutaneous changes in the porphyrias: A microscopic study. *Arch. Dermatol.* 107:689, 1973.

Feldaker, M., Montgomery, H., and Brunsting, L. A. Histopathology of porphyria cutanea tarda. *J. Invest. Dermatol.* 24:131, 1955.

Epidermolysis Bullosa

Bauer, E. A., and Briggaman, R. A. The Mechanobullous Diseases (Epidermolysis Bullosa). In T. B. Fitzpatrick et al. (Eds.), *Dermatology in General Medicine* (2d ed.). New York: McGraw-Hill, 1979.

Briggaman, R. A., and Wheeler, C. E., Jr. Epidermolysis bullosa dystrophica-recessive: A possible role of anchoring fibrils in the pathogenesis. *J. Invest. Dermatol.* 65:203, 1975.

Haneke, E., and Anton-Lamprecht, I. Ultrastructure of blister formation in epidermolysis bullosa hereditaria: V. Epidermolysis bullosa simplex localisata type Weber-Cockayne. *J. Invest. Dermatol.* 78:219, 1982.

Lowe, L. B., Jr. Hereditary epidermolysis bullosa. *Arch. Dermatol.* 95:587, 1967.

Pearson, R. W., Potter, B., and Strauss, F. Epidermolysis bullosa hereditaria letalis: Clinical and histological manifestations and course of the disease. *Arch. Dermatol.* 109:349, 1974.

Roenigk, H. H., Jr., Ryan, J. G., and Bergfeld, W. F. Epidermolysis bullosa acquisita. *Arch. Dermatol.* 103:1, 1971.

Yaoita, H., Briggaman, R. A., Lawley, T. J., et al. Epidermolysis bullosa acquisita: Ultrastructural and immunological studies. *J. Invest. Dermatol.* 76:288, 1981.

Chapter 10

Bandlike Infiltrate at the Dermoepidermal Junction

I. Lichen planus
II. Lichen sclerosus et atrophicus
III. Lupus erythematosus
IV. Arthropod bite reaction
V. Lichen planus–like drug eruption
VI. Some persistent light eruptions, including actinic reticuloid
VII. Acrodermatitis chronica atrophicans
VIII. Parapsoriasis
    A. Parapsoriasis variegata
    B. Parapsoriasis en plaques
IX. Poikiloderma vasculare atrophicans
X. Mycosis fungoides
XI. Lichenoid actinic keratosis
XII. Lichenoid keratosis
XIII. Secondary syphilis
XIV. Urticaria pigmentosa: Papular lesion

Several inflammatory disorders of the skin exhibit a bandlike infiltrate that occupies the papillary dermis and may or may not be associated with epidermal changes. Some of those associated with epidermal alterations were already described in Chapters 4, 7, and 9, but are included again here for completeness and contrast.

The Reactive Process and the Disease	Histopathology	Comments
I. Lichen planus (Fig. 10-1; see also Fig. 9-1)	1. Hyperkeratosis 2. Rare parakeratosis 3. **Wedgelike hypergranulosis** 4. Irregular epidermal hyperplasia with **sawtooth** rete ridges 5. Eosinophilic hyaline cell remnants (**Civatte bodies**) in the epidermis and papillary dermis 6. Squamotization of basal cell layer 7. **Vacuolation** of basal cell layer	Differential diagnosis of *bandlike infiltrate:* Lichen planus Lichen sclerosus et atrophicus Lupus erythematosus Arthropod bite reaction Lichen planus–like drug eruption Persistent light eruption Acrodermatitis chronica atrophicans Parapsoriasis Poikiloderma vasculare atrophicans Mycosis fungoides Actinic keratosis Secondary syphilis
	8. Dense bandlike infiltrate of lymphocytes, histiocytes, and macrophages that may obscure the dermoepidermal interface 9. Melanin incontinence common 10. Eosinophils uncommon	See also Ch. 9, I.A, I.B

Fig. **10-1.** *Lichen planus. The bandlike hugging infiltrate with epidermal hyperplasia is distinctive. Note the absence of stratum corneum, indicating the mucosal origin of this biopsy. (× 100). Compare with Figure 9-1, lichen planus.*

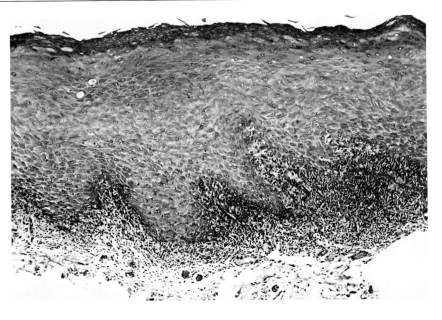

II. Lichen sclerosus et atrophicus (see Fig. 9-4)

1. Variable hyperkeratosis
2. Epidermal atrophy
3. **Edematous homogeneous, broadened papillary dermis**
4. Vacuolation at the dermoepidermal junction
5. Vascular ectasia
6. Bandlike mononuclear cell infiltrate beneath edematous papillary dermis extending around and between venules and into the upper reticular dermis

Subepidermal hemorrhagic bulla occasionally present
See also Ch. 5, IV.E; Ch. 7, I; Ch. 9, I.E

III. Lupus erythematosus (see Fig. 9-3)

1. Hyperkeratosis
2. Follicular plugging
3. Epidermal atrophy
4. Squamotization of basal cell layer
5. Thickened basement membrane zone
6. **Vacuolation along dermoepidermal junction both above and below basement membrane**
7. Edema of papillary dermis
8. Vascular ectasia
9. Bandlike and/or patchy **perivenular and periappendageal lymphohistiocytic dermal infiltrate**
10. Extravasation of erythrocytes

Special stains (see Appendix) are helpful in demonstrating increased acid mucopolysaccharide deposition in the dermis
See also Ch. 7, VI; Ch. 9, I.D, II.D; Ch. 14, I

IV. Arthropod bite reaction (see Fig. 11-2)

1. Variable epidermal spongiosis and microvesicle formation
2. Epidermal necrosis or ulceration occasionally observed at site of bite
3. Bandlike lymphohistiocytic and **eosinophilic infiltrate** may extend into upper reticular dermis
4. Perivascular infiltrate may extend into deep reticular dermis and subcutaneous tissue
5. **Endothelial cell swelling**

The polymorphous infiltrate of insect bites may be bandlike, nodular, perivenular, diffuse, or any combination of these patterns
See also Ch. 4, III.B; Ch. 11, I.F

V. Lichen planus–like drug eruption

1. Variable amount of hyperkeratosis
2. Parakeratosis common
3. Hypergranulosis may not be absent
4. Variable number of Civatte bodies
5. Vacuolation and squamotization of basal layer may be focal
6. Hyperplastic epidermis assumes sawtooth rete pattern
7. Dermal infiltrate containing **eosinophils** and rare neutrophils in addition to mononuclear cells
8. Infiltrate may extend more prominently about superficial venules and mid-dermal small veins than along dermoepidermal junction

VI. Some persistent light eruptions, including actinic reticuloid

1. Occasional dyskeratotic cell
2. Occasional epidermal hyperplasia
3. Focal vacuolation of basal cell layer
4. Bandlike dermal infiltrate composed predominantly of lymphocytes
5. Infiltrate may extend into subcutaneous fat

See also Ch. 9, II.K

In actinic reticuloid, the lymphocytes may appear atypical; at times histiocytes, eosinophils, and plasma cells may be observed (see also Ch. 9, II.K)

VII. Acrodermatitis chronica atrophicans

1. **Epidermal atrophy**
2. Grenz zone of normal papillary dermis
3. Lymphohistiocytic bandlike infiltrate
4. Dermal edema
5. **Decreased amount of collagen and elastic fibers**
6. Atrophy of pilosebaceous units

See also Ch. 7, IV; Ch. 18, X

VIII. Parapsoriasis

A. Parapsoriasis variegata	1. Marked hyperkeratosis and focal parakeratosis 2. Epidermal atrophy 3. Epidermis invaded by lymphocytes with variable atypia 4. Rare Pautrier microabscesses 5. Vacuolation of basal cell layer 6. Bandlike lymphohistiocytic infiltrate	Histology of early lesions may show chronic eczematous dermatitis An admixture of eosinophils and plasma cells with occasional atypical mononuclear cells may be observed in lesions of parapsoriasis that are evolving into mycosis fungoides
B. Parapsoriasis en plaques (see Fig. 4-4)	1. Marked hyperkeratosis 2. Mounds of parakeratotic scale either closely adherent to or separated in toto from the underlying epidermis 3. Epidermis may be normal, slightly hyperplastic, or even atrophic 4. Invasion of epidermis by lymphocytes, forming Pautrier-like microabscesses 5. Grenz zone of normal papillary dermis 6. Bandlike lymphohistiocytic infitrate	See also Ch. 4, I.E
IX. Poikiloderma vasculare atrophicans (see Fig. 7-2)	1. Hyperkeratosis 2. Focal parakeratosis 3. Epidermal atrophy with flattening of rete ridges 4. Dyskeratosis 5. Vacuolation along dermoepidermal interface 6. Bandlike lymphohistiocytic dermal infiltrate 7. Vascular ectasia 8. Melanin incontinence may be prominent	See also Ch. 7, V; Ch. 9, II.F
X. Mycosis fungoides (see Fig. 4-6)	1. Psoriasiform epidermal hyperplasia 2. **Epidermal invasion by atypical mononuclear cells, which may form Pautrier microabscesses** 3. Bandlike, nodular, or perivascular infiltrate of variably atypical mononuclear cells admixed with eosinophils, neutrophils, and plasma cells	See also Ch. 4, III.B; Ch. 16, VII.E.1

XI. Lichenoid actinic keratosis (Fig. 10-2)

1. Hyperkeratosis
2. Parakeratosis
3. Squamous cell atypia, variable
4. Loss of cellular polarity
5. Solar elastosis
6. Dense, bandlike infiltrate composed of lymphocytes and plasma cells

See also Ch. 6, III.A.4

XII. Lichenoid keratosis

See also Ch. 9, I.C

XIII. Secondary syphilis (see Fig. 4-7)

1. Hyperkeratosis and parakeratosis
2. **Psoriasiform epidermal hyperplasia** and **vacuolation** along the dermoepidermal junction
3. Perivascular **lymphohistiocytic and plasma cell** infiltrate at times in a bandlike disposition
4. **Endothelial swelling and proliferation**
5. Nodular, granulomalike aggregates formed by endothelial and inflammatory cells sometimes present
6. Occasional epithelioid cell granulomas with or without giant cells
7. Involvement of venules at all levels of the dermis and subcutaneous tissue may be noted

Condylomata lata are mucosal lesions of secondary syphilis with prominent perivascular, lymphohistiocytic, and plasma cell infiltrate and marked epithelial hyperplasia (see also Ch. 4, III.C; Ch. 9, II.L)

Silver stain may demonstrate spirochetes in epidermis and around vessels (see Appendix)

Fig. **10-2.** *Lichenoid actinic keratosis. Parakeratosis overlies atypical proliferating epidermis. The lymphocytic infiltrate is described as lichenoid because of its close apposition to the lower epidermis. (×160)*

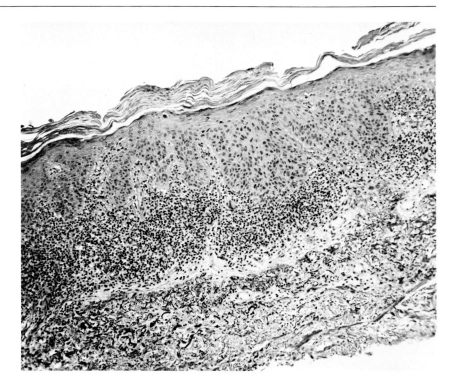

XIV. Urticaria pigmentosa: papular lesion (see Fig. 16-6)

1. Epidermis normal to flattened
2. Increased melanin in basal layer
3. Bandlike infiltrate of **cuboidal or oval mast cells** fills papillary dermis, extending into upper or mid-reticular dermis
4. Variable numbers of eosinophils admixed with mast cells
5. Subepidermal bulla containing mast cells and eosinophils occurs rarely

Grenz zone of uninvolved papillary dermis occasionally observed

Diagnostic metachromatic mast cell granules stain with Giemsa or toluidine blue (see also Ch. 11, IV)

Suggested Reading

Lichen Planus

Altman, J., and Perry, H. O. The variations and course of lichen planus. *Arch. Dermatol.* 84:179, 1961.

Black, M. M. St. John's Hospital Dermatological Society. Symposium on lichen planus, 1977. *Clin. Exp. Dermatol.* 2:303, 1977.

Ellis, F. A. Histopathology of lichen planus based on analysis of one hundred biopsy specimens. *J. Invest. Dermatol.* 48:143, 1967.

Ragaz, A., and Ackerman, A. B. Evolution, maturation and regression of lesions of lichen planus: New observations and correlations of clinical and histologic findings. *Am. J. Dermatopathol.* 3:5, 1981.

Shklar, G. Erosive and bullous oral lesions of lichen planus. *Arch. Dermatol.* 97:411, 1968.

Lichen Sclerosus et Atrophicus

Bergfeld, W. F., and Lesowitz, S. A. Lichen sclerosus et atrophicus. *Arch. Dermatol.* 101:247, 1970.

Steigleder, G. K., and Raab, W. P. Lichen sclerosus et atrophicus. *Arch. Dermatol.* 84:219, 1961.

Lupus Erythematosus

Biesecker, G., Lavin, L., Ziskind, M., and Koffler, D. Cutaneous localization of the membrane attack complex in discoid and systemic lupus erythematosus. *N. Engl. J. Med.* 306:264, 1982.

Brown, M. M., and Yount, W. J. Skin immunopathology in systemic lupus erythematosus. *J.A.M.A.* 243:38, 1980.

Clark, W. H., Reed, R. J., and Mihm, M. C., Jr. Lupus erythematosus: Histopathology of cutaneous lesions. *Hum. Pathol.* 4:157, 1973.

Dubois, E. L. *Lupus Erythematosus: A Review of the Current Status of Discoid and Systemic Lupus Erythematosus and Their Variants* (2nd ed.). Los Angeles: University of Southern California Press, 1974.

McCreight, W. G., and Montgomery, H. Cutaneous changes in lupus erythematosus. *Arch. Dermatol. Syphilol.* 61:1, 1950.

Provost, T. T., Zone, J. J., Synkowski, D., et al. Unusual cutaneous manifestations of systemic lupus erythematosus: I. Urticaria-like lesions. Correlation with clinical and serological abnormalities. *J. Invest. Dermatol.* 75:495, 1980.

Prunieras, M., and Montgomery, H. Histopathology of cutaneous lesions in systemic lupus erythematosus. *Arch. Dermatol.* 74:177, 1956.

Prystowsky, S. D., and Gilliam, J. N. Discoid lupus erythematosus as part of a larger disease spectrum. *Arch. Dermatol.* 111:1448, 1975.

Synkowski, D. R., Reichlin, M., and Provost, T. T. Serum autoantibodies in systemic lupus erythematosus and correlation with cutaneous features. *J. Rheumatol.* 9:380, 1982.

Tuffanelli, D. L., Kay, D., and Fukuyama, K. Dermal-epidermal junction in lupus erythematosus. *Arch. Dermatol.* 99:652, 1969.

Winkelmann, R. K. Spectrum of lupus erythematosus. *J. Cutan. Pathol.* 6:457, 1979.

Lichen Planus–Like (Lichenoid) Drug Eruption

Fry, L. Skin disease from colour developers. *Br. J. Dermatol.* 77:456, 1965.

Penneys, N. S., Ackerman, A. B., and Gottlieb, N. L. Gold dermatitis: A clinical and histopathological study. *Arch. Dermatol.* 109:372, 1974.

Winer, L. H., and Leeb, A. J. Lichenoid eruptions: A histopathological study. *Arch. Dermatol. Syphilol.* 70:274, 1954.

Persistent Light Reactions

Ive, F. A., Magnus, I. A., Warin, R. P., and Jones, E. W. Actinic reticuloid: A chronic dermatosis associated with severe photosensitivity and the histological resemblance to lymphoma. *Br. J. Dermatol.* 81:469, 1969.

Johnson, S. C., Cripps, D. J., and Norback, D. H. Actinic reticuloid: A clinical, pathologic, and action spectrum study. *Arch. Dermatol.* 115:1078, 1979.

Acrodermatitis Chronica Atrophicans

Burgdorf, W. H. C., Worret, W. I., and Schultka, O. Acrodermatitis chronica atrophicans. *Int. J. Dermatol.* 18:595, 1979.

Montgomery, H., and Sullivan, R. R. Acrodermatitis atrophicans chronica. *Arch. Dermatol. Syphilol.* 51:32, 1945.

Parapsoriasis

Bonvalet, D. The different forms of parapsoriasis en plaques. A report of 90 cases. *Acta Derm. Venereol. (Stockh.)* 104:18, 1977.

Hu, C. H., and Winkelmann, R. K. Digitate dermatosis. A new look at symmetrical, small plaque parapsoriasis. *Arch. Dermatol.* 107:65, 1973.

Lambert, W. C. Parapsoriasis. In T. B. Fitzpatrick et al. (Eds.). *Dermatology in General Medicine* (2d ed.). New York: McGraw-Hill, 1979.

Samman, P. D. The natural history of parapsoriasis en plaques (chronic superficial dermatitis) and prereticulotic poikiloderma. *Br. J. Dermatol.* 87:405, 1972.

Sanchez, J. F., and Ackerman, A. B. The patch stage of mycosis fungoides. Criteria for histologic diagnosis. *Am. J. Dermatopathol.* 1:5, 1979.

Poikiloderma Vasculare Atrophicans

Watsky, M. S., and Lynfield, Y. L. Poikiloderma vasculare atrophicans. *Cutis* 17:938, 1976.

Wolf, D. J., and Selmanowitz, V. J. Poikiloderma vasculare atrophicans. *Cancer* 25:682, 1970.

Mycosis Fungoides

Brehmer-Andersson, E. Mycosis fungoides and its relation to Sezary's syndrome, lymphomatoid papulosis, and primary cutaneous Hodgkin's disease. *Acta Derm. Venereol. (Stockh.)* 75 (Suppl. 56):9, 1976.

Degreef, H., Holvoet, C., Van Vloten, W. A., et al. Woringer-Kolopp disease. An epidermotropic variant of mycosis fungoides. *Cancer* 138:2154, 1976.

Jimbow, K., Chiba, M., and Horikoshi, T. Electron microscopic identification of Langerhans cells in the dermal infiltrates of mycosis fungoides. *J. Invest. Dermatol.* 78:102, 1982.

Lutzner, M., Edelson, R., Schein, P., et al. Cutaneous T-cell lymphomas: The Sézary syndrome, mycosis fungoides and related disorders. *Ann. Intern. Med.* 83:534, 1975.

Waldorf, D. S., Ratner, A. C., and Van Scott, E. J. Cells in lesions of mycosis fungoides lymphoma following therapy. Changes in number and type. *Cancer* 21:264, 1968.

Winkelmann, R. K., and Caro, W. A. Current problems in mycosis fungoides and Sézary syndrome. *Annu. Rev. Med.* 28:251, 1977.

Actinic Keratosis

Ackerman, A. B., and Reed, R. J. Epidermolytic variant of solar keratosis. *Arch. Dermatol.* 107:104, 1973.

Pinkus, H. Actinic Keratosis—Actinic Skin. In R. Andrade et al. (Eds.), *Cancer of the Skin.* Philadelphia: Saunders, 1976.

Pinkus, H., and Mehregan, A. H. *A Guide to Dermatohistopathology* (3d ed.). New York: Appleton-Century-Crofts, 1981.

Shapiro, L., and Ackerman, A. Solitary lichen planus–like keratosis. *Dermatologica* 132:386, 1966.

Secondary Syphilis

Abell, E., Marks, R., and Wilson-Jones, E. Secondary syphilis: A clinico-pathological review. *Br. J. Dermatol.* 93:53, 1955.

Jeerapaet, P., and Ackerman, A. B. Histologic patterns of secondary syphilis. *Arch. Dermatol.* 107:373, 1973.

Urticaria Pigmentosa

Burgoon, C. F., Graham, J. H., and McCaffree, D. L. Mast cell disease. A cutaneous variant with multisystem involvement. *Arch. Dermatol.* 98:590, 1968.

Monheit, G. D., Murad, T., and Conrad, M. Systemic mastocytosis and the mastocytosis syndrome. *J. Cutan. Pathol.* 6:42, 1979.

Chapter **11**

Predominantly Perivascular Infiltrate of the Upper Dermis

I. Mixed infiltrate without evidence of vascular damage
  A. Urticaria
  B. Erythema multiforme, drug-induced
  C. Allergic contact dermatitis
  D. Pityriasis rosea—noninflammatory
  E. Drug eruptions
    1. Urticarial
    2. Eczematous
    3. Maculopapular (morbilliform)
  F. Arthropod bite reaction
  G. Secondary syphilis
  H. Acute febrile neutrophilic dermatosis (Sweet's disease)
II. Mixed infiltrate with vascular damage (fibrinoid necrosis)
  A. Cutaneous necrotizing vasculitis (leukocytoclastic vasculitis; allergic cutaneous vasculitis)
  B. Focal embolic lesions in gonococcemia and acute meningococcemia
  C. Chronic meningococcemia
III. Predominantly lymphohistiocytic infiltrate
  A. Lymphocytic infiltration of the skin (Jessner-Kanof)
  B. Superficial annular and figurate erythemas
    1. Erythema annulare centrifugum
    2. Drug-induced figurate erythema
    3. Chronic recurrent figurate erythema
  C. Parapsoriasis, guttate
  D. Photoallergic reaction
  E. Progressive pigmentary purpura
  F. Pityriasis lichenoides et varioliformis acuta (PLEVA, Mucha-Habermann)
  G. Stasis dermatitis
IV. Mast cell infiltrate
  A. Urticaria pigmentosa
    1. Telangiectasia macularis eruptiva perstans and erythrodermic mastocytosis
    2. Macular and papular lesions

The Reactive Process and the Disease	Histopathology	Comments
I. Mixed infiltrate without evidence of vascular damage		
A. Urticaria (see Fig. 14-1)	1. Epidermis normal 2. **Edema** of papillary dermis, demonstrated by separation of collagen bundles and widening of papillary dermis 3. Scant perivascular inflammatory infiltrate	Slight intercellular edema may be present The histologic features of urticaria vary markedly with regard to the intensity and composition of the infiltrate; some lesions exhibit predominantly neutrophils, others exhibit predominantly eosinophils, and still others exhibit only lymphocytes A true necrotizing venulitis may occasionally be seen in chronic urticaria Urticaria is listed in the differential diagnosis of "nothing lesions" (see table, inside back cover, and Ch. 14, I.A)
B. Erythema multiforme, drug-induced	1. Intercellular edema, **dyskeratosis**, and mild to moderate epidermal necrosis 2. Vacuolation at the dermoepidermal junction; occasional **subepidermal bulla** 3. **Lymphocytes with numerous eosinophils** and neutrophils in superficial dermis principally about blood vessels, but also **along the dermoepidermal junction** 4. Prominent endothelial cell swelling 5. Perivascular fibrin exudate; occasional focal fibrinoid necrosis	For the histologic changes seen in the recurrent, Hebra-type erythema multiforme, see Ch. 9, I.G

C. Allergic contact dermatitis (see Fig. 5-1)

1. Variable epidermal hyperplasia
2. Intercellular edema (**spongiosis**)
3. Intraepidermal **spongiotic vesicles**
4. **Epidermis invaded by lymphocytes and often eosinophils**
5. Erythrocytes may be present in the epidermis
6. Perivascular aggregates of lymphocytes with variable numbers of eosinophils
7. Infiltrate sometimes involves venules of the middle to deep reticular dermis
8. Dermal hemorrhage occasionally present

The dermal inflammatory changes described here may occur with minimal epidermal changes in the so-called dermal contact dermatitis

See also Ch. 4, I.B.3; Ch. 5, II.C

Certain oil-soluble haptens affect predominantly the epithelium of hair follicles

D. Pityriasis rosea—noninflammatory (Fig. 11-1)

1. Slight hyperkeratosis
2. Focal parakeratosis ("skipping scale") overlying focal areas of mild intercellular epidermal edema
3. Irregular, mild psoriasiform epidermal hyperplasia
4. Slight exocytosis of lymphocytes, occasionally forming small Pautrier-like microabscesses
5. Slight perivascular lymphohistiocytic infiltrate with a few eosinophils

See also inflammatory pityriasis rosea, Ch. 4, I.H.; Ch. 9, II.I

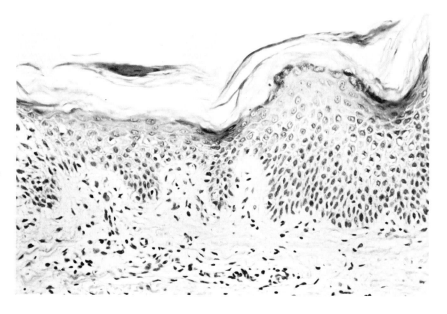

Fig. **11-1.** *Pityriasis rosea. "Skipping" parakeratosis (foci of well-circumscribed, tight parakeratotic scale that frequently appear to be lifting off the epidermis) and a mild superficial perivascular lymphohistiocytic infiltrate are typical but not diagnostic of this disorder. Focal spongiosis and mononuclear cell aggregates within the epidermis are not uncommon. Compare with Figure 9-10, inflammatory pityriasis rosea. Parapsoriasis can exhibit a similar histopathology. (×250)*

E. Drug eruptions

1. Urticarial

1. Epidermis normal
2. **Papillary dermal edema**
3. Slight perivascular infiltrate of lymphocytes, eosinophils, and a few polymorphonuclear leukocytes
4. Perivenular infiltrate may extend to deep venules

2. Eczematous

1. Hyperkeratosis
2. Focal parakeratosis
3. Irregular epidermal hyperplasia
4. Perivascular infiltrate of lymphocytes, histiocytes, eosinophils, and neutrophils

3. Maculopapular (morbilliform)

1. Basal vacuolation
2. Mild to moderately intense perivenular infiltrate, composed of lymphocytes with variable numbers of eosinophils

F. Arthropod bite reaction (Fig. 11-2)

1. Epidermal hyperplasia with variable spongiosis
2. Ulceration or epidermal necrosis may occur at punctum site
3. Edema of the papillary dermis
4. Moderate to dense perivenular lymphohistiocytic and eosinophilic infiltrate

5. Endothelial cell swelling

See also Ch. 4, III.A

The polymorphous infiltrate may occasionally be bandlike, nodular, perivenular, diffuse, or any combination thereof (see Ch. 10, IV; Ch. 14, I.A.2)

G. Secondary syphilis (see Fig. 4-7)

See Ch. 4, III.C

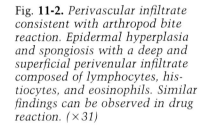

Fig. **11-2.** *Perivascular infiltrate consistent with arthropod bite reaction. Epidermal hyperplasia and spongiosis with a deep and superficial perivenular infiltrate composed of lymphocytes, histiocytes, and eosinophils. Similar findings can be observed in drug reaction. (×31)*

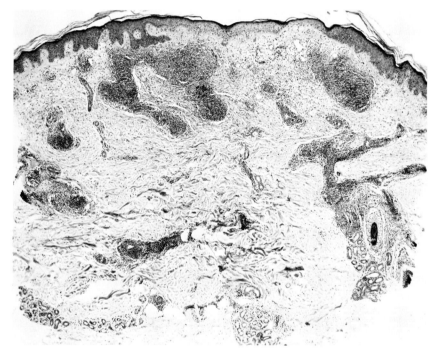

H. Acute febrile neutrophilic dermatosis (Sweet's disease) (Fig. 11-3)

1. Epidermal hyperplasia may be marked
2. Intercellular edema
3. Migration of neutrophils into epidermis
4. **Edema of the papillary dermis, often severe**
5. **Dense perivascular** and diffuse infiltrate made up **predominantly of neutrophils**; infiltrate may extend into the subcutis
6. Nuclear fragments, or "dust," of inflammatory cells
7. Vascular ectasia

See also Ch. 14, I.A.6; Ch. 16, V.C

Fig. **11-3.** *Acute febrile neutrophilic dermatosis (Sweet's disease). Characteristic of this disorder is the perivascular, bandlike, dense dermal infiltrate (A) that contains many neutrophils with little or no vascular damage (B). The degree of edema and epidermal change (A) overlying the infiltrate is variable. (A, ×160; B, ×256)*

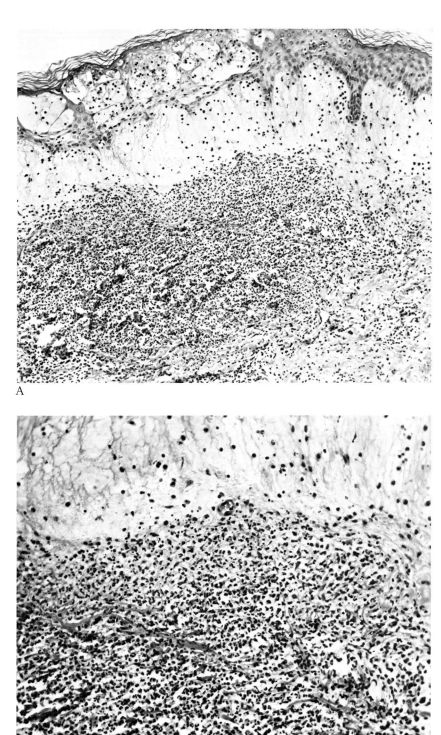

A

B

II. Mixed infiltrate with vascular damage (fibrinoid necrosis)

A. Cutaneous necrotizing vasculitis (leukocytoclastic vasculitis; allergic cutaneous vasculitis) (Fig. 11-4)

1. Perivenular infiltrate of neutrophils, lymphocytes, and eosinophils
2. Invasion of vessel wall by neutrophils
3. Nuclear "dust" (nuclear debris from fragmented, necrotic polymorphonuclear leukocytes)
4. Brightly eosinophilic fibrinoid deposition in and about affected vessels
5. Endothelial cell swelling
6. Extravasation of erythrocytes

Minimal histologic requirements for diagnosis of cutaneous necrotizing venulitis:
  Fibrinoid deposition
  Neutrophils
  Hemorrhage

Necrotizing vasculitis may occur idiopathically or may be seen in association with:

Henoch-Schönlein purpura syndrome
Chronic urticaria
Angioedema
Rheumatoid arthritis, lupus erythematosus, and other collagen-vascular disorders
Lymphoproliferative disorders
Infections
Drug reactions

B. Focal embolic lesions in gonococcemia and acute meningococcemia

1. Necrotic epidermis
2. **Subepidermal pustules**
3. **Vasculitis** with variable fibrinoid necrosis of venules and striking inflammatory infiltrate of lymphocytes, histiocytes, neutrophils, and nuclear dust
4. **Fibrin thrombi in involved vessels**
5. Extravasation of erythrocytes

Fibrin thrombi occur with and without endothelial cell necrosis in disseminated intravascular coagulation (DIC) and may be associated with variable neutrophilic infiltrate

The presence of fibrin thrombi distinguishes septic embolic phenomenon from purely allergic cutaneous vasculitis

Gram-negative intracellular and extracellular organisms are easily demonstrated in acute meningococcemia; organisms are rarely demonstrated in acute gonococcemia

C. Chronic meningococcemia

Histologic picture similar to cutaneous necrotizing venulitis

III. Predominantly lymphohistiocytic infiltrate

A. Lymphocytic infiltration of the skin (Jessner-Kanof)

1. Normal epidermis
2. **Dense circumscribed aggregates of lymphocytes** around blood vessels and appendages
3. Infiltrate characteristically involves papillary and reticular dermis but may extend into subcutaneous tissue
4. Lymphocytes may extend in single-cell array between collagen fibers of the reticular dermis

See also Ch. 14, I.B.3

Fig. **11-4.** *Cutaneous necrotizing vasculitis. The hallmarks of this disorder include fibrinoid change about vessel walls, intramural neutrophilic infiltrates, often with leukocytoclasis, and extravasation of erythrocytes. (B, ×256)*

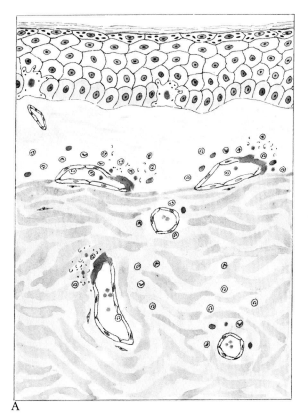

A

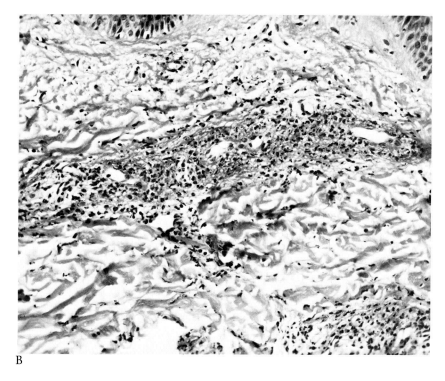

B

B. Superficial annular and figurate erythemas

1. Erythema annulare centrifugum

1. Focal parakeratosis
2. Slight intercellular edema and vacuolation at the dermoepidermal junction
3. **Tight cuff of lymphocytes about vessels** without endothelial swelling

Dermatophytosis is a common cause of figurate erythemas

2. Drug-induced figurate erythema

Irregular disposition of lymphocytes and **eosinophils** about the superficial plexus

3. Chronic recurrent figurate erythema

Lymphocytes and histiocytes in papillary dermis loosely arranged around vessels

C. Parapsoriasis, guttate

1. Hyperkeratosis and focal parakeratosis
2. Slight intercellular edema
3. Slight epidermal hyperplasia

4. Lymphocytes and histiocytes focally may migrate into the epidermis
5. Pautrier-like microabscesses may be present
6. Perivascular lymphohistiocytic infiltrate
7. Endothelial cell swelling

Differential diagnosis:
Subacute eczematous dermatitis
Pityriasis rosea

Parapsoriasis variegata and parapsoriasis en plaques are discussed in Ch. 4, I.E and Ch. 10, VIII

D. Photoallergic reaction

1. Epidermis normal; slight intercellular edema may be present
2. Focal dyskeratosis occasionally observed
3. Vacuolation along the dermoepidermal interface occurs in 40% of plaque-type eruptions
4. Loose perivascular infiltrate of lymphocytes, histiocytes, and rare neutrophils
5. Slight extravasation of erythrocytes
6. Endothelial cell swelling

See also Ch. 14, I.A.4

E. Progressive pigmentary purpura (Fig. 11-5)

1. Epidermis usually unaffected, but rarely may be infiltrated by lymphocytes and show slight intercellular edema
2. **Lymphocytic perivascular infiltrate**
3. **Swollen endothelial cells**
4. **Dermal hemorrhage**
5. Deposition of **hemosiderin** may be prominent

Iron stains will help detect hemosiderin deposition

F. Pityriasis lichenoides et varioliformis acuta (PLEVA, Mucha-Habermann) (see Fig. 9-11)

1. Focal parakeratosis occasionally admixed with nuclei from neutrophils
2. Variable hyperkeratosis
3. Focal epidermal necrosis (**dyskeratosis**) may be prominent
4. Basal **vacuolation**
5. **Exocytosis of lymphocytes and extravasation of erythrocytes into epidermis**
6. Lymphocytes and rarely eosinophils around vessels
7. Marked **endothelial swelling**

8. **Dermal hemorrhage**

Red blood cells in the epidermis may be observed in:

Pityriasis lichenoides et varioliformis acuta
Allergic contact dermatitis
Allograft rejection
Lymphomatoid papulosis
Drug reaction
Pityriasis rosea
Arthropod bites
Eczematous dermatitis
Leukocytoclastic vasculitis
Polymorphous light eruption

Lymphomatoid papulosis may resemble PLEVA clinically and histologically; it is distinguished by the presence of a variable number of markedly atypical mononuclear cells in the dermal infiltrate

See also Ch. 9, II.J; Ch. 14, I.B.5

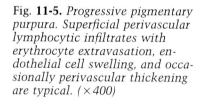
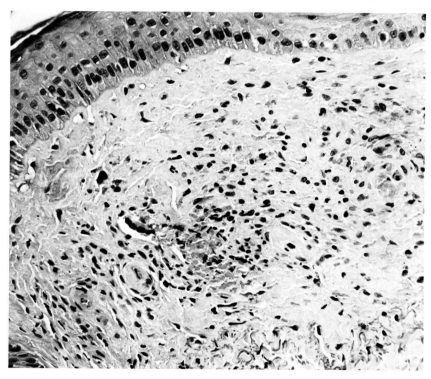

Fig. **11-5.** *Progressive pigmentary purpura. Superficial perivascular lymphocytic infiltrates with erythrocyte extravasation, endothelial cell swelling, and occasionally perivascular thickening are typical. (×400)*

G. Stasis dermatitis (see Fig. 20-15)

1. Atrophic or acanthotic epidermis with flattened rete
2. Mild to moderate intercellular edema
3. Perivascular lymphohistiocytic infiltrate which may be superficial, but often extends into the deep reticular dermis or panniculus
4. **Vascular ectasia; vessel proliferation**
5. **Thickened vessel walls**
6. **Dermal hemorrhage with hemosiderin deposition**
7. **Fibrosis of the reticular dermis**

See also Ch. 14, I.B.7; Ch. 20, XXII

IV. Mast cell infiltrate

A. Urticaria pigmentosa

1. Telangiectasia macularis eruptiva perstans and erythrodermic mastocytosis

1. Perivenular, spindle-shaped **mast cells**
2. Vascular ectasia

The number of mast cells around a given blood vessel is normally not more than five; the finding of more than five perivenular mast cells strongly suggests the diagnosis of urticaria pigmentosa

2. Macular and papular lesions (see Fig. 16-16)

1. Perivenular, oval or spindle-shaped mast cells in papillary and upper reticular dermis
2. Variable number of eosinophils
3. Increased melanin in basal layer

See also Ch. 16, IV.A

Suggested Reading
Urticaria

Lever, W. F., and Schaumburg-Lever, G. *Histopathology of the Skin* (5th ed.). Philadelphia: Lippincott, 1975.
Warin, R. P., and Champion, R. H. *Urticaria*. Philadelphia: Saunders, 1974.

Erythema Multiforme

Ackerman, A. B., Penneys, N. S., and Clark, W. H., Jr. Erythema multiforme exudativum: Distinctive pathological process. *Br. J. Dermatol.* 84:554, 1971.
Bedi, R. R., and Pinkus, H. Histopathological spectrum of erythema multiforme. *Br. J. Dermatol.* 95:243, 1976.
O'Loughlin, S., Schroeter, A. L., and Jordon, R. E. Chronic urticaria-like lesions in systemic lupus erythematosus. A review of 12 cases. *Arch. Dermatol.* 114:879, 1978.
Orfanos, C. E., Schaumburg-Lever, G., and Lever, W. F. Dermal and epidermal types of erythema multiforme. *Arch. Dermatol.* 109:682, 1974.

Allergic Contact Dermatitis

Dvorak, H. F., Mihm, M. C., Jr., Dvorak, A. M., et al. Morphology of delayed type hypersensitivity reactions in man. I. Quantitative description of the inflammatory response. *Lab. Invest.* 31:111, 1974.

Pityriasis Rosea

Bunch, L. W., and Tilley, J. C. Pityriasis rosea. A histologic and serologic study. *Arch. Dermatol.* 84:79, 1961.
Lipman Cohen, E. Pityriasis rosea. *Br. J. Dermatol.* 79:533, 1967.

Drug Eruptions

Mullick, F. G., McAllister, H. A., Jr., Wagner, B. M., and Fenoglio, J. J. Drug related vasculitis. Clinicopathologic correlations in 30 patients. *Hum. Pathol.* 10:313, 1979.

Arthropod Bite Reactions

Fernandez, N., Torres, A., and Ackerman, A. B. Pathologic findings in human scabies. *Arch. Dermatol.* 113:320, 1977.

Goldman, L., Rockwell, E., and Richfield, D. F., III. Histopathological studies on cutaneous reactions to the bites of various arthropods. *Am. J. Trop. Med. Hyg.* 1:514, 1952.

Horen, W. P. Insect and scorpion sting. *J.A.M.A.* 221:894, 1972.

Larrivee, D. H., Benjamini, E., Feingold, B. F., et al. Histologic studies of guinea pig skin: Different stages of allergic reactivity to flea bites. *Exp. Parasitol.* 15:491, 1964.

Steffen, C. Clinical and histopathologic correlation of midge bites. *Arch. Dermatol.* 117:785, 1981.

Thomson, J., Cochran, T., Cochran, R., and McQueen, A. Histology simulating reticulosis in persistent nodular scabies. *Br. J. Dermatol.* 90:421, 1974.

Acute Febrile Neutrophilic Dermatosis

Cooper, P. H., Innes, D. J., Jr., and Greer, K. E. Acute febrile neutrophilic dermatosis (Sweet's syndrome) and myeloproliferative disorders. *Cancer* 51:1518, 1983.

Gunawardena, D. A., Gunawardena, K. A., Ratnayaka R. M. R. S., et al. The clinical spectrum of Sweet's syndrome (acute febrile neutrophilic dermatosis)—a report of eighteen cases. *Br. J. Dermatol.* 92:363, 1975.

Sweet, R. D. An acute febrile neutrophilic dermatosis. *Br. J. Dermatol.* 76:349, 1964.

Sweet, R. D. Acute febrile neutrophilic dermatosis—1978. *Br. J. Dermatol.* 100:93, 1979.

Cutaneous Necrotizing Vasculitis

Copeman, P. W. M., and Ryan, T. J. The problems of classification of cutaneous angiitis with reference to histopathology and pathogenesis. *Br. J. Dermatol.* 82 (Suppl. 5):2, 1970.

Cream, J. J., Gumpel, J. M., and Peachy, R. D. Schönlein-Henoch purpura in the adult: A study of 77 adults with anaphylactoid or Schönlein-Henoch purpura. *Q. J. Med.* 39:461, 1970.

Reed, R. J. *Cutaneous Vasculitides. Immunologic and Histologic Correlations.* Chicago: American Society of Clinical Pathologists, 1977.

Soter, N. A. Chronic urticaria as a manifestation of necrotizing venulitis. *N. Engl. J. Med.* 296:1440, 1977.

Soter, N. A. Necrotizing vasculitis of the skin. In T. B. Fitzpatrick et al. (Eds.), *Dermatology in General Medicine* (2d ed.). New York: McGraw-Hill, 1979.

Gonococcemia and Meningococcemia

Ackerman, A. B., Miller, R. C., and Shapiro L. Gonococcemia and its cutaneous manifestations. *Arch. Dermatol.* 91:227, 1965.

Nielsen, T. Chronic meningococcemia. *Arch. Dermatol.* 102:97, 1970.

Shapiro, L., Teisch, J. A., and Brownstein, M. H. Dermatohistopathology of chronic gonococcal sepsis. *Arch. Dermatol.* 107:403, 1973.

Lymphocytic Infiltration of the Skin (Jessner-Kanof)

Clark, W. H., Mihm, M. C., Reed, R. J., and Ainsworth, A. M. The lymphocytic infiltrates of the skin. *Hum. Pathol.* 5:25, 1974.

Gottlieb, B., and Winkelmann, R. K. Lymphocytic infiltration of the skin. *Arch. Dermatol.* 86:626, 1962.

Jessner, M., and Kanof, N. B. Lymphocytic infiltration of the skin. *Arch. Dermatol. Syphilol.* 68:447, 1953.

Ten Have Opbroek, A. A. W. On the differential diagnosis between chronic discoid lupus erythematodes and lymphocytic infiltration of the skin with emphasis on fluoresence microscopy. *Dermatologica* 132:109, 1966.

Annular and Figurate Erythema

Ellis, F. A., and Friedman, A. A. Erythema annulare centrifugum (Darier's): Clinical and histologic study. *Arch. Dermatol. Syphilol.* 70:496, 1954.

Harrison, P. V. The annular erythemas. *Int. J. Dermatol.* 18:282, 1979.

Maciejewski, W. Annular erythema as an unusual manifestation of chronic disseminated lupus erythematosus. *Arch. Dermatol.* 116:450, 1980.

Thomson, J., and Stankler, L. Erythema gyratum repens: Reports of two further cases associated with carcinoma. *Br. J. Dermatol.* 82:406, 1970.

White, J. W., and Perry, H. O. Erythema perstans. *Br. J. Dermatol.* 81:641, 1969.

Light Eruptions

Epstein, J. H. Polymorphous light eruption. *Ann. Allergy* 24:397, 1966.

Lamb, J. H., Jones, P. E., and Maxwell, T. B. Solar dermatitis. *Arch. Dermatol.* 75:171, 1957.

Panet-Raymond, G., and Johnson, W. C. Lupus erythematous and polymorphous light eruption: Differentiation by histochemical procedures. *Arch. Dermatol.* 108:785, 1973.

Stern, W. K. Evolution of an abnormal light test reaction. *Arch. Dermatol.* 103:154, 1971.

Wright, E. T., and Winer, L. H. Histopathology of allergic solar dermatitis. *J. Invest. Dermatol.* 34:103, 1960.

Pigmented Purpura

Randall, S. J., Kierland, R. R., and Montgomery, H. Pigmented purpuric eruptions. *Arch. Dermatol. Syphilol.* 94:626, 1966.

Stell, J. S., and Moyer, D. G. Schamberg's disease. *Arch. Dermatol.* 94:626, 1966.

Pityriasis Lichenoides et Varioliformis Acuta

Black, M. M., and Marks, R. The inflammatory reaction in pityriasis lichenoides. *Br. J. Dermatol.* 87:533, 1972.

Hood, A. F., and Mark, E. J. Histopathologic diagnosis of pityriasis lichenoides et varioliformis acuta and its clinical correlation. *Arch. Dermatol.* 118:478, 1982.

Marks, R., Black, M., and Wilson-Jones, E. Pityriasis lichenoides: A reappraisal. *Br. J. Dermatol.* 86:215, 1972.

Nigra, T. P., and Soter, N. A. Pityriasis Lichenoides. In T. B. Fitzpatrick et al. (Eds.), *Dermatology in General Medicine* (2d ed.). New York: McGraw-Hill, 1979.

Szymanski, F. J. Pityriasis lichenoides et varioliformis acuta: Histopathological evidence that it is an entity distinct from parapsoriasis. *Arch. Dermatol.* 79:7, 1959.

Lymphomatoid Papulosis

Black, M. M., and Wilson-Jones, E. Lymphomatoid pityriasis lichenoides; a variant with histological features simulating a lymphoma. *Br. J. Dermatol.* 86:329, 1972.

Sina, B., and Burnett, J. W. Lymphomatoid papulosis. Case reports and literature review. *Arch. Dermatol.* 119:189, 1983.

Valentino, L. A., and Helwig, E. B. Lymphomatoid papulosis. *Arch. Pathol.* 96:409, 1973.

Weinman, V. F., and Ackerman, A. B. Lymphomatoid papulosis. A critical review and new findings. *Am. J. Dermatopathol.* 3:129, 1981.

Stasis Dermatitis

Graham, J. H., et al. Stasis Dermatitis. In J. H. Graham, W. C. Johnson, and W. B. Helwig (Eds.), *Dermal Pathology.* Hagerstown, Md.: Harper & Rowe, 1972.

Kulwin, M. H., and Hines, E. A., Jr. Blood vessels of the skin in chronic venous insufficiency: Clinical pathologic study. *Arch. Dermatol. Syphilol.* 62:293, 1950.

Mast Cell Infiltrate

Monheit, G. D., Murad, T., and Conrad, M. Systemic mastocytosis and the mastocytosis syndrome. *J. Cutan. Pathol.* 6:42, 1979.

Parkes-Weber, F. Telangiectasia macularis eruptiva perstans. *Br. J. Dermatol.* 24:372, 1940.

Chapter **12**

Deposition in the Papillary Dermis

The Reactive Process and the Disease	Histopathology	Comments
I. Amyloidosis		
A. Macular amyloidosis (Fig. 12-1)	1. Variable hyperkeratosis 2. Deposition of **eosinophilic acellular globules** of varying sizes in the dermal papillae, occasionally extending to the superficial venular plexus 3. Melanophages in the papillary dermis	Apple-green dichroism of Congophilic deposits examined by polariscopy is characteristic of amyloid Frozen section of unfixed skin stained with Congo red or thioflavin-T is said to be more sensitive than routine methods for detection of amyloid Amyloid fibrils demonstrated by electron microscopy are the most specific findings for the diagnosis of amyloidosis

B. Lichen amyloidosis	1. Hyperkeratosis
	2. **Acanthosis;** elongated rete may be laterally displaced by deposition of **amorphous eosinophilic globules** in papillary dermis and around venules of the superficial plexus
	3. Dermal melanin, free and within macrophages
		See also Ch. 19, I
		
		Differential diagnosis:
		    Colloid milium
		    Solar elastosis

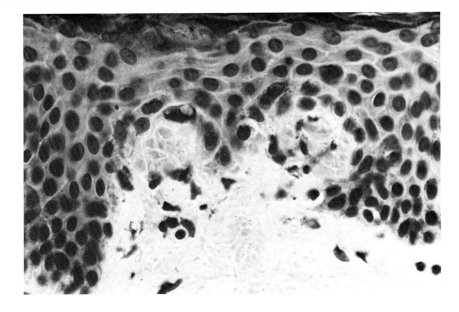

Fig. **12-1.** *Macular amyloidosis. Deposits of glassy eosinophilic and Congophilic cytoid bodies within dermal papillae are associated with melanin-laden macrophages. (approximately ×640)*

II. Colloid milium

1. Hyperkeratosis
2. Flattened to atrophic epidermis
3. Deposition of faintly eosinophilic, amorphous, and homogeneous material that is often **fissured**
4. Material fills and distends dermal papillae
5. Solar elastosis commonly present beneath and adjacent to deposition

Colloid deposits are usually larger than those of amyloidosis but may be histologically and histochemically indistinguishable from amyloid

Suggested Reading
Amyloidosis

Brownstein, M. H., and Helwig, E. B. The cutaneous amyloidoses. I. Localized forms. *Arch. Dermatol.* 102:8, 1970.

Brownstein, M. H., and Helwig, E. B. The cutaneous amyloidoses. II. Systemic forms. *Arch. Dermatol.* 102:20, 1970.

Habermann, M. C., and Montenegro, M. R. Primary cutaneous amyloidosis: Clinical, laboratorial and histopathological study in 25 cases. *Dermatologica* 160:240, 1980.

Kobayashi, H., and Hashimoto, K. Amyloidogenesis in organ-limited cutaneous amyloidosis: An antigenic identity between epidermal keratin and skin amyloid. *J. Invest. Dermatol.* 80:66, 1983.

Vasily, D. B., Bhatia, S. G., and Uhlin, S. R. Familial primary cutaneous amyloidosis. Clinical, genetic, and immunofluorescent studies. *Arch. Dermatol.* 114:1173, 1978.

Chapter 13

Hyperplasia of the Papillary Dermis

I. Fibrous papule

II. Angiofibroma

Fig. **13-1.** *Fibrous papule. Perifollicular fibrosis, numerous small vessels, and fibrosis are characteristic. Large mesenchymal cells (A) are not uncommon. (B, ×100)*

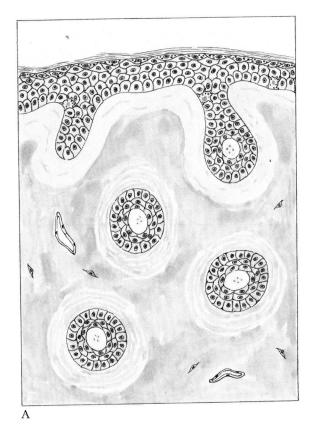

A

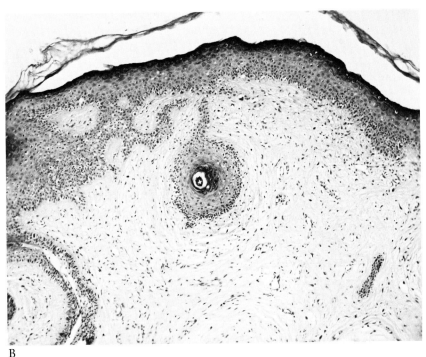

B

The Reactive Process and the Disease	Histopathology	Comments
I. Fibrous papule (Fig. 13-1)	1. Papillary dermal fibrosis with **concentric perifollicular fibrosis** 2. Increased number of spindle-shaped fibroblasts 3. Vascular ectasia and proliferation 4. Bizarre but not dysplastic cells in the dermis, which may be histiocytes or nevocellular nevus cells	A fibrous papule is a flesh-colored, dome-shaped lesion on the nose or face that is often mistaken clinically for a basal cell carcinoma or a nevus
II. Angiofibroma (Fig. 13-2)	1. Fibrovascular hyperplasia of the upper dermis 2. May be histologically indistinguishable from a fibrous papule; usually the concentric perifollicular fibrosis and bizarre cells in the dermis are absent	Angiofibromas occur in tuberous sclerosis; they have variable clinical appearances that include (a) multiple flesh-colored to slightly erythematous papules symmetrically arranged about the nose and mouth and on the cheeks; (b) flesh-colored to reddish-brown papules and nodules under or around the nails Differential diagnosis: Scar Regressed nevus Connective-tissue nevus

Fig. **13-2.** *Angiofibroma. This pattern of delicate fibrosis and vascular ectasia with occasional lymphocytes is typical. These features are similar to those of fibrous papule of the nose (see Fig. 3-1). (×100)*

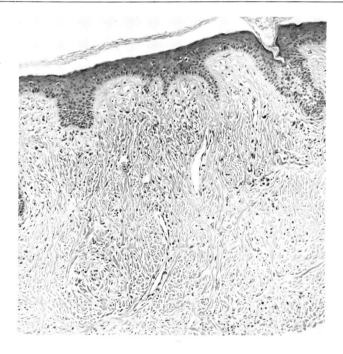

Suggested Reading
Fibrous Papule

Meigel, W. N., and Ackerman, A. B. Fibrous papule of the face. *Am. J. Dermatopathol.* 1:329, 1979.

Willis, W. F., and Garcia, R. L. Giant angiofibroma in tuberous sclerosis. *Arch. Dermatol.* 114:1843, 1978.

Part **IV**

Reticular
Dermis

Chapter 14

Predominantly Perivascular Infiltrate of the Reticular Dermis

I. Perivascular infiltrate without vascular damage
   A. Mixed infiltrate
      1. Urticaria/angioedema
      2. Arthropod bite reaction
      3. Drug reaction, urticarial
      4. Photoallergic reaction
      5. Cellulitis
      6. Acute febrile neutrophilic dermatosis (Sweet's disease)
      7. Secondary syphilis
   B. Lymphohistiocytic infiltrate
      1. Lupus erythematosus
      2. Polymorphous light eruption
      3. Lymphocytic infiltration of the skin (Jessner-Kanof)
      4. Deep figurate or gyrate erythema
      5. Pityriasis lichenoides et varioliformis acuta (PLEVA, Mucha-Habermann)
      6. Lymphomatoid papulosis
      7. Stasis dermatitis
      8. Indeterminate leprosy
II. Perivascular infiltrate with vascular damage—vasculitis
   A. Cutaneous necrotizing vasculitis
   B. Focal septic embolic lesions in gonococcemia and meningococcemia
   C. Granuloma faciale
   D. Erythema elevatum diutinum
      1. Early stage
      2. Late stage
   E. Periarteritis nodosa
      1. Degenerative stage
      2. Inflammatory stage
      3. Granulation stage
      4. Fibrotic stage
   F. Allergic granulomatosis (of Churg and Strauss)
   G. Wegener's granulomatosis
      1. Necrotizing granulomatous inflammation
      2. Necrotizing vasculitis
   H. Lupus erythematosus profundus
   I. Giant-cell (temporal) arteritis
   J. Erythema nodosum leprosum
   K. Tertiary syphilis
III. Perivascular inflammation with thrombosis
   A. Bacterial sepsis
   B. Disseminated intravascular coagulation (DIC)
   C. Superficial migratory thrombophlebitis

The Reactive Process and the Disease	Histopathology	Comments
I. Perivascular infiltrate without vascular damage		
A. Mixed infiltrate		
1. Urticaria/angioedema (Fig. 14-1)	1. Epidermis normal 2. **Edema** of papillary and occasionally reticular dermis 3. Superficial and sometimes deep perivascular infiltrate composed of a variable number and a variable mixture of lymphocytes, neutrophils, and eosinophils	See papillary dermis, Ch. 11, I.A; angioedema exhibits these changes in the deep dermis and subcutis
2. Arthropod bite reaction (see Fig. 11-2)	1. Epidermal changes may include focal spongiosis, hyperplasia, dyskeratosis, necrosis, and ulceration at site of puncta 2. Slight to marked **edema** of the papillary dermis 3. Moderate to heavy **perivascular infiltrate composed of lymphocytes and eosinophils** extending into deep reticular dermis 4. **Endothelial cell swelling** 5. Vascular proliferation common in older lesions	See also Ch. 4, III.B; Ch. 10, IV; Ch. 11, I.F Fibrin deposition may be seen in spider bites Rarely insect parts may be observed in the epidermis or dermis (for example, scabies, tungiasis, myiasis, and bee stings)

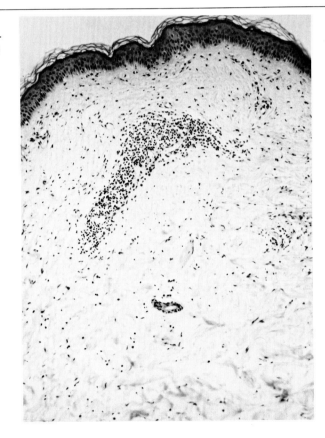

Fig. **14-1.** *Urticaria. Dermal edema as manifested here by separation of collagen bundles is the hallmark of urticaria. Perivascular infiltrates, lymphohistiocytic and eosinophilic, vary from minimal to heavy. Cutaneous necrotizing vasculitis also has been observed in some cases of chronic urticaria. (×160)*

3. Drug reaction, urticarial

1. Normal epidermis
2. Edema of papillary dermis
3. Loose perivascular infiltrate composed of lymphocytes, eosinophils, and a few neutrophils

See also Ch. 11, I.E

4. Photoallergic reaction

1. Focal intercellular edema (spongiosis)
2. Dyskeratosis
3. Basal vacuolization, variable
4. Loose perivascular lymphohistiocytic infiltrate with rare neutrophils
5. Infiltrate predominantly in upper but may extend to mid-reticular dermis
6. Slight extravasation of erythrocytes
7. Endothelial cell swelling

See also Ch. 11, III.D

5. Cellulitis

1. Papillary dermal edema
2. Vascular ectasia
3. Perivascular and diffuse infiltrate composed of neutrophils, lymphocytes, occasional eosinophils, and plasma cells in deep dermis and subcutis
4. Extravasation of erythrocytes

Differential diagnosis: acute febrile neutrophilic dermatosis (Sweet's disease)

6. Acute febrile neutrophilic dermatosis (Sweet's disease) (see Fig. 11-3)

1. Epidermal hyperplasia
2. Intercellular edema
3. Migration of neutrophils into epidermis forming microabscesses
4. Edema of papillary dermis, often severe
5. Dense perivascular and diffuse infiltrate composed predominantly of **neutrophils** with lymphocytes
6. **Nuclear "dust"**
7. Vascular ectasia

Epidermal changes may be absent

See also Ch. 11, I.H; Ch. 16, V.C

The lack of fibrin deposition, hemorrhage, and invasion of blood vessel walls by neutrophils (i.e., necrotizing vasculitis) helps distinguish this entity from erythema elevatum diutinum

7. Secondary syphilis (see Fig. 4-7)

1. Hyperkeratosis and parakeratosis
2. Epidermal hyperplasia and vacuolation at the dermoepidermal junction
3. Dense perivascular lymphohistiocytic and **plasma cell infiltrate,** which may extend to form a bandlike infiltrate in the papillary dermis

See also Ch. 4, III.C; Ch. 11, I.G

Silver stains may demonstrate spirochetes in the epidermis and around vessel walls (see Appendix)

4. **Endothelial cell swelling** with nodular pseudogranulomatous aggregates formed by endothelial cells and inflammatory cells
5. Occasional epithelioid cell granulomas with or without giant cells

B. Lymphohistiocytic infiltrates

1. Lupus erythematosus (see Fig. 9-3)

1. Hyperkeratosis
2. Epidermal **atrophy**
3. Dilated follicles filled with keratin
4. Dyskeratotic cells
5. **Vacuolation and squamotization of basal layer**
6. Basement membrane thickened in older lesions
7. Edema of papillary dermis
8. Vascular ectasia
9. **Perivascular, periappendageal, and occasionally bandlike lymphohistiocytic infiltrate**
10. Extravasation of erythrocytes

See also Ch. 7, VI; Ch. 9, I.D, II.D; Ch. 10, III; Ch. 14, I.B.1; Ch. 22, I.G

Special stains (see Appendix) may demonstrate increased neutral mucopolysaccharides in the basement membrane zone and acid mucopolysaccharide deposition in the dermis

2. Polymorphous light eruption (Fig. 14-2)

1. Focal parakeratosis
2. Intercellular edema (spongiosis)
3. Dyskeratosis
4. Slight basal vacuolation
5. Slight thickening of basement membrane
6. Edema of papillary dermis
7. Loose, perivascular, predominantly lymphohistiocytic infiltrate with occasional neutrophils and rare eosinophils may extend into lower dermis
8. Extravasated erythrocytes
9. Endothelial cell swelling

Differential diagnosis:
Lupus erythematosus
Photoallergic reaction
Drug eruption
Arthropod bite reaction

3. Lymphocytic infiltration of the skin (Jessner-Kanof)

1. Epidermis may appear normal or have flattened rete ridges
2. **Dense, circumscribed aggregates of lymphocytes around vessels and appendages** of the papillary and reticular dermis
3. Lymphocytes may extend in single-cell array between collagen fibers of the dermis
4. Little or no endothelial cell swelling

Differential diagnosis:
Lupus erythematosus
Arthropod bite reaction
Lymphoma cutis
Lymphocytoma cutis

Special stains demonstrate increased acid mucopolysaccharide deposition between collagen fibers in the upper reticular dermis
Normal epidermis helpful in differentiating lymphocytic infiltrate from lupus (see also Ch. 11, III.A)

4. Deep figurate or gyrate erythema

1. Normal epidermis
2. Variable edema of papillary dermis
3. Dense, predominantly lymphocytic infiltrate about vessels throughout reticular dermis
4. Infiltrate may extend around appendages

5. Pityriasis lichenoides et varioliformis acuta (PLEVA, Mucha-Habermann) (see Fig. 9-11)

1. Focal parakeratosis
2. Variable hyperkeratosis
3. Focal **dyskeratosis** may be prominent
4. Exocytosis of lymphocytes into epidermis
5. **Extravasation of erythrocytes into epidermis and dermis**
6. Perivascular infiltrate of lymphocytes, and rarely eosinophils
7. Infiltrate often extends to deep reticular dermis
8. Marked **endothelial cell swelling**

See also Ch. 9, II.J; Ch. 11, III.F

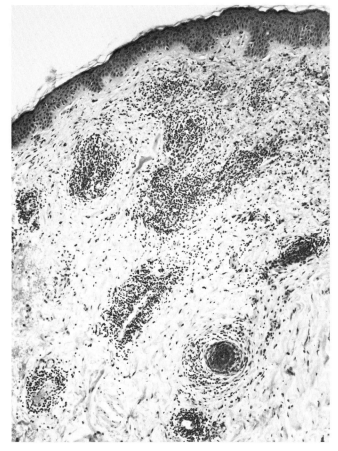

Fig. **14-2.** *Lymphocytic infiltrate consistent with polymorphous light eruption. Perivascular lymphocytic infiltrates disposed somewhat loosely about venules with edema of the papillary dermis and rare dyskeratotic cells within the epidermis (the latter not evident at this power) are characteristic of this disorder. (×160)*

6. Lymphomatoid papulosis (Fig. 14-3)

1. Erosion or ulceration common
2. Parakeratosis, acanthosis, and spongiosis of adjacent epidermis
3. Variable exocytosis and basal vacuolation
4. Dense, polymorphous dermal infiltrate, often perivascular, composed of lymphocytes, histiocytes, and prominent atypical lymphoid cells
5. These cells have extremely bizarre, large nuclei, mitotic figures, and prominent nucleoli
6. Prominent endothelial cell swelling
7. Variable erythrocyte extravasation

Differential diagnosis:
   Hodgkin's disease
   Non-Hodgkin's lymphoma
   Mycosis fungoides
   Arthropod bite reaction

The degree of atypism frequently exceeds that observed in lymphomas and mycosis fungoides

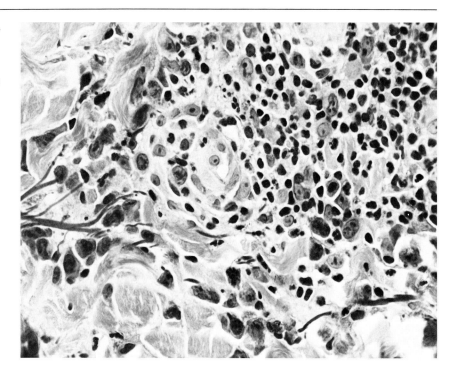

Fig. **14-3.** *Lymphomatoid papulosis. The mix of small, dark lymphocytes and large, extremely atypical lymphoid cells associated with endothelial swelling is typical. These infiltrates frequently are extensive and may be associated with ulceration of the epidermis. (×640)*

7. Stasis dermatitis (see Fig. 20-15)

1. Atrophic or acanthotic epidermis with flattened rete
2. Mild to moderate intercellular edema may be present
3. Perivascular lymphohistiocytic infiltrate which may extend into the subcutaneous tissue
4. **Vascular ectasia and proliferation**
5. **Vessel walls often thickened**
6. Dermal **hemorrhage and hemosiderin** disposition
7. **Fibrosis** of reticular dermis

See also Ch. 11, III.G; Ch. 20, XXII

Differential diagnosis:
   Progressive pigmentary purpura
   Kaposi's sarcoma

8. Indeterminate leprosy

1. Normal epidermis
2. Slight lymphohistiocytic perivascular and **perineural** infiltrate

Special acid-fast stains (see Appendix) may demonstrate organisms within nerves

II. Perivascular infiltrate with vascular damage—vasculitis

A. Cutaneous necrotizing vasculitis (see Fig. 11-4)

See Ch. 11, II.A

B. Focal septic embolic lesions in gonococcemia and acute meningococcemia

See Ch. 11, II.B

C. Granuloma faciale (see Fig. 16-7)

1. Normal epidermis
2. **Grenz zone** of uninvolved papillary and adventitial dermis separates epidermis and adnexal structures from infiltrate
3. Perivascular nodular and diffuse aggregates of lymphocytes, histiocytes, and variable but usually **prominent eosinophils** (up to 90%) plus neutrophils, plasma cells, and mast cells
4. Infiltrate usually confined to upper and middle dermis but may extend to subcutaneous tissue
5. **Leukocytoclastic vasculitis** with endothelial cell swelling, neutrophils within vessel walls, nuclear debris, and fibrinoid deposition in and around vessels
6. Extravasation of erythrocytes
7. Hemosiderin-laden macrophages
8. Variable fibrosis

Grenz zone commonly seen in:

Granuloma faciale
Leukemia cutis
Lymphoma cutis
Parapsoriasis en plaques
Sarcoidosis
Acrodermatitis chronica atrophicans
Lepromatous leprosy

See Ch. 16, V.A

D. Erythema elevatum diutinum

1. Early stage

1. Epidermal hyperplasia and invasion by neutrophils
2. Occasional subepidermal bulla
3. **Nodular aggregates** of inflammatory cells with up to 90% **neutrophils**
4. **Leukocytoclastic vasculitis** involving superficial and deep vessels of dermis with fibrinoid deposition in and around vessels, nuclear debris, and extravasation of erythrocytes

Lack of Grenz zone and predominance of neutrophils separate erythema elevatum diutinum from granuloma faciale

2. Late stage

1. Infiltrate less pronounced but still predominantly neutrophils
2. Fibrinoid deposition may be replaced by fibrous thickening of vessel walls
3. Extracellular and/or intracellular **lipid (cholesterol) deposition** in dermis

Polariscopic examination of formalin-fixed frozen sections will reveal doubly refractile cholesterol esters in the dermis

E. Periarteritis nodosa

Small- and medium-sized vessels at junction of dermis and subcutaneous fat are affected

1. Degenerative stage

Segmental medial or adventitial necrosis extending into the intima

2. Inflammatory stage

Necrotic area densely infiltrated by neutrophils, eosinophils, and mononuclear cells; thrombosis may occur

Vessels of the superficial vascular plexus may show thrombosis and necrosis of the capillary walls with or without inflammation

3. Granulation stage

Granulation tissue replaces the necrotic areas; intimal proliferation leads to partial or complete luminal occlusion

Cutaneous ulceration may follow arterial occlusion

4. Fibrotic stage

Scarring of vascular wall; lumen shows narrowing, obliteration, or recanalization

Subcutaneous hemorrhage may occur secondarily to aneurysm formation

If granulomas are seen, consider allergic granulomatosis or Wegener's granulomatosis

F. Allergic granulomatosis (of Churg and Strauss)

1. The type of vessels involved and the histopathology are similar to those of periarteritis nodosa with the addition of intramural and extravascular granulomatous inflammation
2. **Granulomatous inflammation** consists of a central core of collagen admixed with fibrinoid material and **eosinophilic cellular debris;** a radial arrangement of epithelioid and giant cells surrounds the necrotic area

The following are necessary findings for the diagnosis of allergic granulomatosis:
1. Respiratory involvement, i.e., pulmonary infiltrates or involvement of lung
2. Eosinophilia circulating and within lesions

Differential diagnosis:
Eosinophilic cellulitis
Periarteritis nodosa
Wegener's granulomatosis

G. Wegener's granulomatosis

1. Necrotizing granulomatous inflammation

1. Confluent, variably sized areas of vessel wall necrosis
2. Granulomatous inflammation with giant cells and an infiltrate of neutrophils, lymphoid cells, and plasma cells surrounds necrotic vessels
3. Few eosinophils are present

Differential diagnosis:
Periarteritis nodosa
Allergic granulomatosis

2. Necrotizing vasculitis (see Fig. 11-4)

1. Deep and/or superficial small arteries and veins in the dermis are affected
2. Fibrinous exudate and polymorphous infiltrate
3. Thrombosis of the lumen may be seen
4. Intimal proliferation may be marked

Epidermal ulcers may form as a result of vascular obliteration and/or granulomatous inflammation

Necrotizing vasculitis is seen often in biopsies from patients with Wegener's granulomatosis but is *not* diagnostic; more specific (but less commonly observed) are the granulomatous inflammation and necrosis described above

H. Lupus erythematosus profundus

1. Fibrosis of deep dermal vessel walls with onionskin pattern
2. Intramural and perivascular lymphocytic infiltrates
3. Lobular panniculitis with infiltrate of lymphocytes, plasma cells, and histiocytes
4. One also may find septal fibrosis and hyalinization, mucinous changes, foci of calcification, and altered collagen with fibrinoid deposits in adjacent tissue

The term *onionskin pattern* refers to concentric lamellar perivascular fibrosis

Overlying epidermis may show characteristic features of lupus erythematosus with hyperkeratosis, atrophy, dyskeratosis, and basal vacuolation

I. Giant-cell (temporal) arteritis (Fig. 14-4)

1. Degeneration of internal elastic lamella with phagocytosis by macrophages and multinucleated foreign-body giant cells
2. Intimal fibrosis and fibrinoid degeneration
3. Mononuclear and plasma cell infiltrate between intima and media

Elastic tissue stains demonstrate fragmentation of internal elastic lamella

J. Erythema nodosum leprosum

1. Deep dermal vessels show neutrophilic vasculitis with endothelial cell swelling, fibrinoid material in and around vessel walls, and the perivascular disposition of neutrophils and macrophages
2. Special stains (see Appendix) disclose many bacilli in macrophages, vessel walls, and lumens

K. Tertiary syphilis

1. Deep dermal vessels show endothelial cell swelling and an infiltrate of intramural plasma cells and lymphoid cells
2. Caseation necrosis is marked in tissue adjacent to vessels

Spirochetes difficult to demonstrate

See also Ch. 15, III.H; Ch. 17, V

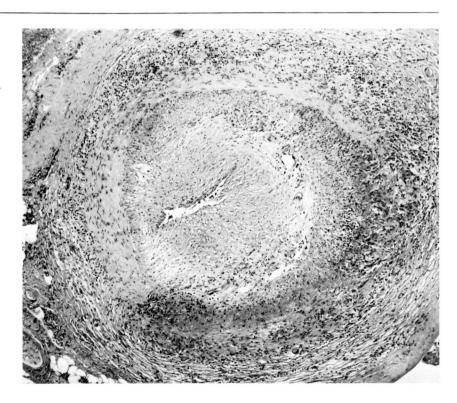

Fig. **14-4.** *Giant-cell (temporal) arteritis. Histiocytic and giant-cell inflammation replace the internal elastic lamella and the media from 2 to 7 o'clock. In addition, marked intimal fibrosis and adventitial lymphocytic infiltrate are seen. (×100)*

III. Perivascular inflammation
with thrombosis

A. Bacterial sepsis

1. **Intraepidermal and subepidermal pustules,** frequently with necrosis of overlying epidermis
2. **Leukocytoclastic vasculitis** with fibrinoid deposition, neutrophils within vessel walls, nuclear debris, and extravasation of erythrocytes
3. **Fibrin thrombi**

Examples include gonococcemia, acute meningococcemia, staphylococcemia

B. Disseminated intravascular coagulation (DIC) (Fig. 14-5)

Fibrin thrombi occur with and without endothelial cell necrosis and variable neutrophilic infiltrate

C. Superficial migratory thrombophlebitis

1. Normal epidermis
2. Inflammation around and within walls of a large vessel in the deep reticular dermis; infiltrate may be predominantly neutrophilic or mononuclear cells depending on age of lesion
3. **Occlusion of lumen by thrombus**

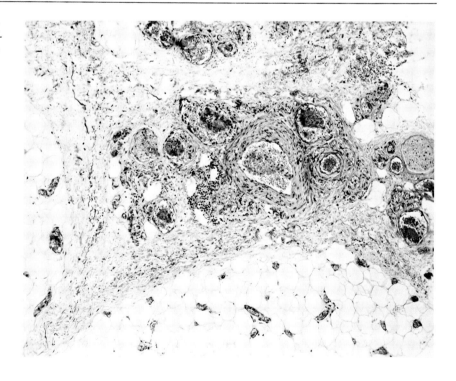

Fig. **14-5.** *Disseminated intravascular coagulation (purpura fulminans). Subcutaneous vessels contain fibrin thrombi and blood. (×100)*

Suggested Reading
Urticaria

Lever, W. F., and Schaumburg-Lever, G. *Histopathology of the Skin* (6th ed.). Philadelphia: Lippincott, 1983. P. 136.

Warin, R. P., and Champion, R. H. *Urticaria.* Philadelphia: Saunders, 1974.

Insect Bite Reactions

Goldman, L., Rockwell, E., and Richfield, D. F. Histopathological studies on cutaneous reactions to the bites of various arthropods. *Am. J. Trop. Med. Hyg.* 1:514, 1952.

Thomson, J., Cochrane, T., Cochran, R., and McQueen, A. Histology simulating reticulosis in persistent nodular scabies. *Br. J. Dermatol.* 90:421, 1974.

Winer, L. H., and Strakosch, E. A. Tick bite—*Dermacentor variabilis* (Say). *J. Invest. Dermatol.* 4:249, 1941.

Photoallergic Reaction

Emmett, E. A. Drug photoallergy. *Int. J. Dermatol.* 17:370, 1978.

Acute Febrile Neutrophilic Dermatosis

Gunawardena, D. A., Gunawardena, K. A., Ratnayaka, R. M. R. S., et al. The clinical spectrum of Sweet's syndrome (acute febrile neutrophilic dermatosis)—A report of eighteen cases. *Br. J. Dermatol.* 92:363, 1975.

Sweet, R. D. An acute febrile neutrophilic dermatosis. *Br. J. Dermatol.* 76:349, 1964.

Sweet, R. D. Acute febrile neutrophilic dermatosis—1978. *Br. J. Dermatol.* 100:93, 1979.

Secondary Syphilis

Abell, E., Marks, R., and Wilson-Jones, E. Secondary syphilis: A clinicopathological review. *Br. J. Dermatol.* 93:53, 1975.

Jeerapaet, P., and Ackerman, A. B. Histologic patterns of secondary syphilis. *Arch. Dermatol.* 107:373, 1973.

Lupus Erythematosus

Biesecker, G., Lavin, L., Ziskind, M., and Koffler, D. Cutaneous localization of the membrane attack complex in discoid and systemic lupus erythematosus. *N. Engl. J. Med.* 306:264, 1982.

Brown, M. M., and Yount, W. J. Skin immunopathology in systemic lupus erythematosus. *J.A.M.A.* 243:38, 1980.

Clark, W. H., Reed, R. J., and Mihm, M. C., Jr. Lupus erythematosus: Histopathology of cutaneous lesions. *Hum. Pathol.* 4:157, 1973.

Dubois, E. L. *Lupus Erythematosus: A Review of the Current Status of Discoid and Systemic Lupus Erythematosus and Their Variants* (2nd ed.). Los Angeles: University of Southern California Press, 1974.

McCreight, W. G., and Montgomery, H. Cutaneous changes in lupus erythematosus. *Arch. Dermatol. Syphilol.* 61:1, 1950.

Provost, T. T., Zone, J. J., Synkowski, D., et al. Unusual cutaneous manifestations of systemic lupus erythematosus: I. Urticaria-like lesions. Correlation with clinical and serological abnormalities. *J. Invest. Dermatol.* 75:495, 1980.

Prunieras, M., and Montgomery, H. Histopathology of cutaneous lesions in systemic lupus erythematosus. *Arch. Dermatol.* 74:177, 1956.

Prystowsky, S. D., and Gilliam, J. N. Discoid lupus erythematosus as part of a larger disease spectrum. *Arch. Dermatol.* 111:1448, 1975.

Synkowski, D. R., Reichlin, M., and Provost, T. T. Serum autoantibodies in systemic lupus erythematosus and correlation with cutaneous features. *J. Rheumatol.* 9:380, 1982.

Tuffanelli, D. L., Kay, D., and Fukuyama, K. Dermal-epidermal junction in lupus erythematosus. *Arch. Dermatol.* 99:652, 1969.

Winkelmann, R. K. Spectrum of lupus erythematosus. *J. Cutan. Pathol.* 6:457, 1979.

Polymorphous Light Reaction

Epstein, J. H. Polymorphous light eruption. *Ann. Allergy* 24:397, 1966.

Panet-Raymond, G., and Johnson, W. C. Lupus erythematosus and polymorphous light eruption: Differentiation by histochemical procedures. *Arch. Dermatol.* 108:785, 1973.

Stern, W. K. Evolution of an abnormal light test reaction. *Arch. Dermatol.* 103:154, 1971.

Wright, E. T. and Winer, L. H. Histopathology of allergic solar dermatitis. *J. Invest. Dermatol.* 34:103, 1960.

Lymphocytic Infiltration of the Skin (Jessner-Kanof)	Clark, W. H., Mihm, M. C., Jr., Reed, R. J., and Ainsworth, A. M. The lymphocytic infiltrates of the skin. *Hum. Pathol.* 5:25, 1974.
	Gottlieb, B., and Winkelman, R. K. Lymphocytic infiltration of the skin. *Arch. Dermatol.* 86:626, 1962.
	Jessner, M., and Kanof, N. B. Lymphocytic infiltration of the skin. *Arch. Dermatol. Syphilol.* 68:447, 1953.
	Ten Have Opbroek, A. A. W. On the differential diagnosis between chronic discoid lupus erythematodes and lymphocytic infiltration of the skin with emphasis on fluorescence microscopy. *Dermatologica* 132:109, 1966.
Figurate Erythema	Ellis, F. A., and Friedman, A. A. Erythema annulare centrifugum (Darier's): Clinical and histologic study. *Arch. Dermatol. Syphilol.* 70:496, 1954.
	Harrison, P. V. The annular erythemas. *Int. J. Dermatol.* 18:282, 1979.
	Maciejewski, W. Annular erythema as an unusual manifestation of chronic disseminated lupus erythematosus. *Arch. Dermatol.* 116:450, 1980.
	Thomson, J., and Stankler, L. Erythema gyratum repens: Reports of two further cases associated with carcinoma. *Br. J. Dermatol.* 82:406, 1970.
	White, J. W., and Perry, H. O. Erythema perstans. *Br. J. Dermatol.* 81:641, 1969.
Pityriasis Lichenoides et Varioliformis Acuta	Black, M. M., and Marks, R. The inflammatory reaction in pityriasis lichenoides. *Br. J. Dermatol.* 87:533, 1972.
	Hood, A. F., and Mark, E. J. Histopathologic diagnosis of pityriasis lichenoides et varioliformis acuta and its clinical correlation. *Arch. Dermatol.* 118:478–482, 1982.
	Marks, R., Black, M. M., and Wilson-Jones, E. Pityriasis lichenoides: A reappraisal. *Br. J. Dermatol.* 86:215, 1972.
	Nigra, T. P., and Soter, N. A. Pityriasis Lichenoides. In T. B. Fitzpatrick et al. (Eds.), *Dermatology in General Medicine* (2d ed.). New York: McGraw-Hill, 1979.
	Szymanski, F. J. Pityriasis lichenoides et varioliformis acuta: Histopathological evidence that it is an entity distinct from parapsoriasis. *Arch. Dermatol.* 79:7, 1959.
Lymphomatoid Papulosis	Black, M. M., and Wilson-Jones, E. Lymphomatoid pityriasis lichenoides; a variant with histological features simulating a lymphoma. *Br. J. Dermatol.* 86:329, 1972.
	Sina, B., and Burnett, J. W. Lymphomatoid papulosis. Case reports and literature review. *Arch. Dermatol.* 119:189, 1983.
	Valentino, L. A., and Helwig, E. B. Lymphomatoid papulosis. *Arch. Pathol.* 96:409, 1973.
	Weinman, V. F., and Ackerman, A. B. Lymphomatoid papulosis. A critical review and new findings. *Am. J. Dermatopathol.* 3:129, 1981.
Leprosy	Azulay, R. D. Histopathology of skin lesions in leprosy. *Int. J. Lepr.* 39:244, 1971.
	Fasal, P. Histopathology of leprosy. *Cutis* 18:66, 1976.
	Ridley, D. S. Histological classification and the immunological spectrum of leprosy. *Bull. W.H.O.* 51:451, 1974.
	Ridley, D. S., and Jopling, W. H. Classification of leprosy according to immunity. A five-group system. *Int. J. Lepr.* 34:255, 1966.
	Williams, R. C., Sr. Symposium on leprosy. *South. Med. J.* 69:969, 1976.
Cutaneous Necrotizing Vasculitis	Copeman, P. W. M., and Ryan, T. J. The problems of classification of cutaneous angiitis with reference to histopathology and pathogenesis. *Br. J. Dermatol.* 82 (Suppl. 5):2, 1970.
	Cream, J. J., Gumpel, J. M., and Peachey, R. D. Schönlein-Henoch purpura in the adult: A study of 77 adults with anaphylactoid or Schönlein-Henoch purpura. *Q. J. Med.* 39:461, 1970.
	Reed, R. J. *Cutaneous Vasculitides. Immunologic and Histologic Correlations.* Chicago: American Society of Clinical Pathologists, 1977.
	Soter, N. A. Chronic urticaria as a manifestation of necrotizing venulitis. *N. Engl. J. Med.* 296:1440, 1977.
	Soter, N. A. Necrotizing Vasculitis of the Skin. In T. B. Fitzpatrick et al. (Eds.), *Dermatology in General Medicine* (2d ed.). New York: McGraw-Hill, 1979.

Gonococcemia and Meningococcemia	Ackerman, A. B., Miller, R. C., and Shapiro, L. Gonococcemia and its cutaneous manifestations. *Arch. Dermatol.* 91:227, 1965. Nielsen, T. Chronic meningococcemia. *Arch. Dermatol.* 102:97, 1970. Shapiro, L., Teisch, J. A., and Brownstein, M. H. Dermatohistopathology of chronic gonococcal sepsis. *Arch. Dermatol.* 107:403, 1973.
Granuloma Faciale	Johnson, W. C., Higdon, R. S., and Helwig, E. B. Granuloma faciale. *Arch. Dermatol.* 79:42, 1959. Okun, M. R., Bauman, L., and Minor, D. Granuloma faciale with lesions on the face and hand. *Arch. Dermatol.* 92:78, 1965. Pedace, F. J., and Perry, H. O. Granuloma faciale: A clinical and histopathologic review. *Arch. Dermatol.* 94:387, 1966.
Erythema Elevatum Diutinum	Cream, J. J., Levene, G. M., and Calnan, C. D. Erythema elevatum diutinum. *Br. J. Dermatol.* 84:393, 1971. Haber, H. Erythema elevatum diutinum. *Br. J. Dermatol.* 67:121, 1955. Laymon, C. W. Erythema elevatum diutinum. *Arch. Dermatol.* 85:22, 1962.
Periarteritis Nodosa	Arkin, A. A clinical and pathological study of periarteritis nodosa. *Am. J. Pathol.* 6:401, 1930. Borrie, P. Cutaneous polyarteritis nodosa. *Br. J. Dermatol.* 87:87, 1972. Diaz-Perez, J. L., and Winkelmann, R. K. Cutaneous periarteritis nodosa. *Arch. Dermatol.* 110:407, 1974. Zeek, P. M., Smith, C. C., and Weeter, J. C. Studies on periarteritis nodosa. III. The differentiation between the vascular lesions of periarteritis nodosa and of hypersensitivity. *Am. J. Pathol.* 24:889, 1948.
Allergic Granulomatosis	Burton, J. L., and Burton, P. A. Pulmonary eosinophilia associated with vasculitis and extra-vascular granulomata. *Br. J. Dermatol.* 87:412, 1972. Chumbley, L. C., Harrison, E. G., and DeRemee, R. A. Allergic granulomatosis and angiitis (Churg-Strauss syndrome) *Mayo Clin. Proc.* 52:477, 1977. Churg, J., and Strauss, L. Allergic granulomatosis, allergic angiitis and periarteritis nodosa. *Am. J. Pathol.* 27:277, 1951.
Wegener's Granulomatosis	Godman, G. C., and Churg, J. Wegener's granulomatosis: Pathology and review of the literature. *Arch. Pathol.* 58:533, 1954. Reed, W. B., Jenson, A. K., Konwaler, B. E., et al. The cutaneous manifestations in Wegener's granulomatosis. *Acta. Derm. Venereol. (Stockh.)* 43:250, 1968.
Lupus Erythematosus Profundus	Fountain, R. B. Lupus erythematosus profundus. *Br. J. Dermatol.* 80:571, 1968. Tuffanelli, D. L. Lupus erythematosus panniculitis (profundus). *Arch. Dermatol.* 103:231, 1971.
Erythema Nodosum Leprosum	Jolliffe, D. S. Leprosy reactional states and their treatment. *Br. J. Dermatol.* 97:345, 1977. Ridley, D. S. Reactions in leprosy. *Lepr. Rev.* 40:77, 1969.
Tertiary Syphilis	Johnson, W. C. Venereal Diseases and Treponemal Infections. In J. H. Graham, W. C. Johnson, and W. B. Helwig (Eds.), *Dermal Pathology.* Hagerstown, Md.: Harper & Row, 1972.
Bacterial Sepsis	Alpert, J. S., Krous, H. F., Dalen, J. E., et al. Pathogenesis of Osler's nodes. *Ann. Intern. Med.* 85:471, 1976.
Disseminated Intravascular Coagulation	DiCato, M. A., and Ellman, L. Coumadin-induced necrosis of breast, disseminated intravascular coagulation, and hemolytic anemia. *Ann. Intern. Med.* 83:233, 1975. Robboy, S. J., Mihm, M. C., Jr., Colman, R. W., et al. The skin in disseminated intravascular coagulation: Prospective analysis of thirty-six cases. *Br. J. Dermatol.* 88:221, 1973.
Superficial Migratory Thrombophlebitis	Rossman, R. E., and Freeman, R. G. Chest wall thrombophlebitis (Mondor's disease). *Arch. Dermatol.* 87:475, 1963.

Chapter 15

Granulomas and Granulomatous Inflammation

I. Palisading granulomas
    A. Granuloma annulare
    B. Necrobiosis lipoidica
    C. Rheumatoid nodule
    D. Rheumatic fever nodule
    E. Pseudorheumatoid nodule
II. Epithelioid cell granulomas
    A. Tuberculosis
        1. Primary inoculation
        2. Lupus vulgaris
        3. Tuberculosis verrucosa cutis
        4. Scrofuloderma
        5. Orificial tuberculosis (tuberculosis cutis orificialis)
        6. Miliary tuberculosis
    B. "Tuberculids"
        1. Lupus miliaris disseminatus faciei
        2. Lichen scrofulosorum
        3. Erythema induratum
        4. Papulonecrotic tuberculid
    C. Tuberculoid leprosy
    D. Sarcoidosis
    E. Granulomatous rosacea
    F. Zirconium granuloma and cutaneous lesions of systemic berylliosis
    G. Inoculation beryllium granuloma
    H. Cheilitis granulomatosa (Miescher-Melkersson-Rosenthal)
    I. Miscellaneous foreign-body granulomas
III. Granulomatous inflammation
    A. North American blastomycosis (cutaneous nodule or verrucous plaque associated with systemic infection)
    B. South American blastomycosis (mucosal or cutaneous lesions)
    C. Chromoblastomycosis
        1. Dermal lesions
        2. Subcutaneous lesions
    D. Sporotrichosis
        1. Primary lesion
        2. Secondary cutaneous nodules
    E. Coccidioidomycosis
        1. Early primary cutaneous lesions
        2. Late primary cutaneous lesions; secondary (disseminated) cutaneous lesions
        3. Subcutaneous abscesses
    F. Cryptococcosis
        1. Granulomatous reaction
        2. Gelatinous reaction
    G. Swimming pool granuloma
        1. Early lesions
        2. Late lesions
    H. Tertiary syphilis
    I. Cat-scratch disease

Histologically, a *granuloma* is defined as a space-occupying lesion composed of aggregates of histiocytic cells. Granulomatous disorders are divided into three categories according to the disposition and arrangement of the histiocytes within the dermis: (1) palisading granulomas: histiocytes and lymphocytes with long axis arranged perpendicular to ("palisading") areas of altered collagen; (2) epithelioid cell granulomas: focal aggregates of epithelioid histiocytes with or without necrosis; and (3) granulomatous inflammation: diffuse infiltration of histiocytes admixed with other inflammatory cells without discrete granuloma formation.

The Reactive Process and the Disease	Histopathology	Comments
I. Palisading granulomas		
A. Granuloma annulare (Fig. 15-1)	1. Normal epidermis (except in perforating variant)	See Table 15-1 for comparison of various palisading granulomas
	2. Small or large foci of altered collagen, most frequently in upper and mid dermis but occasionally in deep dermis or subcutaneous tissue	Very earliest lesions are said to have leukocytoclastic vasculitis in area of collagen alteration
	3. Early **collagen alteration** consists of:	
	a. Fragmentation of collagen fibers	Early lesions may show very subtle changes, best appreciated at low power by a faint focal bluish tinctorial change in the dermis
	b. **Infiltration of histiocytes and lymphocytes between collagen bundles**	
	c. Deposition of **acid mucopolysaccharides** on and between collagen fibers	Staining for acid mucopolysaccharide (see Appendix) is often helpful in identifying areas of altered collagen
	4. Later lesions show well-defined areas of dermal degeneration characterized by foci of relatively acellular, homogeneous, or amorphous collagen	
	5. Scant numbers of histiocytes and lymphocytes surround abnormal collagen	
	6. Giant cells and/or aggregates of epithelioid cells occasionally present	

Table **15-1.** *Comparison of Histologic Findings in Palisading Granulomas*

Disease	Area of collagen alteration "necrobiosis"	Type and degree of collagen alteration	Acid mucopoly-saccharide deposition	Extracellular fat in dermis	Vascular changes
Granuloma annulare	Upper to mid-reticular dermis; rarely, subcutaneous tissue	Focally altered collagen alternating with normal collagen	Common	Rare	None
Necrobiosis lipoidica	Entire reticular dermis	Larger confluent areas of altered collagen	Rare	Common	Endothelial cell hypertrophy and proliferation
Rheumatoid nodule	Deep reticular dermis; subcutaneous tissue	Large areas with fibrinoid alteration	Variable	Variable	Variable
Rheumatic fever nodule	Subcutaneous tissue	Large areas of fibrinoid alteration	Variable	Variable	Vessel proliferation
Pseudorheumatoid nodule	Mid- to deep reticular dermis and subcutaneous tissue	Large confluent areas of altered collagen	Common	Variable	Variable

Fig. **15-1.**

A. *Comparison of granuloma annulare and necrobiosis lipoidica.* Left: *Granuloma annulare. Areas of necrobiosis are usually (but not always) smaller and the infiltrate is patchier than in necrobiosis lipoidica; granulomas and vasculitis are absent.* Right: *Necrobiosis lipoidica. Necrobiotic areas are usually larger and show variable staining, indicating necrobiosis of collagen; inflammatory infiltrates are typically organized into granulomas and vasculitis.*

B. *Granuloma annulare. A central zone of necrobiotic collagen is surrounded by histiocytes, lymphocytes, and a few scattered multinucleate giant cells. A portion of another palisading granuloma is present at the extreme right of the field. (×64).*

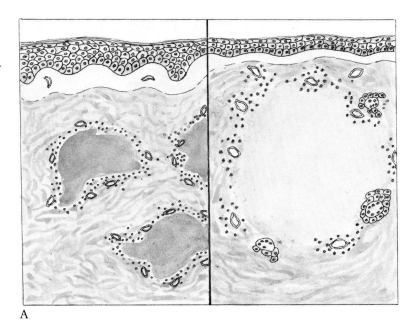

A

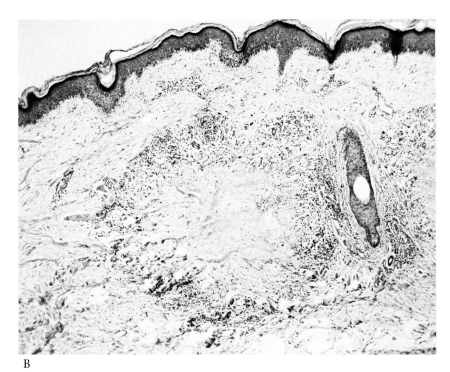

B

B. Necrobiosis lipoidica (Figs. 15-1A, 15-2)

1. Epidermal **atrophy,** occasionally with ulceration
2. Ectatic venules in compressed papillary dermis
3. One or more areas of altered collagen that initially show fragmentation and clumping of collagen fibers and later become **hyalinized, eosinophilic, and relatively acellular (necrobiosis)**
4. Altered collagen surrounded by a zone of palisading histiocytes, epithelioid cells, and lymphocytes
5. Inflammatory infiltrate composed of lymphocytes, plasma cells, lipid-laden histiocytes, and giant cells is present around altered collagen or scattered throughout dermis
6. **Vessel walls thickened** by endothelial proliferation

Frozen sections stained for fat (see Appendix) often reveal abundant lipid globules within areas of collagen alteration

Epidermal atrophy, thickened vessel walls, extracellular fat in the dermis, and the presence of plasma cells in the infiltrate help differentiate necrobiosis lipoidica from granuloma annulare; however, at times it may be impossible to histologically distinguish these two entities, and the use of the generic term *palisading granuloma* is preferable

Vascular changes are often prominent in lesions from the leg but may be absent or mild in lesions from other areas

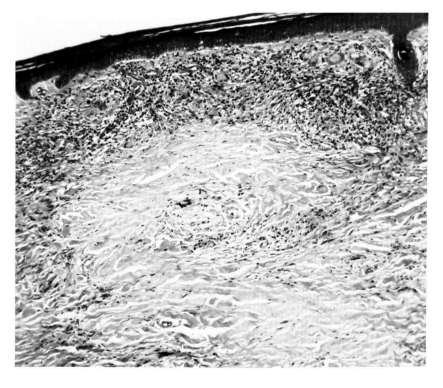

Fig. **15-2.** *Necrobiosis lipoidica. Lymphohistiocyte infiltrates with multinucleate cells surround large areas of collagen necrobiosis. The palisading granulomas and necrobiosis extend well beyond the field of this micrograph. (×160)*

C. Rheumatoid nodule
(Fig. 15-3)

1. Normal epidermis
2. In the subcutaneous tissue and/or deep reticular dermis are large, well-demarcated areas of eosinophilic, **relatively amorphous, fibrinoid material**
3. A zone of histiocytes and lymphocytes surrounds fibrinoid material
4. Vascular proliferation often observed peripheral to altered collagen

Special stains (see Appendix) reveal fibrin deposition in areas of collagen degeneration

Differential diagnosis:
Other palisading granulomas
Epithelioid cell sarcoma

D. Rheumatic fever nodule

In the deep dermis and subcutaneous tissue are areas of edematous altered collagen admixed with **neutrophils** and surrounded by loosely aggregated palisading histiocytes and other mononuclear cells

E. Pseudorheumatoid nodule

Deep dermal or subcutaneous areas of altered collagen with peripheral palisading of histiocytes and lymphocytes

Most commonly appearing in young individuals without any evidence of rheumatoid disease, these lesions are now thought to be subcutaneous granuloma annulare

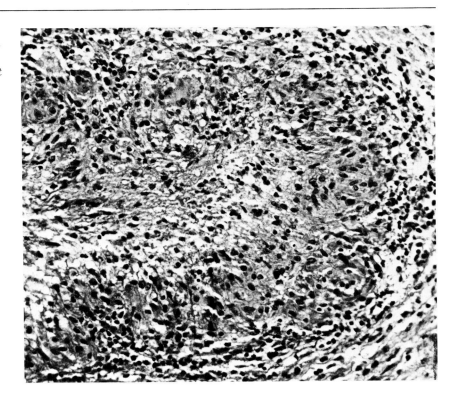

Fig. **15-3.** *Rheumatoid nodule. This biopsy from the subcutis exhibits palisading of histiocytes admixed with lymphocytes about a central zone of fibrinoid necrosis. Only a portion of the rheumatoid nodule is present in this field. (×400)*

II. Epithelioid cell granulomas

A. Tuberculosis

1. Primary inoculation: 1 to 14 days 1 to 6 weeks	1. Suppurative inflammation of dermis 2. Appearance of epithelioid cells with subsequent granuloma formation and chronic inflammation	In early suppurative lesions, numerous tubercle bacilli may be observed with acid-fast stains; in the granulomatous phase, organisms may be more difficult to demonstrate

2. Lupus vulgaris	1. Epidermal changes vary from atrophy and ulceration to marked hyperplasia
	2. Sharply demarcated epithelioid cell granulomas with Langhans giant cells are located in upper third of dermis
	3. Numerous histiocytes and lymphocytes surround granulomas
	4. Caseation variably present
	5. Fibrosis of reticular dermis variably present
		Differential diagnosis:
		  Sarcoidosis
		  Rosacea
		  Lupus miliaris disseminatus faciei
		  Foreign-body reaction (e.g., zirconium)
		  Deep fungal infection
		
		Acid-fast bacilli difficult to demonstrate with special stains

3. Tuberculosis verrucosa cutis	1. Hyperkeratosis and epidermal hyperplasia with papillomatosis
	2. Intraepidermal microabscesses containing neutrophils may be present
	3. Edema of papillary and upper reticular dermis
	4. Diffuse inflammatory infiltrate in upper dermis composed of neutrophils, lymphocytes, and histiocytes
	5. Dermal abscesses often present
	6. Epithelioid cell granulomas in mid-dermis admixed with neutrophils and lymphocytes
	7. Variable caseation
		Differential diagnosis:
		  Atypical mycobacteria (especially *M. marinum*)
		  Sporotrichosis
		  Deep fungal infections
		
		Acid-fast bacilli often difficult to demonstrate

4. Scrofuloderma	1. Epidermal ulceration
	2. Track of necrotic tissue lined by an inflammatory infiltrate composed of lymphocytes, histiocytes, neutrophils, and occasional plasma cells
	3. Caseating epithelioid cell granulomas
	4. Fibrosis of adjacent dermis
		Scrofuloderma refers to tuberculous lymphadenitis extending to overlying skin
		
		Differential diagnosis:
		  Subcutaneous coccidioidomycosis
		  Actinomycosis
		  Gummatous tertiary syphilis
		
		Acid-fast bacilli readily demonstrable

5. Orificial tuber-culosis (tuberculosis cutis orificialis)	1. Mucosal ulceration 2. Polymorphous inflammatory infiltrate composed of neutro-phils, lymphocytes, histio-cytes, and poorly formed epithelioid cell granulomas at base of ulcer	Acid-fast bacilli readily demon-strable Differential diagnosis: Crohn's disease South American blastomycosis Histoplasmosis
6. Miliary tuberculosis	Focal zone of neutrophils, debris, epithelioid cells, and histio-cytes in mid-dermis	Numerous acid-fast bacilli pres-ent

B. "Tuberculids"

1. Lupus miliaris dis-seminatus faciei	1. Epithelioid cell granulomas located in the upper third of the dermis surrounded by his-tiocytes and lymphocytes 2. Necrosis within granulomas variable	Tuberculids are currently be-lieved to be *unrelated* to tuberculosis and are thought to be manifestations of other diseases (e.g., lupus miliaris disseminatus faciei is probably a form of acne rosacea); by definition acid-fast bacilli are not demonstrable in tuber-culids Differential diagnosis: Lupus vulgaris Rosacea Sarcoidosis
2. Lichen scrofulosorum	1. Parakeratosis, epidermal atro-phy, and occasionally follicu-lar plugs 2. Noncaseating epithelioid cell granulomas 3. Langhans giant cells and lym-phocytes around and between hair follicles	
3. Erythema in-duratum	See also Ch. 24, III.A	
4. Papulonecrotic tuberculid	1. Focal epidermal necrosis and ulceration 2. Aggregates of histiocytes and epithelioid cells sometimes observed at base of ulcer 3. Perivenular lymphocytic and histiocytic infiltrate 4. Endothelial swelling often marked 5. Scattered erythrocytes in der-mis 6. Dermal fibrosis	Differential diagnosis: Pityriasis lichenoides et varioliformis acuta Allergic granulomatosis

C. Tuberculoid leprosy (Fig. 15-4)

1. Epidermis usually normal
2. Epithelioid cell granulomas throughout entire dermis admixed with lymphocytes, and occasional giant cells
3. **Tubercles (granulomas) often arranged in "cords" around nerves and vessels**
4. Granulomatous infiltrate often extends upward and "hugs" the epidermis
5. Invasion of nerve and/or arrector pili muscle by granulomatous infiltrate common
6. Atrophy of pilosebaceous units

Acid-fast bacilli, when present, are found more frequently within granulomas, nerves, or arrector pili muscles

Differential diagnosis: sarcoidosis

Nerve involvement is quite characteristic of tuberculoid leprosy; bodian or other silver stains may demonstrate a nerve in the center of a granuloma

Fig. **15-4.** *Leprosy, tuberculoid or borderline type. Numerous tuberculoid granulomas are present throughout the dermis. Some of these granulomas appear elongated (B), presumably because of their disposition along nerves. (A, ×45; B, ×160)*

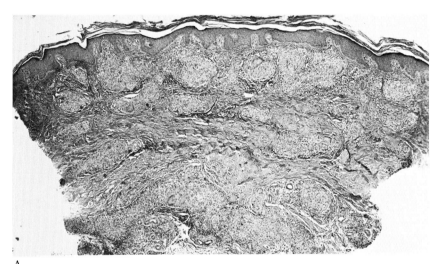

A

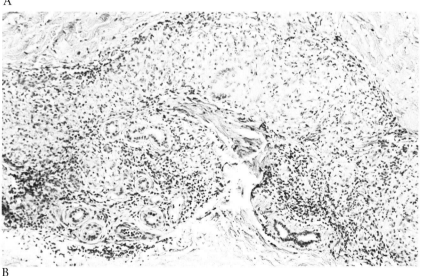

B

D. Sarcoidosis (Figs. 15-5, 15-6)

1. Epidermis usually normal but may show parakeratosis, atrophy, or even basal vacuolation
2. **Epithelioid cell granulomas** of variable size scattered throughout the papillary dermis, reticular dermis, and/or subcutaneous tissue
3. Granulomas and granulomatous inflammation may extend upward to hug the epidermis
4. Granulomas often contain giant cells and lymphocytes
5. Central "caseation" or necrosis may be present but is rarely extensive

Differential diagnosis:
   Zirconium granuloma
   Silica granuloma
   Beryllium granuloma
   Tuberculoid leprosy
   Lupus vulgaris and tuberculids
   Certain deep fungal infections
   Certain atypical mycobacterial infections
   Cheilitis granulomatosa
   Crohn's disease
   Rosacea

Histologic changes observed in a positive Kveim test are similar to those of sarcoid

Reticulum stain demonstrates compressed fibers that surround and outline granuloma

6. Schaumann bodies (round, laminated, calcified inclusions) and asteroid bodies (stellate eosinophilic inclusions surrounded by a clear zone) occasionally present in giant cells

Schaumann and *asteroid* bodies may be found in:
Sarcoidosis
Tuberculosis
Leprosy
Berylliosis
Foreign-body reaction

E. Granulomatous rosacea

1. Epidermis may be normal or atrophic
2. Small, epithelioid cell granulomas with or without focal necrosis frequently present around follicles
3. Variable infiltrate of lymphocytes and histiocytes

Differential diagnosis:
   Lupus vulgaris
   Sarcoidosis

See also II.B.1

F. Zirconium granuloma and cutaneous lesions of systemic berylliosis

1. Epidermis usually normal
2. Noncaseating epithelioid cell granulomas accompanied by a few giant cells and slight lymphocytic infiltrate

Polaroscopy is negative in these disorders; however, spectrographic analysis identifies both zirconium and beryllium

Differential diagnosis:
   Sarcoidosis
   Silica granuloma

G. Inoculation (local) beryllium granuloma

1. Epidermal acanthosis
2. Epithelioid cell granulomas throughout dermis and subcutaneous fat
3. Eosinophilic, **hyalinized necrosis** prominent

Diffuse hyalinization of granulomas is specific for this disorder

Differential diagnosis:
   Necrobiosis lipoidica
   Rheumatoid nodule

H. Cheilitis granulomatosa (Miescher-Melkersson-Rosenthal)

1. Epidermis and mucosal epithelium normal
2. Edema of dermis and submucosa
3. Epithelioid cell granulomas
4. Infiltrate of plasma cells and lymphocytes

Differential diagnosis: sarcoidosis

By definition this disorder usually occurs on the lip
Granulomas may occasionally be absent

Fig. **15-5.** *Granulomas. Aggregates of epithelioid histiocytes and multinucleate giant cells (as well as an asteroid body, left) can be seen in a variety of granulomatous disorders including sarcoid.*

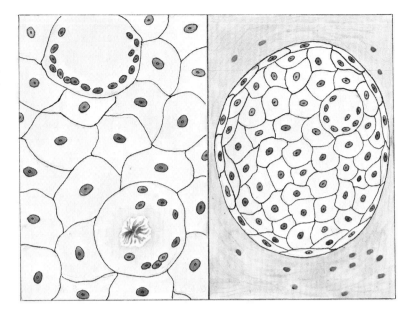

Fig. **15-6.** *Sarcoidosis. Granulomas within the dermis are associated with numerous etiologies such as infections, physical agents, and so on. These causes must be ruled out and the clinical status of the patient evaluated before a diagnosis of sarcoidosis can be rendered. (×100)*

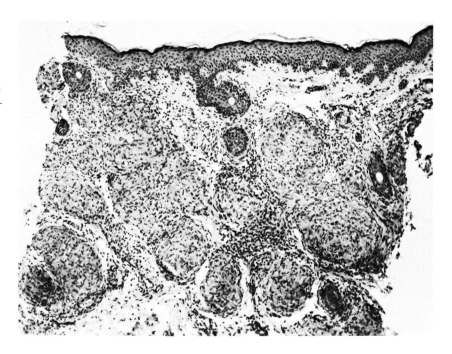

I. Miscellaneous foreign-body granulomas

1. Diffuse epithelioid cell granulomas and granulomatous inflammation
2. Granulomas or giant cells may contain **foreign bodies** such as suture material, talc, starch, keratin, hair, tattoo pigment

Silica particles (soil, talc), wood, and suture material are birefringent with polarized light

III. Granulomatous inflammation

A. North American blastomycosis (cutaneous nodule or verrucous plaque associated with systemic infection)

1. **Marked epidermal hyperplasia** with papillomatosis (pseudoepitheliomatous hyperplasia)
2. Intraepidermal neutrophilic **microabscesses**
3. Dense dermal infiltrate composed of histiocytes, epithelioid cells, giant cells, lymphocytes, and many neutrophils
4. Collections of dermal neutrophils frequently surrounded by epithelioid and giant cells
5. Organisms usually numerous and found within neutrophilic abscesses, within giant cells or free in dermis

Intraepidermal neutrophilic microabscesses may be seen in:

Deep mycotic infections
Sporotrichosis
Granuloma inguinale
Swimming pool granuloma
Tuberculosis verrucosa cutis
Impetigo
Candidiasis
Bromoderma
Iododerma
Psoriasis

Causative organism: *Blastomyces dermatitidis*
Thick-walled spores measure 8 to 15 μm with budding forms occasionally seen; the neck where budding occurs is wide, in contrast to the narrow neck of Cryptococcus; although organisms can be seen in H&E stained sections, visualization is facilitated by use of PAS stain or Gomori's methenamine silver stain

Differential diagnosis:
    Chromoblastomycosis
    Cryptococcosis
    Coccidioidomycosis and other deep fungal infections
    Tuberculosis verrucosa cutis
    Swimming pool granuloma
    Squamous cell carcinoma
    Bromoderma

Primary cutaneous inoculation blastomycosis is characterized by a predominantly neutrophilic dermal infiltrate with numerous organisms

B. South American blastomycosis (mucosal or cutaneous lesions)

1. **Marked epidermal** or **epithelial hyperplasia**
2. Granulomatous infiltrate with epithelioid and giant cells admixed with **neutrophilic abscesses**
3. Organisms are numerous and found within abscesses and giant cells
4. Diagnostic multiple budding organisms, so-called "**marine pilot's wheel,**" may be difficult to detect

Causative organism: *Paracoccidioidomycosis brasiliensis*
Spherules with or without single buds measure 5 to 20 μm in diameter; those with multiple buds measure up to 60 μm; PAS or methenamine silver stains helpful in identifying organism

Differential diagnosis:
  North American blastomycosis
  Coccidioidomycosis
  Cryptococcosis
  Tuberculosis verrucosa cutis

C. Chromoblastomycosis

1. Dermal lesions

1. **Marked epidermal hyperplasia** with papillomatosis (pseudoepitheliomatous hyperplasia)
2. Spongiosis
3. **Intraepidermal abscesses** filled with neutrophils and mononuclear cells
4. Dense dermal infiltrate composed of histiocytes, giant cells, epithelioid cells, lymphocytes, plasma cells, and neutrophils
5. Dermal neutrophilic abscesses common
6. Epithelioid cell granulomas sometimes present
7. **Brown, thick-walled "copper penny" organisms** are present in giant cells and in abscesses or are free in tissue

Causative organisms include:
  Phialophora verrucosa
  Cladosporium carrionii
  Fonsecaea pedrosoi
  Fonsecaea compactum

For differential diagnosis, see North American blastomycosis (III.A)

Special stains *not* required to see organism

2. Subcutaneous lesions

1. Subcutaneous abscess composed of necrotic debris and eosinophils
2. Epithelioid and giant cells surround abscesses
3. Fibrous capsule
4. Organisms found within abscess or in giant cells

Causative organism: *Cladosporium gougerotti*

D. Sporotrichosis

1. Primary lesion

1. Epidermal hyperplasia with papillomatosis adjacent to ulceration
2. Intraepidermal neutrophilic microabscesses
3. Dermal infiltrate composed of many lymphocytes, plasma cells, and variable numbers of giant and epithelioid cells
4. Small dermal neutrophilic abscesses often present
5. Organism notoriously difficult to find

Causative organism: *Sporotrichum schenckii*
Very early lesions may only show a nonspecific lymphohistiocytic infiltrate with plasma cells and neutrophils
Organisms best visualized with PAS stain after diastase digestion; round to oval budding spores measure 3 to 8 μm in diameter; characteristic cigar-shaped oval organism measures 4 to 5 μm in length and 1 to 2 μm in diameter
Asteroid spores with peripherally radiating eosinophilic extensions occasionally are seen in cases from tropical countries
Culture of lesions often necessary to confirm diagnosis

2. Secondary cutaneous nodules

1. Epidermis usually normal but may be ulcerated
2. Deep dermal and/or subcutaneous infiltrate, characteristically with three zones of inflammation:
   a. Central zone: necrosis, debris, and neutrophils
   b. Middle zone: epithelioid cells and giant multinucleate cells
   c. Outer zone: lymphocytes and plasma cells with vascular proliferation

Secondary cutaneous nodules occur either locally over draining lymphatic channels or secondary to disseminated hematogenous or lymphatic spread

Differential diagnosis: tularemia

E. Coccidioidomycosis

1. Early primary cutaneous lesions

1. Diffuse dermal infiltrate composed predominantly of neutrophils and lymphocytes
2. Epithelioid cells and giant cells rare to absent
3. Abundant organisms

Causative organism: *Coccidioides immitis*

Differential diagnosis:
Primary cutaneous tuberculosis
Sporotrichosis

2. Late primary cutaneous lesions; secondary (disseminated) cutaneous lesions	1. Marked epidermal hyperplasia with papillomatosis (pseudoepitheliomatous hyperplasia) 2. Neutrophilic abscesses within the epidermis and dermis 3. Dense dermal infiltrate composed of lymphocytes, plasma cells, histiocytes, many neutrophils, with variable numbers of epithelioid and giant cells 4. Organisms present in histiocytes and giant cells or free in tissue	Large, thick-walled spores measuring 10 to 80 μm in diameter contain either granular cytoplasm or a variable number of endospores; endospores measure 2 to 10 μm in diameter Number of organisms varies with host immunity
3. Subcutaneous abscesses	1. Central necrosis 2. Lymphocytes, histiocytes, plasma cells, epithelioid cells, and a few giant cells surrounding an area of necrosis 3. Numerous organisms	Differential diagnosis: Scrofuloderma Rheumatoid nodule Tertiary syphilis
F. Cryptococcosis		Causative organism: *Cryptococcus neoformans*
1. Granulomatous reaction	1. Epidermal hyperplasia adjacent to ulceration 2. Dense dermal infiltrate of lymphocytes, histiocytes, epithelioid cells, giant cells, and plasma cells 3. Neutrophils uncommon 4. Organisms present within histiocytes and giant cells and free in tissue	Both the granulomatous and gelatinous reactions to infection may be seen in the same lesion Spherical to oval organism measures 5 to 10 μm in diameter and is surrounded by a clear halo; capsule visualized with special stains (see Appendix); staining tissue with both alcian blue and PAS results in organism with red or magenta cell wall and blue capsule; budding of yeast forms typically occurs with a narrow neck in comparison to *Blastomyces dermatitidis*
2. Gelatinous reaction	Abundant numbers of organisms with minimal inflammatory response	
G. Swimming pool granuloma		Causative organism: *Mycobacterium marinum*
1. Early lesions	Dermal infiltrate of neutrophils admixed with variable numbers of lymphocytes and histiocytes	Acid-fast organisms usually can be detected in earlier lesions

2. Late lesions

1. Hyperkeratosis, parakeratosis
2. Epidermal hyperplasia often adjacent to ulceration
3. Neutrophilic epidermal microabscesses
4. Edema of papillary and upper reticular dermis
5. Diffuse dermal infiltrate composed of lymphocytes, histiocytes, plasma cells, epithelioid cells, and giant cells
6. Epithelioid cell granulomas frequently seen in lower reticular dermis of older lesions
7. Vascular ectasia and proliferation
8. Dermal fibrosis

Because the number of organisms may be small, diagnosis may be difficult to establish without culture

H. Tertiary syphilis

1. Normal, flattened, or ulcerated epidermis
2. Edema of papillary dermis
3. Nodular or diffuse dermal infiltrate in reticular dermis composed of lymphocytes, histiocytes, epithelioid cells, giant cells, and **plasma cells**
4. Variable dermal necrosis
5. **Endothelial cell proliferation** may produce occlusion of vessel lumen
6. Proliferation of fibroblasts common in older lesions

Deep dermal infiltrate, extensive necrosis, and ulceration are characteristic of gummatous lesion
Plasma cell infiltrate usually prominent

See also Ch. 14, II.K; Ch. 17, V

Spirochetes not demonstrable

I. Cat-scratch disease

1. Variable epidermal changes, sometimes including necrosis
2. Dermal "granulomatous abscess," i.e., central necrosis peppered with neutrophils and karyorrhectic material is surrounded by histiocytes, giant cells, and lymphocytes
3. The dermal process is sometimes described as "stellate abscess" because the overall contours may appear folded or stellate rather than round or oval

The histology within lymph nodes is identical

Suggested Reading
Palisading Granulomas

Bennett, G. A., Zeller, J. W., and Bauer, W. Subcutaneous nodules of rheumatoid arthritis and rheumatic fever: A pathologic study. *Arch. Pathol.* 30:70, 1940.

Dahl, M. V., Ullman, S., and Goltz, R. W. Vasculitis in granuloma annulare. *Arch. Dermatol.* 113:463, 1977.

Gray, H. R., Graham, J. H., and Johnson, W. C. Necrobiosis lipoidica: A histopathological and histochemical study. *J. Invest. Dermatol.* 44:369, 1965.

Muller, S. A., and Winkelmann, R. K. Necrobiosis lipoidica diabeticorum: Histopathologic study of 98 cases. *Arch. Dermatol.* 94:1, 1966.

Owens, D. W., and Freeman, R. G. Perforating granuloma annulare. *Arch. Dermatol.* 103:64, 1971.

Reed, R. J., Clark, W. H., and Mihm, M. C. The cutaneous collagenoses. *Hum. Pathol.* 4:165, 1973.

Rubin, M., and Lynch, F. W. Subcutaneous granuloma annulare: Comment on familial granuloma annulare. *Arch. Dermatol.* 93:416, 1966.

Umbert, P., and Winkelmann, R. K. Histologic, ultrastructural, and histochemical studies of granuloma annulare. *Arch. Dermatol.* 113:1681, 1977.

Wood, M. G., and Beerman, H. Necrobiosis lipoidica, granuloma annulare and rheumatoid nodule. *J. Invest. Dermatol.* 34:139, 1960.

Epithelioid Cell Granulomas (Tuberculosis and Tuberculids)

Jetton, R. L., and Coker, W. L. Tuberculosis verrucosa cutis. *Arch. Dermatol.* 100:380, 1969.

Minkowitz, S., Brandt, L. J., Rapp, Y., and Raudlauer, C. B. ''Prospector's wart'' (cutaneous tuberculosis) in a medical student. *Am. J. Clin. Pathol.* 51:260, 1969.

Mitchell, P. C. Tuberculosis verrucosa cutis among Chinese in Hong Kong. *Br. J. Dermatol.* 66:444, 1954.

Montgomery, H. Histopathology of various types of cutaneous tuberculosis. *Arch. Dermatol. Syphilol.* 35:698, 1937.

Morrison, J. G. L., and Fourie, E. D. The papulonecrotic tuberculide. From arthus reaction to lupus vulgaris. *Br. J. Dermatol.* 91:263, 1974.

Moschella, S. L. Mycobacterial Infections of the Skin. In S. L. Moschella (Ed.), *Dermatology Update.* New York: Elsevier, 1979.

Schermer, D. R., Simpson, C. G., Haserick, J. R., et al. Tuberculosis cutis miliaris acuta generalisata. *Arch. Dermatol.* 99:64, 1969.

Smith, N. P., Ryan, T. J. Sanderson, K. V., et al. Lichen scrofulosorum. A report of four cases. *Br. J. Dermatol.* 94:319, 1976.

Van Der Lugt, L. Some remarks about tuberculosis of the skin and tuberculids. *Dermatologica* 131:266, 1965.

Wolf, K. Mycobacterial Diseases: Tuberculosis. In T. B. Fitzpatrick et al. (Eds.), *Dermatology in General Medicine* (2d ed.). New York: McGraw-Hill, 1979.

Wong, K. O., Lee, K. P., and Chiu, S. F. Tuberculosis of the skin in Hong Kong (a review of 160 cases). *Br. J. Dermatol.* 80:424, 1968.

Leprosy

Azulay, R. D. Histopathology of skin lesions in leprosy. *Int. J. Lepr.* 39:244, 1971.

Fasal, P. Histopathology of leprosy. *Cutis* 18:66, 1976.

Ridley, D. S. Histological classification and the immunological spectrum of leprosy. *Bull. W.H.O.* 51:451, 1974.

Ridley, D. S., and Jopling, W. H. Classification of leprosy according to immunity. A five group system. *Int. J. Lep.* 34:255, 1966.

Williams, R. C., Sr. Symposium on leprosy. *South. Med. J.* 69:969, 1976.

Sarcoidosis

Elgart, M. L. Cutaneous lesions of sarcoidosis. *Primary Care* 5:249, 1978.

James, D. G. Dermatological aspects of sarcoidosis. *Q. J. Med.* 28:108, 1959.

James, D. G., et al. Pathobiology of sarcoidosis. *Pathobiol. Annu.* 7:31, 1977.

Mitchell, D. N., Scadding, J. G., Heard, B. E., and Hinson, K. F. W. Sarcoidosis: Histopathological definition and clinical diagnosis. *J. Clin. Pathol.* 30:395, 1977.

Sitzbach, L. E. (Ed.). Seventh international conference on sarcoidosis and other granulomatous disorders. *Ann. N.Y. Acad. Sci.* Vol. 278, 1976.

Steigleder, G. K., Silva, A., Jr., and Nelson, C. T. Histopathology of the Kveim test. *Arch. Dermatol.* 84:828, 1961.

Rosacea

Marks, R., and Harcourt-Webster, J. N. Histopathology of rosacea. *Arch. Dermatol.* 100:683, 1969.

Mullanax, M. G., and Kierland, R. R. Granulomatous rosacea. *Arch. Dermatol.* 101:206, 1970.

Zirconium Granuloma

Epstein, W. L., and Allen, J. R. Granulomatous hypersensitivity after use of zirconium-containing poison oak lotions. *J.A.M.A.* 190:940, 1964.

Epstein, W. L., Skahen, J. R., and Krasnobrod, H. The organized epithelioid cell granuloma: Differentiation of allergic (zirconium) from colloidal (silica) types. *Am. J. Pathol.* 43:391, 1963.

Beryllium Granuloma

Grier, R. S., et al. Skin lesions in persons exposed to beryllium compounds. *J. Ind. Hyg. Toxicol.* 30:228, 1948.

Hardy, H. L., and Tabershaw, I. R. Delayed chemical pneumonitis occuring in workers exposed to beryllium compounds. *J. Ind. Hyg. Toxicol.* 28:197, 1946.

Neave, H. J., Frank, S. B., and Tolmach, J. A. Cutaneous granuloma following laceration by fluorescent light bulbs. *Arch. Dermatol. Syphilol.* 61:401, 1950.

Pyre, J., and Oatway, W. H., Jr. Beryllium granulomatosis. *Ariz. Med.* 4:21, 1947.

Cheilitis Granulomatosa (Miescher-Melkersson-Rosenthal Syndrome)

Hornstein, O. P. Melkersson-Rosenthal syndrome: A neuro-mucocutaneous disease of complex origin. *Curr. Probl. Dermatol.* 5:117, 1973.

Laymon, C. W. Cheilitis granulomatosa and Melkersson-Rosenthal syndrome. *Arch. Dermatol.* 83:112, 1961.

Granulomatous Inflammation

Binford, C. H., and Connor, D. H. *Pathology of Tropical and Extraordinary Diseases*, Vols. I and II. Washington, D.C.: Armed Forces Institute of Pathology, 1976.

Emmons, C. W., Binford, C. H., Utz, J. P., and Kwon-Chung, K. J. *Medical Mycology* (3d ed.). Philadelphia: Lea & Febiger, 1977.

Blastomycosis

Busey, J. F. Blastomycosis. I. A review of 198 collected cases in Veterans Administration hospitals. *Am. Rev. Respir. Dis.* 89:659, 1969.

Hashimoto, K., Kaplan, R. J., Daman, L. A., et al. Pustular blastomycosis. *Int. J. Dermatol.* 16:277, 1977.

Landay, M. E., and Schwarz, J. Primary cutaneous blastomycosis. *Arch. Dermatol.* 104:408, 1971.

Chromoblastomycosis

Carrion, A. L. Chromoblastomycosis and related infections. *Int. J. Dermatol.* 14:27, 1975.

Vollum, D. I. Chromomycosis: A review. *Br. J. Dermatol.* 96:454, 1977.

Sporotrichosis

Lurie, H. I. Histopathology of sporotrichosis. *Arch. Pathol.* 75:421, 1963.

Coccidioidomycosis

Basler, R. S., and Lagomarsino, S. L. Coccidioidomycosis: Clinical review and treatment update. *Int. J. Dermatol.* 18:104, 1979.

Harvey, W. C., and Greendyke, W. H. Skin lesions in acute coccidioidomycosis. *Am. Fam. Physician* 2:81, 1970.

Levan, N. E., and Huntington, R. W. Primary cutaneous coccidioidomycosis in agricultural workers. *Arch. Dermatol.* 92:215, 1965.

Cryptococcosis

Noble, R. C., and Fajardo, L. F. Primary cutaneous cryptococcosis: Review and morphologic study. *Am. J. Clin. Pathol.* 57:13, 1972.

Sarosi, G. A., Silberfarb, P. M., and Tosh, F. E.: Cutaneous cryptococcosis. A sentinel of disseminated disease. *Arch. Dermatol.* 104:1, 1971.

Schupbach, C. W., Wheeler, C. E., Briggaman, R. A., et al. Cutaneous manifestations of disseminated cryptococcosis. *Arch. Dermatol.* 112:1734, 1976.

Swimming Pool Granuloma

Adams, R. M., Remington, J. S., Steinberg, J., et al. Tropical fish aquariums—A source of *Mycobacterium marinum* infections resembling sporotrichosis. *J.A.M.A.* 211:457, 1970.

Feldman, R. A., Long, M. W., and David, H. L. *Mycobacterium marinum:* A leisure-time pathogen. *J. Infect. Dis.* 129:618, 1974.

Owens, D. W. Atypical mycobacteria. *Int. J. Dermatol.* 17:180, 1978.

Philpott, J. A., Woodburne, A. R., Philpott, O. S., et al. Swimming pool granuloma—A study of 290 cases. *Arch. Dermatol.* 88:158, 1963.

Zeligman, I. *Mycobacterium marinum* granuloma. *Arch. Dermatol.* 106:26, 1972.

Cat-Scratch Disease

Johnson, W. T., and Helwig, E. B. Cat-scratch disease. Histopathologic changes in the skin. *Arch. Dermatol.* 100:148, 1969.

Chapter 16

Diffuse Infiltrate

I. Predominantly histiocytes
   A. Xanthelasma
   B. Eruptive xanthoma
   C. Tuberous and tendon xanthoma
   D. Lepromatous leprosy
   E. Histiocytosis X
   F. Juvenile xanthogranuloma
   G. Reticulohistiocytic granuloma (reticulohistiocytoma) and multicentric reticulohistiocytosis
   H. Leishmaniasis
II. Predominantly lymphocytes
   A. Lymphoma cutis (non-Hodgkin's type), monomorphous infiltrate
   B. Leukemia cutis (lymphocytic type)
III. Predominantly plasma cells
   A. Plasmacytoma, primary lesions; lesions associated with multiple myeloma
IV. Predominantly mast cells
   A. Urticaria pigmentosa
V. Predominantly neutrophils
   A. Granuloma faciale
   B. Erythema elevatum diutinum
   C. Acute febrile neutrophilic dermatosis (Sweet's disease)
   D. Cellulitis
VI. Predominantly eosinophils
   A. Eosinophilic cellulitis (Well's syndrome)
VII. Mixed infiltrate
   A. Chancroid
   B. Primary syphilis
   C. Rhinoscleroma
   D. Granuloma inguinale
   E. Lymphoma cutis, polymorphous infiltrate
      1. Hodgkin's disease
      2. Mycosis fungoides

The Reactive Process and the Disease	Histopathology	Comments
I. Predominantly histio-cytes		
A. Xanthelasma (Fig. 16-1)	1. Flattened, occasionally atrophic epidermis 2. Perivascular and diffuse infiltrate of **foam cells** in up-per and middle reticular der-mis 3. Inflammation and fibrosis minimal to absent	Lipid-laden histiocytes or foam cells have a round to oval, dark-staining nucleus sur-rounded by pale, vacuolated, or reticulated cytoplasm
B. Eruptive xanthoma (Fig. 16-2)	1. Normal epidermis 2. Lipid-laden histiocytes ad-mixed with lymphocytes, his-tiocytes, and neutrophils	
C. Tuberous and tendon xanthoma	1. Normal epidermis 2. Sheets of lipid-laden histio-cytes throughout the reticular dermis 3. Multinucleate giant cells common 4. Early lesions have variable lymphohistiocytic and neutro-philic infiltrates admixed with foam cells 5. Older lesions characterized by dermal fibrosis	Differential diagnosis: Histiocytosis X Granular cell tumor Balloon cell nevus Lepromatous leprosy

Fig. **16-1.** *Xanthelasma. Histio-cytes with foamy cytoplasm aggregate around vessels. (×400)*

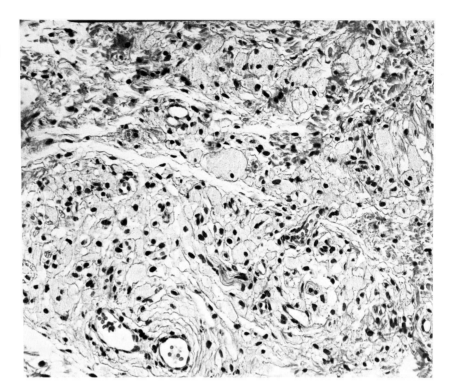

Fig. **16-2.** *Eruptive xanthoma. Histiocytic aggregates, including foamy histiocytes, are associated with inflammatory cells including lymphocytes and neutrophils. (approximately ×256)*

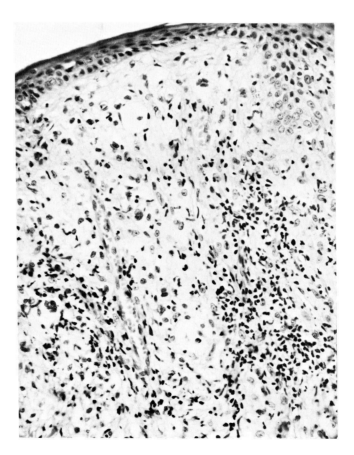

D. Lepromatous leprosy (Fig. 16-3)

1. Normal to flattened epidermis
2. Grenz zone of uninvolved papillary dermis
3. Aggregates and sheets of foamy histiocytes admixed with lymphocytes and occasional plasma cells extending throughout reticular dermis and into subcutaneous fat
4. Destruction and loss of appendages

Numerous acid-fast organisms found within foamy histiocytes, nerves, blood vessel walls, arrector pili muscles, and follicular epithelium

E. Histiocytosis X

1. Epidermis may be normal, focally invaded by histiocytes, or ulcerated
2. Infiltrate of **characteristic histiocytic cells** admixed with variable numbers of lymphocytes, eosinophils, neutrophils, and plasma cells with multinucleate giant cells of either foreign body or Touton type
3. Distribution of infiltrate may be:
   a. Perivenular, with extension into papillary dermis
   b. Bandlike and periappendageal
   c. Diffuse, extending from the epidermis into the subcutaneous fat
4. Proliferation of fibroblasts common
5. Extravasation of erythrocytes often present

Subclassification of the histiocytosis X group of diseases (Letterer-Siwe disease, Hand-Schüller-Christian disease, eosinophilic granuloma) depends on correlation of histologic and clinical findings

The characteristic cell of the histiocytosis X group is a large histiocyte 15 to 25 μm in diameter with a round, oval, notched, or bean-shaped nucleus containing one or more fine, dotlike nucleoli; the abundant cytoplasm is pale pink or clear, and the cell margins may blend to form a syncytium; the cytoplasm of cells in older lesions is often quite foamy or vacuolated secondary to accumulation of lipid

Differential diagnosis:
Lymphoma cutis (histiocytic type)
Hodgkin's disease
Mycosis fungoides
Xanthomas
Nodular lesions of urticaria pigmentosa
Histiocytic medullary reticulosis

Fig. **16-3.** *Lepromatous leprosy.*
A. *These histiocytes with granular cytoplasm (called* lepra cells) *aggregate around vessels. (×640)*
B. *Wade-Fite stains usually are employed to demonstrate the lepra bacilli which are often not as acid-fast or alcohol-resistant as other mycobacteria. (×640)*

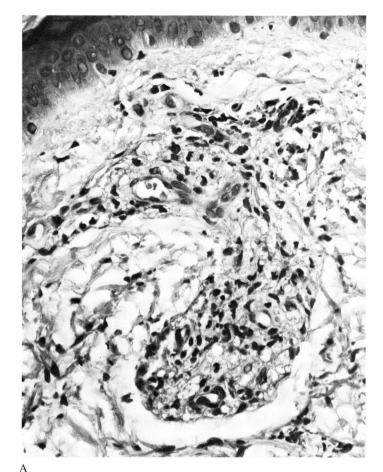

A

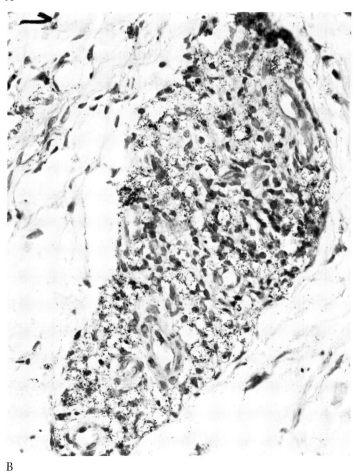

B

F. Juvenile xantho-
granuloma (Fig. 16-4)

1. Normal, acanthotic, or atrophic epidermis
2. Patchy or diffuse infiltrate
composed of:
   a. Histiocytes, many of
   which are lipid-laden and
   foamy
   b. Lymphocytes, eosinophils,
   fibroblasts, and multinucleate giant cells
   c. **Touton giant cells**

The presence of Touton giant
cells with their "perfect
wreath" of nuclei surrounded
by foamy cytoplasm is a characteristic feature of juvenile
xanthogranuloma

3. The infiltrate usually involves
both the papillary and reticular dermis and rarely extends
into subcutaneous tissue

Differential diagnosis:
Xanthoma
Dermatofibroma
Histiocytosis X

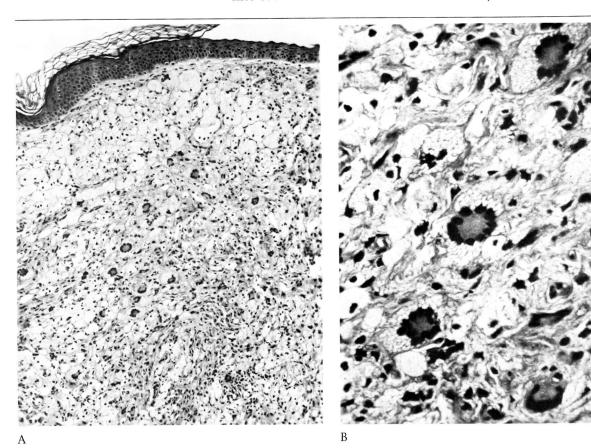

A   B

Fig. **16-4.** *Juvenile xanthogranuloma.*
A. *The upper and middle dermis
is filled with histiocytes
(many with foamy cyto-
plasm), Touton giant cells,
and lymphocytes. (×160)*

B. *Note the foamy appearance of
the cytoplasm and the
"wreathed nuclei" of Touton
giant cells. The latter are considered to be the distinctive
cell of juvenile xanthogranuloma; however, similar giant
cells can be seen in other disorders. (×640)*

G. Reticulohistiocytic granuloma (reticulo-histiocytoma) and multicentric re-ticulohistiocytosis

1. Normal or acanthotic epidermis
2. Dense, diffuse dermal infiltrate composed of:
   a. Histiocytes, lymphocytes, neutrophils, some plasma cells, and eosinophils
   b. Characteristic giant cells with abundant homogeneous eosinophilic **ground glass or "muddy rose" cytoplasm** and one or more distinctive **vesicular nuclei** with prominent nucleoli

H. Leishmaniasis

1. Epidermis may be normal, flattened, hyperplastic, or ulcerated
2. Dense infiltrate composed primarily of histiocytes admixed with epithelioid cells, lymphocytes, plasma cells, and occasional giant cells
3. Edematous stroma with proliferation and ectasia of vessels
4. Variable fibrosis
5. Organisms more frequently found in deep dermis within histiocytes and epithelioid cells and free in tissue

2 to 3 μm in diameter, round to oval organisms with thin cell wall, large nucleus, and rod-shaped paranucleus (kineto-plast) are visible in sections stained with H&E; Giemsa stain accentuates nucleus and kinetoplast

Late lesions may show epithelioid cell granuloma and few organisms

Differential diagnosis:
  Lepromatous leprosy
  Xanthoma
  Histoplasmosis
  Cryptococcosis and other deep mycoses

II. Predominantly lympho-cytes

A. Lymphoma cutis (non-Hodgkin's type), monomorphous infiltrate (see Fig. 17-2)

1. Epidermis usually normal
2. Papillary dermis spared (Grenz zone)
3. Dense nodular aggregates, patchy aggregates, or diffuse dermal infiltration of lymphoid cells throughout entire reticular dermis, often extending into subcutaneous fat
4. Nuclear atypia and atypical mitoses characteristic, though quantitatively variable
5. Cells often infiltrate between collagen fibers in an "Indian file" fashion
6. Nuclei packed tightly together appear distorted and "smudged"
7. Absence of endothelial cell hyperplasia and vascular proliferation

See also Ch. 17, IV.A

Differential diagnosis:
  Histiocytosis X
  Lymphomatoid papulosis
  Actinic reticuloid
  Leukemia cutis
  Lymphocytoma cutis
  Lymphocytic infiltrate
  Arthropod bite reaction
  Mycosis fungoides
  Urticaria pigmentosa

B. Leukemia cutis (lymphocytic type)

1. Normal epidermis
2. Grenz zone of uninvolved papillary dermis
3. Diffuse or nodular aggregates of immature leukocytes extending throughout the reticular dermis, often into the subcutaneous tissue
4. Cells infiltrate between collagen bundles
5. Cells tightly packed together and sometimes appear "smudged"

The cells of cutaneous leukemic infiltrates usually have the morphology of the circulating leukemic cells; granulocytic leukemia cells may be distinguished from lymphocytic leukemia cells by the presence of chloracetate esterase positive cytoplasmic granules (Fig. 16-5)

Differential diagnosis: lymphoma cutis

III. Predominantly plasma cells

A. Plasmacytoma, primary lesions, and lesions associated with multiple myeloma

1. Normal or flattened epidermis
2. Dense infiltrate of atypical plasma cells in reticular and often papillary dermis
3. Atypical mitoses common

Differential diagnosis: lymphoma cutis

Round, homogeneous, eosinophilic PAS-positive Russell bodies may be present intracellularly and extracellularly

Methyl green-pyronine (MGP) stain will help differentiate plasma cells from lymphoreticular cells

IV. Predominantly mast cells

A. Urticaria pigmentosa (Fig. 16-6) (papules, nodules, or diffuse infiltrative lesions)

1. Epidermis normal or flattened
2. Increased melanin in basal layer
3. Infiltrate of cuboidal **mast cells** fills papillary dermis and upper and mid-reticular dermis, occasionally extending into subcutaneous tissue
4. Variable number of eosinophils admixed with mast cells

See also Ch. 11, IV.A

The cuboidal mast cell with its distinct cell walls and round to oval, dense, basophilic nucleus has a "fried egg" appearance
Diagnostic metachromatic cytoplasmic granules may be demonstrated with either Giemsa or toluidine blue stain

Differential diagnosis:
Histiocytosis X
Dermal nevus
Leukemia cutis
Lymphoma cutis

Fig. **16-5.** *Involvement of the subcutis by chronic myelogenous leukemia. Numerous atypical megakaryocytes, immature myeloid cells, and rare neutrophils are present in this biopsy. (×640)*

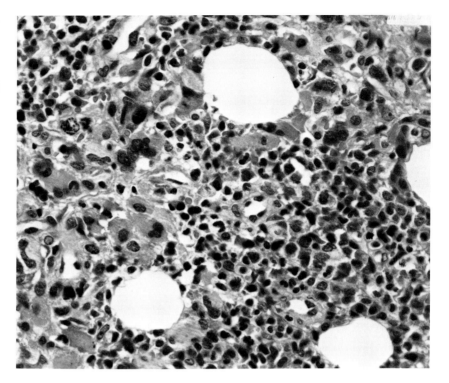

Fig. **16-6.** *Urticaria pigmentosa. The mast cell infiltrate is present in the mid and upper dermis. Mast cells may be mistaken for lymphocytes, but their nuclei stain less intensely and more uniformly than those of lymphocytes. Mast cells also have more cytoplasm and better demarcated cytoplasmic borders than lymphocytes. Giemsa stains demonstrate metachromasia of mast cell granules. (approximately ×940)*

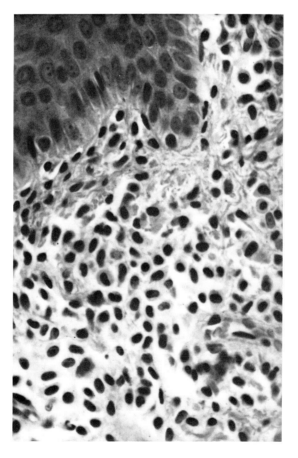

V. Predominantly neutrophils

    A. Granuloma faciale (Fig. 16-7)

        1. Normal epidermis

        2. Grenz zone of uninvolved papillary or adventitial dermis separates epidermis and adnexal structures from infiltrate

        3. Nodular and diffuse aggregates of lymphocytes and **eosinophils** (up to 90%) plus neutrophils, plasma cells, and mast cells

        4. Infiltrate usually confined to upper and middle dermis but may extend to subcutaneous tissue

        5. **Leukocytoclastic vasculitis** with endothelial cell swelling, neutrophils within vessel walls, and nuclear debris often observed

        6. Fibrin deposition in and around vessels

        7. Extravasation of erythrocytes

        8. Hemosiderin-laden macrophages

        9. Variable fibrosis

See also Ch. 14, II.C

    B. Erythema elevatum diutinum

See Ch. 14, II.D

    C. Acute febrile neutrophilic dermatosis (Sweet's disease) (see Fig. 11-3)

See Ch. 11, I.H;

    D. Cellulitis

See Ch. 14, I.A.5

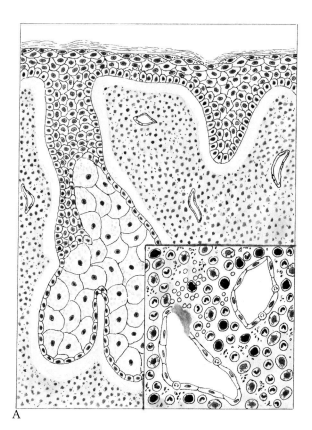

A

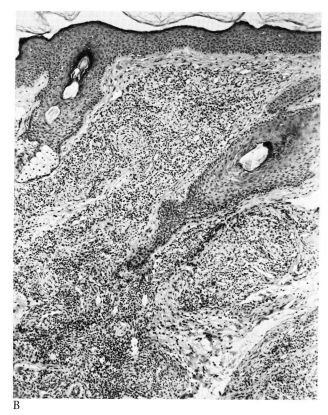

B

Fig. **16-7.** *Granuloma faciale.*
A. *The diffuse polymorphous infiltrate including neutrophils, eosinophils, and lymphocytes spares the upper papillary dermis (the Grenz zone). Changes suggestive of vasculitis frequently are present. The inset illustrates the polymorphous nature of the infiltrate and vascular damage.*
B. *Photomicrograph for comparison. The low-power pattern of the Grenz zone and numerous eosinophils is distinctive. (×100)*

VI. Predominantly
eosinophils

    A. Eosinophilic cellulitis (Well's syndrome)

1. Normal epidermis
2. Edema of reticular dermis may be marked
3. Perivascular and diffuse infiltrate composed predominantly of eosinophils admixed with lymphocytes, histiocytes, and occasional giant multinucleate cells
4. Eosinophil granules scattered loosely in dermis
5. **Focal areas of altered collagen surrounded by eosinophils,** eosinophil granules, and histiocytes (so-called **flame figure**)
6. Infiltrate may extend through panniculus, fascia, and muscle

> *Flame figures* have also been observed in:
> Bullous pemphigoid
> Eczema
> Prurigo
> Dermatophytosis

VII. Mixed infiltrate

    A. Chancroid

1. Epithelial hyperplasia adjacent to central ulceration
2. **Three relatively distinct zones** of inflammation present at base of ulcer
   a. *Superficial zone:* thin band of neutrophils admixed with extravasated erythrocytes, fibrin, and necrotic debris
   b. *Middle zone:* wide band of markedly edematous stroma containing many thin-walled, dilated, vertically oriented blood vessels with variable necrosis of vessel walls and variable inflammatory infiltrate
   c. *Deep zone:* dense perivascular and diffuse infiltrate composed predominantly of plasma cells and lymphocytes

Causative organism:
Haemophilus ducreyi

Short, 1 to 2-μm, rodlike organisms in clusters or chains often demonstrable in superficial zone with either Giemsa (organisms blue) or Brown-Brenn (organisms red) stains

B. Primary syphilis

1. Erosion, ulceration, or epidermal hyperplasia with variable spongiosis and invasion by neutrophils
2. Dense, diffuse, and perivascular infiltrate composed of plasma cells, lymphocytes, and histiocytes
3. Neutrophils prominent only in infiltrate beneath ulceration
4. Marked vascular proliferation with endothelial swelling

Silver stains (see Appendix) demonstrate numerous spirochetes around vessels and occasionally within epithelium

C. Rhinoscleroma

1. Epithelial hyperplasia may be extreme
2. Dense infiltrate of many plasma cells, with histiocytes, lymphocytes, and neutrophils
3. Large (100–200 μm) vacuolated histiocytes called **Mikulicz cells** contain organisms
4. Round, eosinophilic, homogeneous extracellular and intracellular **Russell bodies** may be prominent
5. Fibrosis common in older lesions

Causative organism: *Klebsiella rhinoscleromatis*

Cutaneous involvement restricted to nose

2 to 3 μm, oval to round, rod-shaped, encapsulated organisms within Mikulicz cells are best visualized with Warthin-Starry or Giemsa stains

Differential diagnosis:
Leishmaniasis
Histoplasmosis
Granuloma inguinale
Squamous cell carcinoma
Lepromatous leprosy
Syphilis

Plasma cells conspicuous in:

Syphilis
Rhinoscleroma
Granuloma inguinale
Chronic folliculitis
Plasmacytoma
Zoon's balanitis
Syringocystadenoma papilliferum
Inflammatory infiltrates in and around body orifices

D. Granuloma inguinale

1. Epithelium adjacent to ulceration commonly hyperplastic with spongiosis and intraepithelial neutrophilic abscesses
2. Dense, dermal or submucosal infiltrate with **neutrophilic microabscesses surrounded by** plasma cells, histiocytes, and lymphocytes

Causative organism: *Calymmatobacterium granulomatis*

Intracytoplasmic inclusion (Donovan) bodies visible as either 1- to 2-μm, black, oval to rod-shaped structures with silver stains or as encapsulated bipolar ("safety pin") bodies with Giemsa stain; these organisms are better visualized in smears or touch preps from biopsy material rather than tissue section

Differential diagnosis:
Syphilis
Squamous cell carcinoma

Obligate *intrahistiocytic organisms* occur in:

Granuloma inguinale (E)*
Leishmaniasis
Histoplasmosis
Rhinoscleroma (E)

E. Lymphoma cutis, polymorphous infiltrate

1. Hodgkin's disease

1. Epidermis usually normal
2. Grenz zone of spared papillary dermis
3. Nodular or diffuse infiltrate throughout the reticular dermis composed of:
   a. **atypical mononuclear cells** admixed with histiocytes, lymphocytes, and variable numbers of neutrophils, eosinophils, plasma cells, and multinucleate giant cells
   b. **Reed-Sternberg cells,** which are large cells with abundant cytoplasm, bilobed nuclei, and prominent nucleoli, giving an "owl's eye" appearance

Differential diagnosis:
Lymphomatoid papulosis
Arthropod bite reaction
Mycosis fungoides

See also Ch. 17, IV.B.1

---

*(E) = encapsulated organisms.

2. Mycosis fungoides
(see Fig. 4-6)

1. Epidermal changes variable and include psoriasiform hyperplasia, atrophy, or ulceration with or without Pautrier microabscesses

2. Dense accumulations of atypical mononuclear cells (*mycosis cells*) characterized by convoluted or cerebriform, hyperchromatic large nuclei; these atypical cells are admixed with lymphocytes, histiocytes, eosinophils, and plasma cells

If epidermal involvement is absent, a careful search for appendageal infiltrate may be helpful
See also Ch. 4, III.A; Ch. 17, IV.B.2
Atypical cells comprise 10 to 20% of infiltrate

Differential diagnosis:
Hodgkin's disease
Histiocytosis X
Lymphoma cutis
Lymphomatoid papulosis
Actinic reticuloid

Suggested Reading

Xanthomas

Montgomery, H., and Osterberg, A. E. Xanthomatosis. Correlation of clinical, histopathologic and chemical studies of cutaneous xanthoma. *Arch. Dermatol. Syphilol.* 37:373, 1938.
Winkelmann, R. K. Cutaneous syndromes of non-X histiocytosis. A review of the macrophage-histiocyte diseases of the skin. *Arch. Dermatol.* 117:667, 1981.

Leprosy

Azulay, R. D. Histopathology of skin lesions in leprosy. *Int. J. Lep.* 39:244, 1971.
Fasal, P. Histopathology of leprosy. *Cutis* 18:66, 1976.
Ridley, D. S. Histological classification and the immunological spectrum of leprosy. *Bull. W.H.O.* 5:451, 1974.
Ridley, D. S., and Jopling, W. H. Classification of leprosy according to immunity. A five group system. *Int. J. Lep.* 34:255, 1966.
Williams, R. C., Sr. Symposium on leprosy. *South. Med. J.* 69:969, 1976.

Histiocytosis X

Altman, J., and Winkelmann, R. K. Xanthomatous cutaneous lesions of histiocytosis X. *Arch. Dermatol.* 87:164, 1963.
Mihm, M. C., Jr., Clark, W. H., and Reed, R. J. The histiocytic infiltrates of the skin. *Hum. Pathol.* 5:45, 1974.

Juvenile Xanthogranuloma

Helwig, E. B., and Hackney, V. C. Juvenile xanthogranuloma (nevoxanthoendothelioma). *Am. J. Pathol.* 30:625, 1954.
Rodriguez, J., and Ackerman, A. B. Xanthogranuloma in adults. *Arch. Dermatol.* 112:43, 1976.
Webster, S. B., Reister, H. C., and Harman, L. E. Juvenile xanthogranuloma with extracutaneous lesions. *Arch. Dermatol.* 93:71, 1966.

Reticulohistiocytic Granuloma

Caro, M. R., and Senear, F. E. Reticulohistiocytoma of the skin. *Arch. Dermatol. Syphilol.* 65:701, 1952.
Goltz, R. W., and Laymon, C. W. Multicentric reticulohistiocytosis of the skin and synovia. *Arch. Dermatol. Syphilol.* 69:717, 1954.

Leishmaniasis

Dowlati, T. Cutaneous leishmaniasis. *Int. J. Dermatol.* 18:362, 1979.
Farah, F. S., and Malak, J. A. Cutaneous leishmaniasis. *Arch. Dermatol.* 103:467, 1971.
Nicolis, G. D., Tosca, A. D., Stratigos, J. D., et al. A clinical and histological study of cutaneous leishmaniasis. *Acta Derm. Venereol. (Stockh.)* 58:521, 1978.

Lymphoma Cutis

Cozzutto, C., DeBernardi, B., Comelli, A., and Mori, I. Primary cutaneous lymphoma with a nodular pattern in infancy. *Cancer* 45:603, 1980.

Evans, H. L., Winkelmann, R. K., and Banks, P. M. Differential diagnosis of malignant and benign cutaneous lymphoid infiltrates. *Cancer* 44:699, 1979.

Lukes, R. J. The immunologic approach to the pathology of malignant lymphomas. *Am. J. Clin. Pathol.* 72:657, 1979.

Smith, J. L., and Butler, J. J. Skin involvement in Hodgkin's disease. *Cancer* 45:354, 1980.

Wolk, B. H. Primary malignant lymphoma cutis. *Can. Med. Assoc. J.* 117:750, 1977.

Plasmacytoma

Mikhail, G. R., Spindler, A. C., and Kelly, A. P. Malignant plasmacytoma cutis. *Arch. Dermatol.* 101:59, 1970.

Wuepper, K. D., and MacKenzie, M. R. Cutaneous extramedullary plasmacytomas. *Arch. Dermatol.* 100:155, 1969.

Urticaria Pigmentosa

Burgoon, C. F., Graham, J. H., and McCaffree, D. L. Mast cell disease: A cutaneous variant with multisystem involvement. *Arch Dermatol.* 98:590, 1968.

Monheit, G. D., Murad, T., and Conrad, M. Systemic mastocytosis and the mastocytosis syndrome. *J. Cutan. Pathol.* 6:42, 1979.

Eosinophilic Cellulitis

Spigel, G. T., and Winkelmann, R. K. Well's syndrome. Recurrent granulomatous dermatitis with eosinophilia. *Arch. Dermatol.* 115:611, 1979.

Wells, G. C., and Smith, N. P. Eosinophilic cellulitis. *Br. J. Dermatol.* 100:101, 1979.

Chancroid

Gaisin, A., and Heaton, C. L. Chancroid: Alias the soft chancre. *Int. J. Dermatol.* 14:188, 1975.

Margolis, R. J., and Hood, A. F. Chancroid: Diagnosis and treatment. *J. Am. Acad. Dermatol.* 6:493, 1982.

Sheldon, W. H., and Weyman, A. Studies on chancroid. I. Observations on the histology with an evaluation of biopsy as a diagnostic procedure. *Am. J. Pathol.* 22:415, 1946.

Rhinoscleroma

Hyams, V. J. Rhinoscleroma. In C. H. Binford and D. H. Connor (Eds.), *Pathology of Tropical and Extraordinary Diseases*, Vol. I. Washington: Armed Forces Institute of Pathology, 1976. Pp. 187–189.

Granuloma Inguinale

Davis, C. M. Granuloma inguinale: A clinical, histological and ultrastructural study. *J.A.M.A.* 211:632, 1970.

Hodgkin's Disease

Smith, J. L., and Butler, J. J. Skin involvement in Hodgkin's disease. *Cancer* 45:354, 1980.

Mycosis Fungoides

Brehmer-Andersson, E. Mycosis fungoides and its relation to Sézary's syndrome, lymphomatoid papulosis, and primary cutaneous Hodgkin's disease. *Acta Dermatol. Venereol. (Stockh.)* 56 (Suppl. 75):9, 1976.

Degreef, H., Holvoet, C., Van Vloten, W. A., et al. Woringer-Kolopp disease. An epidermotropic variant of mycosis fungoides. *Cancer* 38:2154, 1976.

Jimbow, K., Chiba, M., and Horikoshi, T. Electron microscopic identification of Langerhans cells in the dermal infiltrates of mycosis fungoides. *J. Invest Dermatol.* 78:102, 1982.

Lutzner, M., Edelson, R., Schein, P., et al. Cutaneous T-cell lymphomas: The Sézary syndrome, mycosis fungoides and related disorders. *Ann. Intern. Med.* 83:534, 1975.

Waldorf, D. S., Ratner, A. C., and Van Scott, E. J. Cells in lesions of mycosis fungoides lymphoma following therapy. Changes in number and type. *Cancer* 21:264, 1968.

Winkelmann, R. K., and Caro, W. A. Current problems in mycosis fungoides and Sézary syndrome. *Annu. Rev. Med.* 28:251, 1977.

Chapter 17

Nodular Infiltrate

I. Lymphocytoma cutis (reactive lymphoid hyperplasia, cutaneous lymphoplasia, pseudolymphoma of Spiegler-Fendt)
II. Arthropod bite reaction
III. Angiolymphoid hyperplasia with eosinophilia
IV. Lymphoma cutis
    A. Monomorphous infiltrate (non-Hodgkin's lymphoma)
    B. Polymorphous infiltrate
        1. Hodgkin's disease
        2. Mycosis fungoides
V. Tertiary syphilis

The Reactive Process and the Disease	Histopathology	Comments

I. Lymphocytoma cutis (reactive lymphoid hyperplasia, cutaneous lymphoplasia, pseudolymphoma of Spiegler-Fendt)	1. Normal or sometimes atrophic epidermis
	2. Sparing of the upper dermis (Grenz zone)
	3. Dense nodular aggregates of lymphocytes and histiocytes admixed with occasional eosinophils
	4. Infiltrate extends throughout reticular dermis, occasionally in a perivascular perifollicular array
	5. **Germinal centers (lymphoid follicles)** often present
	6. Hyperplasia of venular endothelial cells
	7. Proliferation of fibroblasts
		Absence of psoriasiform hyperplasia helps differentiate lymphocytoma from insect bite reaction
		
		Differential diagnosis:
		  Lymphoma cutis
		  Arthropod bite reaction
		  Angiolymphoid hyperplasia with eosinophilia
		
		Lymphoid follicles are made up of a collection of large, pale lymphoblasts and macrophages surrounded by small, mature lymphocytes; the presence of lymphoid follicles helps differentiate lymphocytoma from lymphoma
		
		Lymphoid follicles may be seen in:
		
		Lymphocytoma cutis
		Insect bite reaction
		Angiolymphoid hyperplasia with eosinophilia

II. Arthropod bite reaction (see Fig. 11-2)	1. Hyperkeratosis and/or crust 2. Epidermal hyperplasia may be marked 3. Ulceration at site of puncta 4. Bandlike or nodular, polymorphous infiltrate composed of lymphocytes and many **eosinophils** with variable numbers of plasma cells 5. Occasional germinal center formation 6. Prominent endothelial cell swelling and vascular proliferation	See also Ch. 4, III.A; Ch. 10, IV; Ch. 14, I.A.2 Histologically may be indistinguishable from lymphocytoma cutis Lesions may be localized to subcutis

III. Angiolymphoid hyperplasia with eosinophilia (Fig. 17-1)

1. Epidermis normal
2. Aggregates of lymphocytes with histiocytes and eosinophils; **eosinophils** and plasma cells scattered between collagen fibers throughout dermis
3. Lymphoid follicles may be present
4. Dermal hemorrhage and hemosiderin deposition common
5. Sheetlike cellular aggregates composed of histiocytes and/or endothelial cells
6. Numerous **prominent vessels,** occasionally branching and stellate
7. Plump endothelial cells protrude into vascular lumen ("hobnail" appearance)
8. Proliferation of delicate reticulin fibers and deposition of acid mucopolysaccharide around vessels

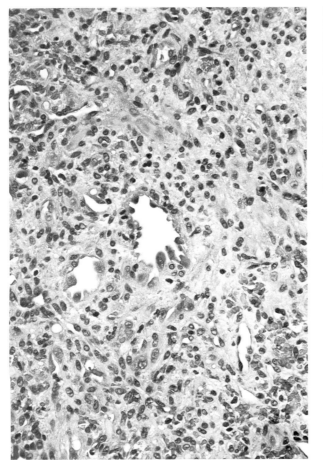

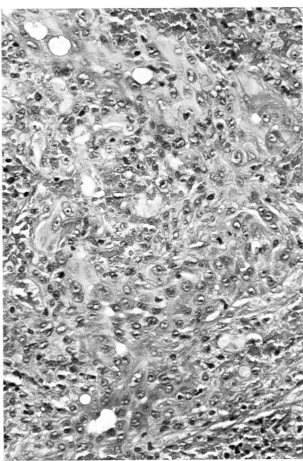

A

B

Fig. **17-1.** *Angiolymphoid hyperplasia with eosinophilia.*

A. *Vascular channels may be
   numerous and ectatic; endothelial cells appear to protrude into the lumen. (×400)*

B. *Sheetlike cellular aggregates
   with mitoses appear to arise
   from endothelial cells (plump
   endothelial cells surround vessel lumens in the upper and
   lower left portions of the
   field). (×400)*

C. *Inflammation with numerous
   lymphocytes and eosinophils
   is also typical. Lymphoid follicles (not illustrated here) may
   be present. (×400)*

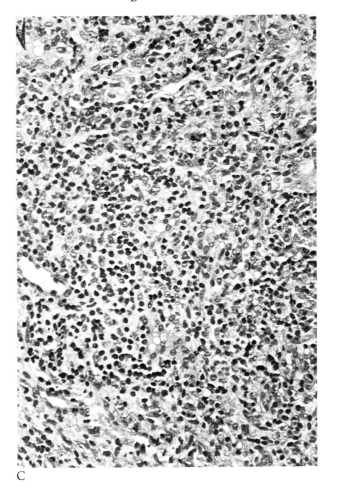

C

IV. Lymphoma cutis

A. Monomorphous infiltrate (non-Hodgkin's lymphoma) (Fig. 17-2)

1. Epidermis usually normal
2. Papillary dermis spared (Grenz zone)
3. Dense nodular aggregates, patchy aggregates, or diffuse dermal infiltration of lymphoid cells throughout entire reticular dermis, often extending into subcutaneous fat
4. Nuclear atypia and atypical mitoses characteristic, though quantitatively variable
5. Cells often infiltrate between collagen fibers in an "Indian file" fashion
6. Nuclei, packed tightly together, appear distorted and "smudged"
7. Absence of endothelial cell hyperplasia and vascular proliferation

Histologic classification of lymphomas (Rappaport):
Monomorphous
Undifferentiated
Lymphocytic, well differentiated
Lymphocytic, poorly differentiated
Mixed lymphocytic-histiocytic
Histiocytic
Polymorphous
Hodgkin's disease
Mycosis fungoides

Luke's immunologic classification for malignant lymphoma:
1. Null cell (undefined)
2. T cell
   a. Small lymphocyte
   b. Convoluted lymphocyte
   c. Cerebriform cell (of Sézary's syndrome and mycosis fungoides)
   d. Lymphoepithelioid cell
   e. Immunoblastic sarcoma
3. B cell
   a. Small lymphocyte
   b. Plasmacytoid lymphocyte
   c. Follicular center cell (FCC) types:
      (1) Small cleaved
      (2) Small noncleaved
      (3) Large cleaved
      (4) Large noncleaved
   d. Immunoblastic sarcoma
4. Histiocytic
5. Cell of uncertain origin: Hodgkin's disease
6. Unclassifiable (for technical reasons)

Differential diagnosis:
Histiocytosis X
Lymphomatoid papulosis
Actinic reticuloid
Leukemia cutis
Lymphocytoma cutis
Lymphocytic infiltrate
Arthropod bite reaction
Mycosis fungoides
Urticaria pigmentosa
Absence of (1) eosinophils and plasma cells, (2) vascular reactivity, and (3) lymphoid follicles helps differentiate malignant lymphoma from benign reactive inflammatory processes
See also Ch. 16, II.A

Fig. **17-2.** *Lymphoma cutis.*
A. *The massive infiltrate of atypical lymphocytes fills the dermis, sparing only the uppermost papillary dermis (Grenz zone). In the absence of systemic disease, the diagnosis is difficult to make with certainty. (×37)*
B. *The high magnification exhibits the monomorphous atypical appearance of the infiltrate. (×640)*

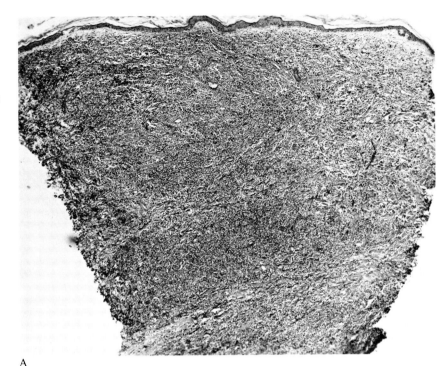

A

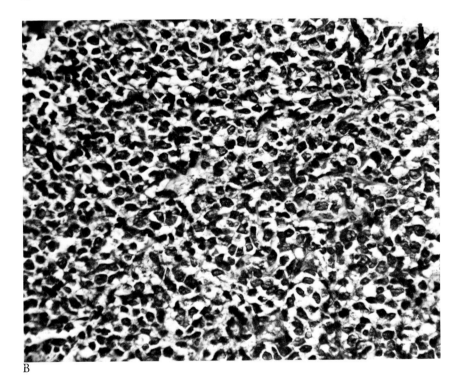

B

B. Polymorphous infiltrate

1. Hodgkin's disease	1. Epidermis usually normal
	2. Grenz zone of spared papillary dermis
	3. Nodular or diffuse infiltrate throughout the reticular dermis composed of:
	   a. Atypical mononuclear cells admixed with histiocytes and variable numbers of neotrophils, eosinophils, plasma cells, and multinucleate giant cells
	   b. Reed-Sternberg cells—large cells with abundant cytoplasm, binucleate or bilobed nuclei, and prominent nucleoli, giving an "owl's eye" appearance
		See also Ch. 16, VII.E.1
		
		Systemic involvement in Hodgkin's disease almost always precedes cutaneous involvement
		
		Differential diagnosis:
		  Lymphomatoid papulosis
		  Arthropod bite reaction
		  Mycosis fungoides

2. Mycosis fungoides (see Fig. 4-6)	1. Epidermal changes variable and include psoriasiform hyperplasia, atrophy, or ulceration with or without Pautrier microabscesses
	2. Dense accumulations of atypical mononuclear cells (so-called mycosis cells) characterized by convoluted or cerebriform, hyperchromatic nuclei admixed with lymphocytes, histiocytes, eosinophils, and plasma cells
		If epidermal involvement is absent, a careful search for appendageal infiltrate may be helpful
		
		See also Ch. 4, III.A; Ch. 16, VII.E.2
		Tumor-type lesions usually composed of 15 to 20% atypical cells
		
		Differential diagnosis:
		  Hodgkin's disease
		  Histiocytosis X
		  Lymphoma cutis
		  Lymphomatoid papulosis
		  Actinic reticuloid

V. Tertiary syphilis	1. Epidermis normal, flattened, or ulcerated 2. Edema of papillary dermis with mild perivascular lymphohistiocytic and plasma cell infiltrate 3. Perivascular and periappendageal nodular infiltrate composed of aggregates of epithelioid and giant cells surrounded by lymphocytes, histiocytes, and plasma cells 4. Endothelial cell proliferation prominent and may produce narrowing and/or obliteration of vessel lumen	Differential diagnosis: lupus vulgaris See also Ch. 14, II.K; Ch. 15, III.H Spirochetes not demonstrable

Suggested Reading

Lymphocytoma Cutis

Caro, W. A., and Helwig, E. B. Cutaneous lymphoid hyperplasia. *Cancer* 24:487, 1969.

Clark, W. H., Mihm, M. C., Jr., Reed, R. J., and Ainsworth, A. M. The lymphocytic infiltrates of the skin. *Hum. Pathol.* 5:25, 1974.

Evans, H. L., Winkelmann, R. K., and Banks, P. M. Differential diagnosis of malignant and benign cutaneous lymphoid infiltrates. *Cancer* 44:699, 1979.

Mach, K. W., and Wilgram, G. F. Characteristic histopathology of cutaneous lymphoplasia (lymphocytoma). *Arch. Dermatol.* 94:26, 1966.

Arthropod Bite Reaction

Fernandez, N., Torres, A., and Ackerman, A. B. Pathologic findings in human scabies. *Arch. Dermatol.* 113:320, 1977.

Goldman, L., Rockwell, E., and Richfield, D. F., III. Histopathological studies on cutaneous reactions to the bites of various arthropods. *Am. J. Trop. Med. Hyg.* 1:514, 1952.

Horen, W. P. Insect and scorpion sting. *J.A.M.A.* 221:894, 1972.

Larrivee, D. H., Benjamini, E., Feingold, B. F., et al. Histologic studies of guinea pig skin: Different stages of allergic reactivity to flea bites. *Exp. Parasitol.* 15:491, 1964.

Steffen, C. Clinical and histopathologic correlation of midge bites. *Arch. Dermatol.* 117:785, 1981.

Thomson, J., Cochran, T., Cochran, R., and McQueen, A. Histology simulating reticulosis in persistent nodular scabies. *Br. J. Dermatol.* 90:421, 1974.

Angiolymphoid Hyperplasia

Henry, P. G., and Burnett, J. W. Angiolymphoid hyperplasia with eosinophilia. *Arch. Dermatol.* 114:1168, 1978.

Lymphoma Cutis

Cozzutto, C., DeBernardi, B., Comelli, A., and Mori, P. Primary cutaneous lymphoma with a nodular pattern in infancy. *Cancer* 54:603, 1980.

Evans, H. L., Winkelmann, R. K., and Banks, P. M. Differential diagnosis of malignant and benign cutaneous lymphoid infiltrates. *Cancer* 44:699, 1979.

Lukes, R. J. The immunologic approach to the pathology of malignant lymphomas. *Am. J. Clin. Pathol.* 72:657, 1979.

Smith, J. L., and Butler, J. J. Skin involvement in Hodgkin's disease. *Cancer* 45:354, 1980.

Wolk, B. H. Primary malignant lymphoma cutis. *Can. Med. Assoc. J.* 117:750, 1977.

Mycosis Fungoides

Brehmer-Andersson, E. Mycosis fungoides and its relation to Sézary's syndrome, lymphomatoid papulosis, and primary cutaneous Hodgkin's disease. *Acta Derm. Venereol. (Stockh.)* 75:(Suppl. 56):9, 1976.

Degreef, H., Holvoet, C., Van Vloten, W. A., et al. Woringer-Kolopp disease. An epidermotropic variant of mycosis fungoides. *Cancer* 38:2154, 1976.

Jimbow, K., Chiba, M., and Horikoshi, T. Electron microscopic identification of Langerhans cells in the dermal infiltrates of mycosis fungoides. *J. Invest. Dermatol.* 78:102, 1982.

Lutzner, M., Edelson, R., Schein, P., et al. Cutaneous T-cell lymphomas: The Sézary syndrome, mycosis fungoides and related disorders. *Ann. Intern. Med.* 83:534, 1975.

Waldorf, D. S., Ratner, A. C., and Van Scott, E. J. Cells in lesions of mycosis fungoides lymphoma following therapy. Changes in number and type. *Cancer* 21:264, 1968.

Winkelmann, R. K., and Caro, W. A. Current problems in mycosis fungoides and Sézary syndrome. *Annu. Rev. Med.* 28:251, 1977.

Chapter 18

Degenerative Disorders of Collagen and Connective Tissue

I. Radiodermatitis
   A. Early state
   B. Late stage
II. Morphea
   A. Early stage
   B. Late stage
III. Progressive systemic sclerosis (scleroderma)
IV. Solar elastosis
V. Pseudoxanthoma elasticum
VI. Ehlers-Danlos syndrome
VII. Cutis laxa
VIII. Angiofibroma
IX. Anetoderma
   A. Inflammatory, idiopathic type (Jadassohn)
      1. Inflammatory stage
      2. Late stage
   B. Noninflammatory, idiopathic type (Schweninger and Buzzi)
X. Acrodermatitis chronica atrophicans (atrophic stage)

The Reactive Process and the Disease	Histopathology	Comments
I. Radiodermatitis		
A. Early stage	1. Frequent epidermal necrosis, even ulceration 2. Prominent edema of dermis 3. Fibroblasts in dermis often with pyknotic nuclei 4. Variable polymorphous inflammatory infiltrate throughout dermis, especially in perivenular distribution 5. Swelling and occasional necrosis of endothelial cells	See also Ch. 9, III.C

B. Late stage (Figs. 18-1, 18-2)	1. Hyperkeratosis and parakeratosis associated with epidermal hyperplasia and/or epidermal atrophy
	2. Epidermal atypism with dyskeratosis frequent
	3. Variable ulceration
	4. Increased melanin in basal layer
	5. **Ectatic vessels** in upper dermis
	6. Focal pigment incontinence with melanin free and within macrophages
	7. Medium-size arteries and veins exhibit fibrotic thickening of walls with frequent endothelial cell hyperplasia and luminal occlusion
	8. Hyalinized collagen **usually uniformly eosinophilic** from basement membrane zone to subcutaneous fat
	9. Collagen fibers irregularly fragmented and often hyalinized
	10. Fibroblasts exhibit irregular, large, variably pyknotic nuclei with variable shape; abundant cytoplasm of the so-called **radiation fibroblasts** is frequently vacuolated
	11. Pilosebaceous units and eccrine glands atrophic
		Differential diagnosis:
		    Lichen sclerosus et atrophicus
		    Lupus erythematosus
		    Scleroderma
		
		Invasive squamous cell carcinoma may arise in areas of radiodermatitis

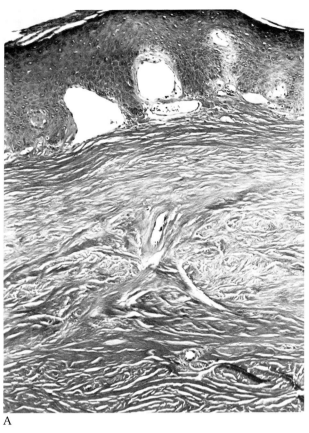

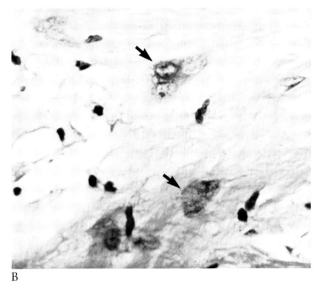

A   B

Fig. **18-1.** *Chronic radiodermatitis. Superficial vascular ectasia with dense dermal fibrosis (A) and bizarre fibroblasts (B, arrows). (A, ×100; B, ×1000)*

Fig. **18-2.** *Comparison of normal skin, scleroderma, and chronic radiodermatitis. Left, Normal skin: note the thickness of normal epidermis, the presence of pilosebaceous follicles and eccrine glands, and the appearance of normal collagen and periec-crine gland fat. Middle, Scleroderma: loss of appendages, swollen and/or sclerotic collagen bundles, and "entrapped" eccrine glands are typical. Right, Chronic radiodermatitis: epidermal atrophy, hyalinized sclerotic collagen, vascular ectasia, loss of appendages, and bizarre "radiation fibroblasts" (inset) are characteristic.*

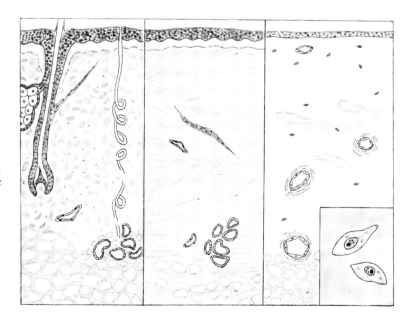

II. Morphea

A. Early stage
(Fig. 18-3)

1. Closely packed, new collagen fibers in lower dermis that run parallel to long axis of epidermis; normal pattern of interlacing collagen bundles in lower dermis is lost
2. Moderately intense mononuclear cell infiltrate at junction of reticular dermis and subcutis
3. Prominent inflammation and widening of septa of subcutaneous fat by new collagen fibers
4. Rarely plasma cells predominate in inflammatory infiltrate

Formalin-fixed skin biopsies typically exhibit a tapered or "cone" shape; thickened or sclerotic collagen produces a rectangular or square biopsy

---

Differential diagnosis of a *"square" biopsy:*

Normal back
Morphea/progressive systemic sclerosis
Scar
Chronic graft-versus-host reaction
Radiodermatitis
Connective-tissue nevus
Scleredema

B. Late stage

1. Epidermal atrophy
2. Bundles of dermal collagen fibers appear closely packed or **hyalinized** because of loss of interbundle space
3. Marked decrease in cellularity of dermis

Aggregations of inflammatory cells may be prominent in areas of fibrosis; these aggregates may persist many years; the presence of inflammation favors the diagnosis of morphea over progressive systemic sclerosis

---

Fig. **18-3.** *Morphea. Swelling of collagen bundles in the deep dermis is characteristic. Note also the trapped eccrine glands near the base of the field. The amount of inflammatory infiltrate is a variable feature in biopsies of this disorder. (×64)*

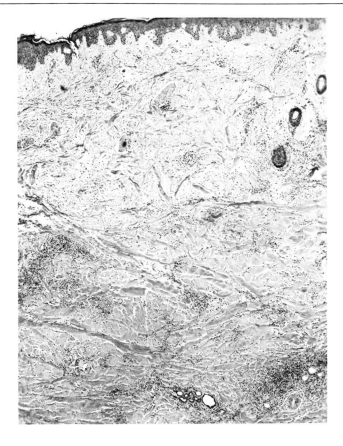

	4. Appendages completely surrounded and **entrapped** by collagen with loss of adventitial fat	
	5. Inflammation present in subcutis; slight to absent elsewhere	Differential diagnosis: scar
III. Progressive systemic sclerosis (scleroderma) (Figs. 18-2, 18-3)	Changes similar to those described in morphea except inflammation is usually minimal or absent	Systemic scleroderma in its early stages shows a mild inflammatory infiltrate
		Late systemic scleroderma exhibits diminished vessels with frequent hyalinization of vessel walls and frequent luminal obliteration
IV. Solar elastosis (see Fig. 6-10B)	1. Epidermal changes variable 2. Grenz zone of normal papillary dermis 3. Individual and clumped, wavy, faintly basophilic fibers intermingled with collagen of upper reticular dermis or admixed with relatively homogeneous gray-blue material 4. Vessels in upper dermis often ectatic	Fibers and amorphous material stain positive with elastic tissue stain
V. Pseudoxanthoma elasticum (Fig. 18-4)	1. Epidermis normal 2. Grenz zone (normal papillary and reticular dermis) 3. **Swollen, fragmented and irregularly clumped basophilic** (and sometimes eosinophilic) **fibers** in lower two-thirds of dermis	Abnormal fibers stain both with elastic tissue and calcium stains (see Appendix) Basophilia is due to calcium uptake by the fibers Foreign-body giant cells occasionally admixed with elastic fibers

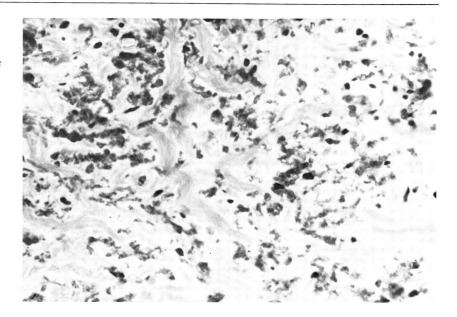

Fig. **18-4.** *Pseudoxanthoma elasticum. Elastic fibers exhibit this characteristic frizzy appearance. Special stains (see Appendix) are recommended for optimal visualization of elastic fibers. (approximately ×400)*

VI. Ehlers-Danlos syndrome	No abnormal light microscopic findings
VII. Cutis laxa (Fig. 18-5)	1. **Reduced number of elastic fibers,** especially in papillary dermis 2. Elastic fibers exhibit granular degeneration
VIII. Angiofibroma (see Fig. 13-2)	See Ch. 13, II
IX. Anetoderma	
A. Inflammatory, idiopathic type (Jadassohn)	
1. Inflammatory stage	1. Normal epidermis 2. Superficial perivenular infiltrate of lymphocytes and histiocytes 3. Nuclear debris occasionally present 4. Edema of papillary dermis

Fig. **18-5.**

A. *Cutis laxa. The elastic fibers exhibit attenuation and a granular, beaded appearance. (×400)*

B. *Control (adjacent normal) skin. The normal appearance of elastic fibers for comparison. (×400) (Both are van Gieson stained.)*

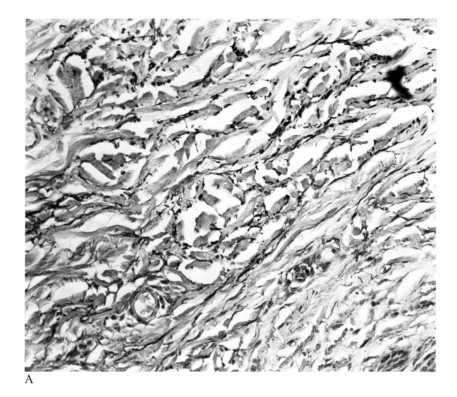

A

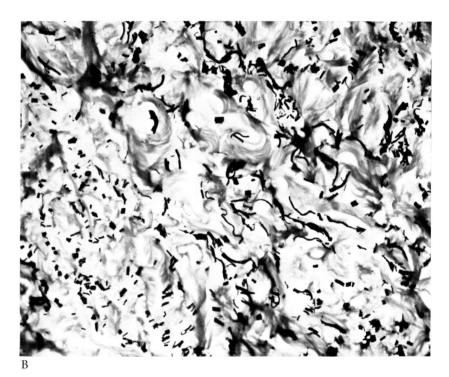

B

2. Late stage

1. **Partial to complete loss of elastic fibers** in dermis with retention of elastica of vessels
2. **Apparent diminution in dermal thickness** when compared with normal skin

Differential diagnosis:
    Striae distensae
    Cutis laxa
    Connective-tissue nevus

Evaluation of elastic fiber abnormalities requires comparison of appropriately stained biopsies of normal and affected skin (see Appendix)

B. Noninflammatory, idiopathic type (Schweninger and Buzzi) (Fig. 18-6)

See late-stage Jadassohn-type

X. Acrodermatitis chronica atrophicans (atrophic stage)

1. Epidermal atrophy with flattening of rete ridges
2. Grenz zone (normal papillary dermis)
3. Bandlike and perivascular mononuclear cell infiltrate
4. Dermal edema
5. **Diminution of collagen, elastic fibers, and subcutaneous fat**
6. Atrophy of pilosebaceous units; preservation of eccrine glands

See also Ch. 7, IV; Ch. 10, VII

Fig. **18-6.**
A. *Anetoderma. Elastic fibers are reduced in number and size (×400)*
B. *Control (normal) skin. The normal appearance of elastic fibers is demonstrated here. (×400) (Both are van Gieson stained.)*

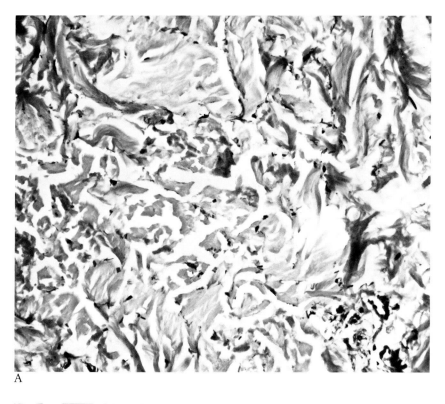

A

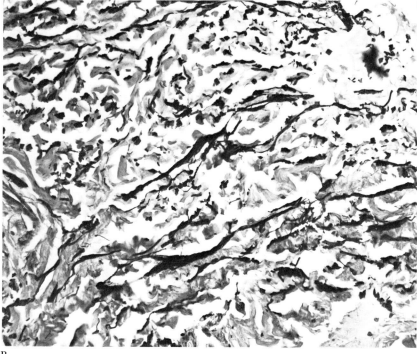

B

Suggested Reading
Radiodermatitis

Epstein, E. *Radiodermatitis.* Springfield, Ill.: Thomas, 1972.

Teloh, H. A., Mason, M. L., and Wheelock, M. C. A histopathologic study of radiation injuries of the skin. *Surg. Gynecol. Obstet.* 90:335, 1950.

Morphea

Fleischmajer, R., and Nedwich, A. Generalized morphea. I. Histology of the dermis and subcutaneous tissue. *Arch. Dermatol.* 106:509, 1972.

O'Leary, P. A., Montgomery, H., and Ragsdale, W. E., Jr. Dermatohistopathology of various types of scleroderma. *Arch. Dermatol.* 75:78, 1957.

Progressive Systemic Sclerosis (Scleroderma)

Barnett, A. J. *Scleroderma (Progressive Systemic Sclerosis).* Springfield, Ill.: Thomas, 1974.

Fleischmajer, R., Damiano, V., and Nedwich, A. Alteration of subcutaneous tissue in systemic sclerosis. *Arch. Dermatol.* 105:59, 1972.

Fleischmajer, R., Perlish, J. S., and Reeves, J. R. Cellular infiltrates in scleroderma skin. *Arthritis Rheum.* 20:975, 1977.

Piper, W. N., and Helwig, E. B. Progressive systemic sclerosis. *Arch. Dermatol.* 72:535, 1955.

Pseudoxanthoma Elasticum

Goodman, R. M., Smith, E. W., Paton, D., et al. Pseudoxanthoma elasticum: A clinical and histopathological study. *Medicine* 42:297, 1963.

Lund, H. Z., and Gilbert, C. F. Perforating pseudoxanthoma elasticum. Its distinction from elastosis perforans serpiginosa. *Arch. Pathol. Lab. Med.* 100:544, 1976.

Ehlers-Danlos Syndrome

Sulica, V. I., Cooper, P. H., Pope, F. M., et al. Cutaneous histologic features in Ehlers-Danlos syndrome. *Arch. Dermatol.* 115:40, 1979.

Cutis Laxa

Goltz, R. W., Hult, A. M., Goldfarb, M., et al. Cutis laxa. *Arch. Dermatol.* 92:373, 1965.

Tuberous Sclerosis

Nickel, W. R., and Reed, W. B. Tuberous sclerosis. *Arch. Dermatol.* 85:209, 1962.

Anetoderma

Feldman, S. Macular atrophy (Schweninger and Buzzi type). *Arch. Dermatol. Syphilol.* 38:117, 1938.

Varadi, D. P., and Saqueton, A. C. Perifollicular elastolysis. *Br. J. Dermatol.* 83:143, 1970.

Verhagen, A. R., and Woerdeman, M. J. Post-inflammatory elastolysis and cutis laxa. *Br. J. Dermatol.* 92:183, 1975.

Acrodermatitis Chronica Atrophicans

Burdorf, W. H. C., Worret, W. I., and Schultka, O. Acrodermatitis chronica atrophicans. *Int. J. Dermatol.* 18:595, 1979.

Montgomery, H., and Sullivan, R. R. Acrodermatitis atrophicans chronica. *Arch. Dermatol. Syphilol.* 51:32, 1945.

Chapter 19

Diseases Recognized Histologically by Deposition of Material in the Dermis

I. Amyloidosis
  A. Systemic amyloidosis
    1. Primary
    2. Secondary
  B. Localized amyloidosis
    1. Nodular amyloidosis
II. Mucinoses
  A. Focal mucinosis; cutaneous myxoma
  B. Digital mucous cyst; myxoid cyst
  C. Mucous cyst of oral mucosa
  D. Myxedema
  E. Pretibial myxedema
  F. Papular mucinosis; lichen myxedematosus; scleromyxedema
  G. Scleredema of Buschke
III. Gouty tophus
IV. Calcinosis cutis (metastatic, dystrophic, idiopathic)
V. Ochronosis
VI. Hemochromatosis
VII. Tattoo
VIII. Argyria
IX. Lipoid proteinosis

The Reactive Process and the Disease	Histopathology	Comments
I. Amyloidosis		
A. Systemic amyloidosis		

1. Primary	1. Epidermal changes range from atrophy to hyperkeratosis and acanthosis
	2. Grenz zone (normal papillary dermis) may be present
	3. Pale eosinophilic, homogeneous, acellular, sometimes fissured material deposited in the dermis
	4. Deposition of amyloid usually in upper and mid reticular dermis but may extend up to the epidermis or down to involve the subcutaneous fat
	5. Extravasation of erythrocytes common when amyloid is present within vessel walls
	6. Deposition of amyloid around individual fat cells produces characteristic "amyloid rings"
		Frozen sections of unfixed skin stained with either Congo red or thioflavin-T optimally demonstrate amyloid deposition
		Amyloid deposits also may be seen in arrector pili muscles and lamina propria of sweat ducts and glands
		
		Differential diagnosis:
		  Colloid milium
		  Lipoid proteinosis
		  Solar elastosis
		  Scleroderma

2. Secondary	Amyloid sometimes observed around appendages and fat cells	Biopsy of clinically normal skin or subcutaneous fat from abdomen may reveal amyloid deposition
B. Localized amyloidosis		
1. Nodular amyloidosis	1. Epidermis flattened and often atrophic 2. Large masses of amyloid deposited in papillary dermis, reticular dermis, and subcutaneous fat 3. Amyloid deposited in vessel walls and eccrine glands and around fat cells 4. Variable lymphohistiocytic, plasma cell, and giant-cell infiltrate around amyloid deposits 5. Foci of calcification occasionally present	Nodular amyloidosis cannot be distinguished histologically from systemic amyloidosis (see also I.A) Two other diseases—macular amyloidosis and lichen amyloidosis—are characterized by amyloid deposition limited to the papillary dermis (see also Ch. 12, I)

II. Mucinoses

This group of disorders is characterized by the dermal deposition of mucin (usually the acid mucopolysaccharide, hyaluronic acid), which can be seen as faint, wispy basophilic threads and granules with H&E stained sections; it is better demonstrated with colloidal iron, alcian blue, or toluidine blue stains

A. Focal mucinosis; cutaneous myxoma

1. Epidermis normal to flattened
2. Mucin deposition displaces and replaces collagen fibers of reticular dermis
3. Proliferation of fibroblasts in areas of mucin deposition
4. Small cystic spaces may occur

B. Digital mucous cyst; myxoid cyst

1. Elevated, dome-shaped lesion with flattened epidermis
2. Variable mucin deposition:
   a. Between collagen fibers
   b. Within fissures or cleftlike spaces in the dermis
   c. Within large cystic spaces which may fill entire dermis
3. Proliferation of fibroblasts in and around areas of mucin deposition

Early lesions may resemble focal mucinosis

C. Mucous cyst of oral mucosa

1. Normal mucosa
2. Submucosal cystic space or spaces filled with amorphous, pale eosinophilic material
3. Cystic space is lined by histiocytes, lymphocytes, macrophages, and fibroblasts

The material in mucous cysts of the oral mucosa is sialomucin, which contains acid and neutral mucopolysaccharides; sialomucin will stain with PAS as well as alcian blue and colloidal iron

D. Myxedema

1. Variable hyperkeratosis, follicular plugging with keratin, and follicular atrophy
2. **Mucin deposited about venules and appendages as well as in the reticular dermis**
3. Slight swelling and separation of collagen fibers

Increased mucin deposition in the papillary and upper reticular dermis may be seen in dermatomyositis and lupus erythematosus

E. Pretibial myxedema (Fig. 19-1)

1. Hyperkeratosis, keratin plugs in follicular openings
2. Grenz zone of normal papillary dermis
3. **Bandlike deposition of mucin throughout upper reticular dermis**
4. Displacement and replacement of collagen fibers by mucin
5. Fibroblast proliferation
6. Increased number of mast cells
7. Mucin frequently deposited between fat cells in subcutaneous tissue

F. Papular mucinosis; lichen myxedematosus; scleromyxedema

1. Flattened epidermis
2. Mucin deposition in papillary dermis and upper reticular dermis
3. Fibroblast proliferation
4. Increased number of mast cells
5. Increased reticulum and elastic fibers

Serum protein immunoelectrophoresis demonstrates the presence of an abnormal IgG, usually with lambda light chains

Differential diagnosis: Granuloma annulare

G. Scleredema of Buschke

1. Normal epidermis
2. Markedly thickened dermis with broad collagen bundles
3. "Entrapment" of appendages
4. Mucin often demonstrable between collagen fibers and fat cells in early lesions

Differential diagnosis: Scleroderma

III. Gouty tophus (see Fig. 2-2)

1. Normal or ulcerated epidermis
2. Variously sized deposits of amphophilic material with characteristic **parallel, needle-shaped clefts** present in dermis and subcutaneous tissue
3. Lymphohistiocytic and **giant-cell infiltrate around urate deposits**
4. Calcification of urate deposits may occur

If tissue is fixed in 100% ethanol instead of formalin, needle-shaped urate crystals may be better visualized

IV. Calcinosis cutis (metastatic, dystrophic, idiopathic)

1. Epidermis normal or occasionally ulcerated
2. Small to massive deposition of dark blue particles in dermis and subcutaneous tissue
3. Foreign-body giant-cell reaction sometimes present adjacent to calcium deposits

Special stains such as Von Kossa or Alizarin red-S may be helpful in confirming the presence of calcium

Fig. **19-1.** *Pretibial myxedema.*
A. *The lightly stained band in the upper reticular dermis indicates the area of acid mucopolysaccharide deposition. (×49)*
B. *The higher magnification shows the loosely cellular nature of the myxedematous zone as well as a dilated lymphatic channel. (×160)*

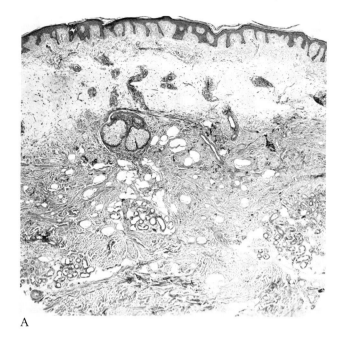

A

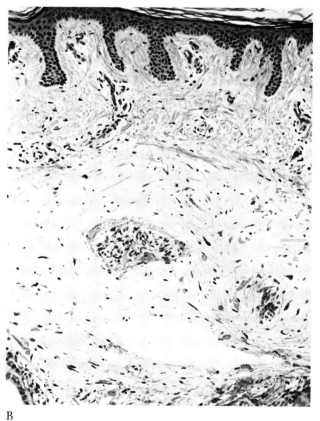

B

V. Ochronosis

1. Normal epidermis
2. Intracellular and extracellular deposition of yellow to **light brown homogentisic acid granules and globules**
3. Particles often seen within endothelial cells and secretory cells of eccrine gland
4. **Large deposits within collagen, and elastic fibers may assume bizarre, irregular shapes**
5. Giant multinucleate cells occasionally present

Homogentisic acid crystals stain black with cresyl violet or methylene blue

Differential diagnosis:
Argyria
Tattoo
Hemochromatosis

VI. Hemochromatosis

1. **Increased melanin** in basal layer
2. Intracellular and extracellular deposition of **golden brown, irregularly shaped** hemosiderin and hemofuscin granules
3. Granules commonly found in and around basement membrane of eccrine units and around blood vessels

Hemosiderin deposition can be demonstrated with the Prussian blue stain

Differential diagnosis:
Venous stasis
Progressive pigmented purpura
Argyria

VII. Tattoo (Fig. 19-2)

1. Epidermis usually normal
2. Dark pigment granules dispersed in the upper and middle reticular dermis, both **free and within macrophages**
3. Most tattoo pigments appear black with routine microscopy but occasionally a reddish hue (cinnabar) or bluish hue (cobalt) is apparent

Rarely eczematous or granulomatous reactions to the injected material may occur

VIII. Argyria (Fig. 19-3)

1. Increased melanin may be present in basal cells
2. Uniform, small, round, brown-black refractile granules deposited intracellularly and extracellularly in papillary and reticular dermis
3. **Granules characteristically deposited in basement membrane of vessels and eccrine glands** and within endothelial cells

Dark-field examination demonstrates particles of heavy metals and emphasizes the uniformity in the size of the silver granules; uniform size of granules helps differentiate argyria from ochronosis, tattoo, hemosiderin, and other heavy-metal deposition

Fig. **19-2.** *Tattoo. Black pigment within and outside of dermal histiocytes is characteristic. (×256)*

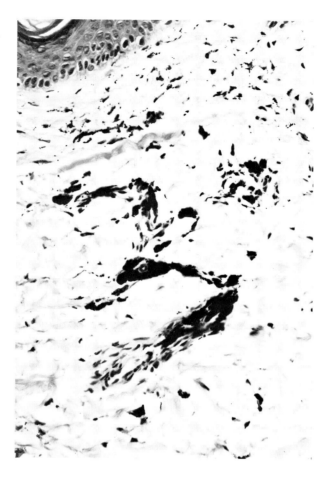

Fig. **19-3.** *Argyria. Deposition of dark, almost refractile granules in the basement membrane zone of these eccrine glands is characteristic of argyria. Deposition of granules about other skin appendages and upon elastic fibers as well as hypermelanosis also occurs in this disorder. (approximately ×1000)*

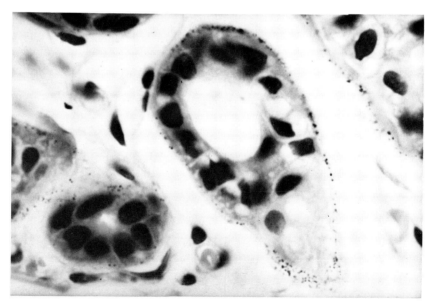

IX. Lipoid proteinosis

1. Hyperkeratosis and papillomatosis
2. **Homogeneous eosinophilic hyaline material deposited in arrays perpendicular to epidermis in papillary dermis**
3. In reticular dermis the material surrounds and deposits in vessel walls, eccrine glands, and arrector pili muscles
4. Elastosis frequently present peripheral to hyaline deposition
5. Increased number of mast cells

The hyaline material, a glycolipoprotein, has the following staining properties:
PAS-positive, diastase-resistant
Alcian blue positive at pH of 3
Slightly positive with Congo red and variably positive with other lipid stains

---

Suggested Reading
Amyloidosis

Brownstein, M. H., and Helwig, E. B. The cutaneous amyloidoses. I. Localized forms. *Arch. Dermatol.* 102:8, 1970.

Brownstein, M. H., and Helwig, E. B. The cutaneous amyloidoses. II. Systemic forms. *Arch. Dermatol.* 102:20, 1970.

Habermann, M. C., and Montenegro, M. R. Primary cutaneous amyloidosis: Clinical, laboratory and histopathological study in 25 cases. *Dermatologica* 160:240, 1980.

Kobayashi, H., and Hashimoto, K. Amyloidogenesis in organ-limited cutaneous amyloidosis: An antigenic identity between epidermal keratin and skin amyloid. *J. Invest. Dermatol.* 80:66, 1983.

Vasily, D. B., Bhatia, S. G., and Uhlin, S. R. Familial primary cutaneous amyloidosis. Clinical, genetic, and immunofluorescent studies. *Arch. Dermatol.* 114:1173, 1978.

Mucinoses

Cohn, B. A., Wheeler, C. E., Jr., and Briggaman, R. A. Scleredema adultorum of Buschke and diabetes mellitus. *Arch. Dermatol.* 101:27, 1970.

Farmer, E. R., Hambrick, G. W., and Shulman, L. E. Papular mucinosis: A clinicopathologic study of four patients. *Arch. Dermatol.* 118:9, 1982.

Johnson, W. C., Graham, J. H., and Helwig, E. B. Cutaneous myxoid cyst: A clinicopathological and histochemical study. *J.A.M.A.* 191:15, 1965.

Johnson, W. C., and Helwig, E. B. Cutaneous focal mucinosis: A clinicopathological and histochemical study. *Arch. Dermatol.* 93:13, 1966.

Lynch, P. J., Maize, J. C., and Sisson, J. C. Pretibial myxedema and nonthyrotoxic thyroid disease. *Arch. Dermatol.* 107:107, 1973.

Montgomery, H., and Underwood, L. J. Lichen myxedematosus (differentiation from cutaneous myxedemas or mucoid states). *J. Invest. Dermatol.* 20:213, 1953.

Reed, R. J., Clark, W. H., and Mihm, M. C. The cutaneous mucinoses. *Hum. Pathol.* 4:201, 1973.

Rudner, E. J., Mehregan, A., and Pinkus, H. Scleromyxedema: A variant of lichen myxedematosus. *Arch. Dermatol.* 93:3, 1966.

Gout

Lichtenstein, L., Scott, H. W., and Levin, M. H. Pathologic changes in gout. *Am. J. Pathol.* 32:871, 1956.

Calcinosis Cutis

Kolton, B., and Pedersen, J. Calcinosis cutis and renal failure. *Arch. Dermatol.* 110:256, 1974.

Whiting, D. A., Simson, I. W., Kalimeyer, J. C., et al. Unusual cutaneous lesions in tumoral calcinosis. *Arch. Dermatol.* 102:465, 1970.

Ochronosis

Lichtenstein, L., and Kaplan, L. Hereditary ochronosis. *Am. J. Pathol.* 30:99, 1954.

O'Brien, W. M., La Du, B. N., and Bunim, J. J. Biochemical, pathologic and clinical aspects of alcaptonuria, ochronosis and ochronotic arthropathy: Review of world literature (1584–1962). *Am. J. Med.* 34:813, 1963.

Hemochromatosis

Cawley, E. P., Hsu, Y. T., Wood, B. T., et al. Hemochromatosis and the skin. *Arch. Dermatol.* 100:1, 1969.

Chevrant-Breton, J., Simon, M., Bourel, M., and Ferrand, B. Cutaneous manifestations of idiopathic hemochromatosis, study of 100 cases. *Arch. Dermatol.* 113:161, 1977.

Perdrup, A., and Poulsen, H. Hemochromatosis and vitiligo. *Arch. Dermatol.* 90:34, 1964.

Tattoo

Rostenberg, A., Jr., Brown, R. A., and Caro, M. R. Discussion of tattoo reactions with report of a case showing a reaction to a green color. *Arch. Dermatol. Syphilol.* 62:540, 1950.

Taaffe, A., Knight, A. G., and Marks, R. Lichenoid tattoo hypersensitivity. *Br. Med. J.* 1:616, 1978.

Argyria

Hill, W. R., and Montgomery, H. Argyria (with special reference to the cutaneous histopathology). *Arch. Dermatol. Syphilol.* 44:588, 1941.

Mehta, A. C., Dawson-Butterworth, K., and Woodhouse, M. A. Argyria. Electron microscopic study of a case. *Br. J. Dermatol.* 78:175, 1966.

Pariser, R. J. Generalized argyria. Clinicopathologic features and histochemical studies. *Arch. Dermatol.* 114:373, 1978.

Lipoid Proteinosis

Caro, I. Lipoid proteinosis. *Int. J. Dermatol.* 17:388, 1978.

Van Der Walt, J. J., and Heyl, T. Lipoid proteinosis and erythropoietic protoporphyria: A histological and histochemical study. *Arch. Dermatol.* 104:501, 1971.

Chapter 20

Hyperplasias and Neoplasms

The Reactive Process and the Disease	Histopathology	Comments

I. Skin tag; acrochordon; soft fibroma	1. Polypoid structure with variable hyperplasia and hyperkeratosis of epidermal surface
	2. Central core composed of fibrovascular or fibrofatty tissue without adnexal structures
		Differential diagnosis:
		  Fibrosed pyogenic granuloma
		  Fibrous papule of the nose
		  Neurofibroma
		  Dermal nevus, pedunculated

II. Hypertrophic scar and keloid (Fig. 20-1)	1. Epidermis normal or flattened 2. Irregularly arranged, hyalinized collagen fibers of markedly variable shapes and sizes 3. Slight perivenular inflammatory infiltrate of lymphocytes and eosinophils at periphery of lesion may be present	

Fig. **20-1.**
A. *Keloid. These large, eosinophilic collagen bundles with a glassy, hyalinized appearance are characteristic. (approximately ×400)*
B. *Hypertrophic scar. The dense fibrous tissue frequently runs parallel to the surface in scars. The histologic patterns of keloid and hypertrophic scar often are mixed within a biopsy. (×400)*

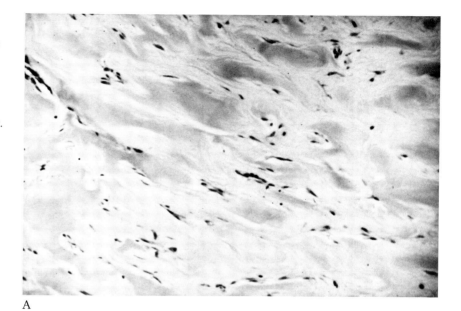

A

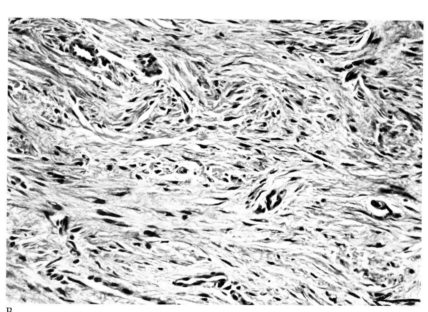

B

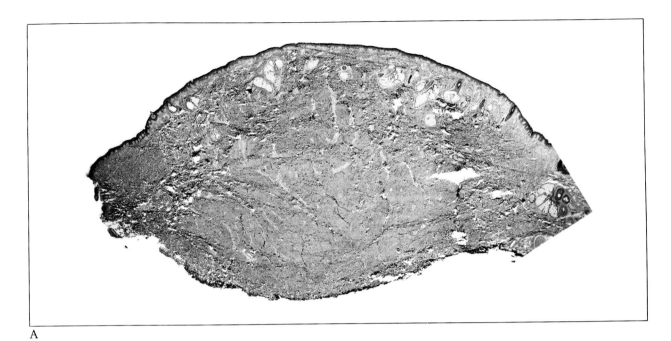

A

Fig. **20-2.** *Connective-tissue
nevus.*
A. *The nodular appearance of this
dermal hamartomatous
growth is evident in this low-
power micrograph. (×10)*
B. *Collagen bundles appear
smaller and vessels more
numerous and thick-walled
than usual. Alterations in collagen and elastic tissue vary in
type and degree in this disorder. (×400)*

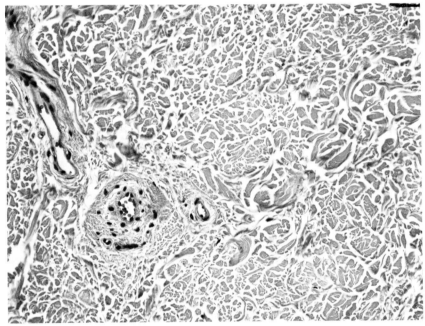

B

III. Connective-tissue nevus (Fig. 20-2)	1. Reticular dermis widened by increased collagen with normal, increased, or decreased number of elastic fibers	This lesion is essentially a hamartoma of connective tissue
IV. Neurofibroma (Fig. 20-3)	1. Discrete but nonencapsulated dermal mass composed of: 2. **Thin, wavy, faintly eosinophilic fibers** lying in loosely textured strands 3. Slender, oval to spindle-shaped, wavy nuclei 4. Focal areas of myxoid change occasionally present 5. Increased number of mast cells often present 6. Few nerves present; no demonstrable nerve trunks	Differential diagnosis: "Neurotized" nevus Neurilemmoma
V. Traumatic or amputation neuroma	1. Large, irregular bundles of peripheral nerves associated with considerable connective-tissue proliferation 2. Organization into bundles is a distinctive feature	Differential diagnosis: Neurofibroma Neurilemmoma Leiomyoma

Fig. **20-3.** *Neurofibroma. The elongated spindle cells have small nuclei that appear to loop and curl. The cells appear smaller than those of leiomyoma. Mucinous and edematous areas (not shown here) are common. (×400)*

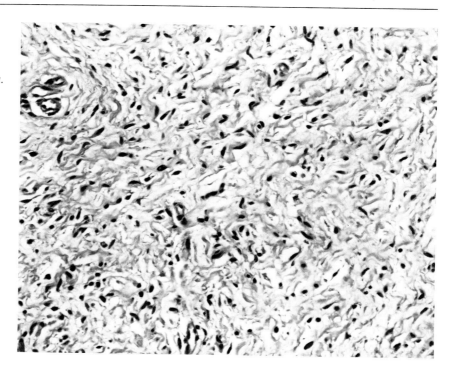

VI. Neurilemmoma;
schwannoma
(Fig. 20-4)

1. Circumscribed spindle cell (Schwann cell) proliferation with a reticulin and collagenous matrix
2. Antoni A and Antoni B areas with Verocay bodies
3. Few nerves present within lesion; however, nerve trunks can be demonstrated adjacent to capsule if included in the excision
4. Mast cells may be numerous

Cells with closely apposed nuclei in parallel array are called Antoni A areas; mucinous edematous stroma with scattered cells is called an Antoni B area; rows of palisaded nuclei that are parallel but separated by an acellular matrix are called Verocay bodies

Bodian stain shows few nerves present

Fig. **20-4.** *Neurilemmoma.*
  A. When well-developed, this spindle cell tumor exhibits Antoni A and B patterns. The former refers to areas of loose, edematous connective tissue; the latter, to foci of nuclear palisading. (×160)
B,C. Two nuclear palisades enclosing a relatively anuclear central area are called a Verocay body. (C, ×400)

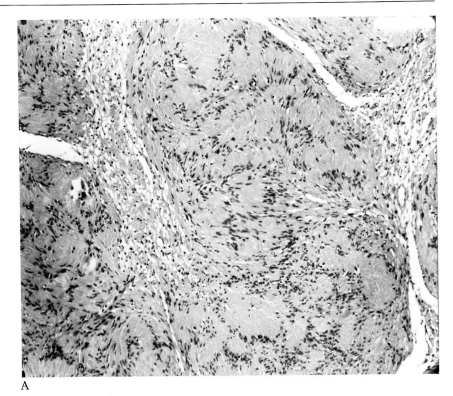

A

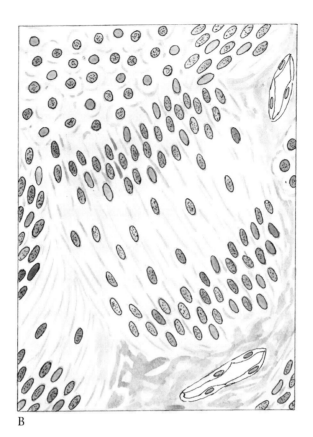

B

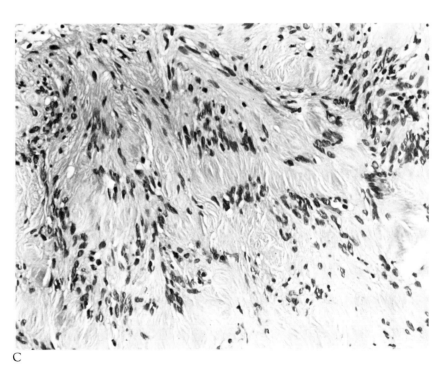

C

VII. Leiomyoma (Fig. 20-5)

1. Bundles of spindle-shaped cells with abundant cytoplasm and oval, cigar-shaped nuclei
2. In cross section, nuclei appear round and in the center of the cell
3. Leiomyomas, as they age, may undergo mucoidedematous changes and fibrosis

Differential diagnosis:
Neurofibroma
Neurilemmoma

Special stains help confirm the diagnosis; with the trichrome stain, smooth muscle appears pink to red and collagen appears blue green; using the van Gieson stain, muscle and nerves appear yellow and collagen appears red

VIII. Dermatofibroma—fibrous histiocytoma group (Fig. 20-6)

1. Overlying epidermis commonly (80%) shows elongated rete ridges and increased melanin in basal layer (so-called "dirty fingers")
2. Tumor composed of spindle cells and histiocytes
3. Cellularity varies; spindle cells often interspersed between collagen bundles
4. Spindle cells commonly arranged in whorled, cartwheel patterns

Differential diagnosis:
Scar
Leiomyoma
Xanthoma
Desmoid tumor
Dermatofibrosarcoma protuberans
Fibrosarcoma
Neurofibroma
Cellular blue nevus
Kaposi's sarcoma

Fig. **20-5.** *Leiomyoma. This spindle cell tumor has abundant eosinophilic cytoplasm and cigar-shaped nuclei. Compared with neurofibroma, these cells are larger, the cytoplasm is more abundant, and the shape of these cells is larger and less contorted. (×400)*

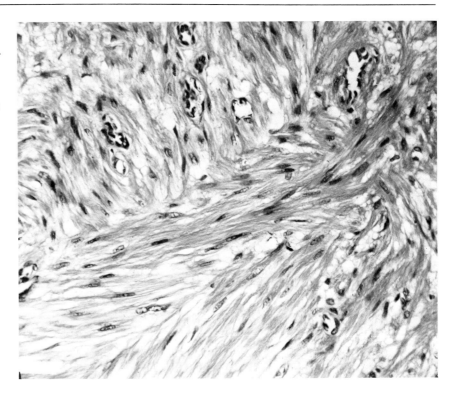

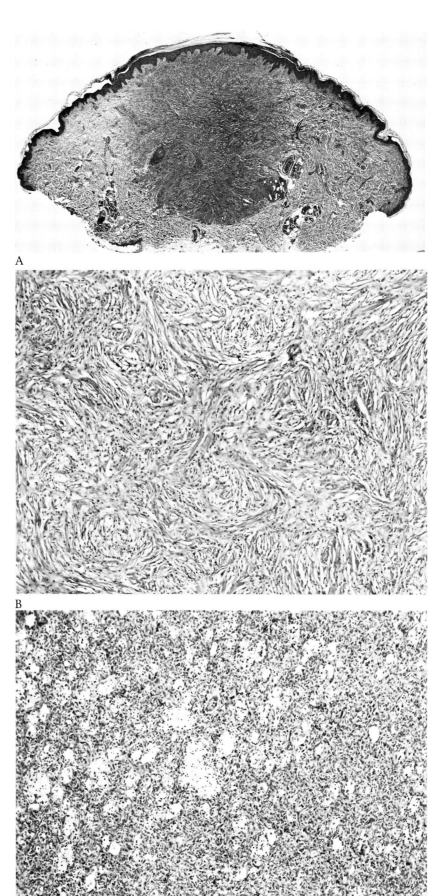

Fig. **20-6.** *Fibrous histiocytoma (and dermatofibroma). The cellular area within the dermis is usually capped by epidermal hyperplasia (A). The dermis exhibits a spindle cell proliferation with a cartwheel or storiform pattern (B) or a dense proliferation of commalike cells, sometimes admixed with foam cells (C). The former pattern is called* fibrous histiocytoma *and the latter,* dermatofibroma, *but the terms often are used interchangeably. (A, ×13; B, ×100; C, ×100)*

A

B

C

	5. Multinucleate giant cells, frequently Touton type, may be present 6. Tumor may involve deep dermis and rarely subcutaneous fat 7. Hemosiderin commonly present within histiocytes	If many histiocytes are present, the lesion can be called a histiocytoma; if numerous vessels are present, the lesion can be called a sclerosing hemangioma; and if many comma-shaped spindle cells are present, the lesion can be called a dermatofibroma

IX. Dermatofibrosarcoma protuberans	1. Epidermis normal, atrophic, or ulcerated
	2. Spindle cells commonly arranged in cartwheel pattern
	3. **Slight to moderate nuclear pleomorphism**
	4. **Mitoses frequently present**
	5. Giant cells and foam cells rare
	6. Lesion present in **deep dermis and subcutaneous tissue** but may involve fascia
		Differential diagnosis:
		  Dermatofibroma
		  Fibrosarcoma

X. Desmoid tumor	1. Dense cellular proliferation of fibroblasts in collagen, which is arranged in interlacing bundles
	2. Rare to moderate mitoses present
	3. Tumor tends to invade surrounding structures, especially skeletal muscle
	4. Mucoid alteration and calcification may be observed
		Desmoid tumors arise from "muscular" aponeurosis and are commonly associated with pregnancy and Gardner's syndrome
		
		Pleomorphism and atypical mitoses are not present in desmoid tumors
		
		Differential diagnosis:
		  Nodular fasciitis
		  Palmar-plantar fibromatosis

XI. Fibrosarcoma		

A. Typical	1. Densely cellular tumor composed of spindle cells
	2. Nuclei are pleomorphic and are arranged in a **herringbone** pattern
	3. Mitoses usually numerous; atypical mitoses often seen
	4. Tumor arises from fascia or deep subcutis and rarely from the reticular dermis
		Reticulin stain frequently reveals many reticulin fibers
		
		Differential diagnosis:
		  Leiomyosarcoma
		  Malignant schwannoma
		  Spindle cell squamous carcinoma
		  Malignant melanoma, desmoplastic type
		  Dermatofibrosarcoma protuberans
		  Desmoid tumor
		  Malignant fibrous histiocytoma

B. Fibroxanthosarcoma; malignant fibrous histiocytoma (Fig. 20-8)	1. Pleomorphic, spindle-shaped cells with cartwheel pattern
	2. Mitoses frequent; some atypical
	3. Bizarre giant cells
	4. Foam cells variably present
		Differential diagnosis:
		  Fibrous histiocytoma
		  Atypical fibroxanthoma (Fig. 20-7)

Fig. **20-7.** *Atypical fibroxan-thoma. This tumor exhibits a proliferation of spindle cells and histiocytes, several with multinucleate and large, bizarre nuclei. (A, ×160; B, ×400)*

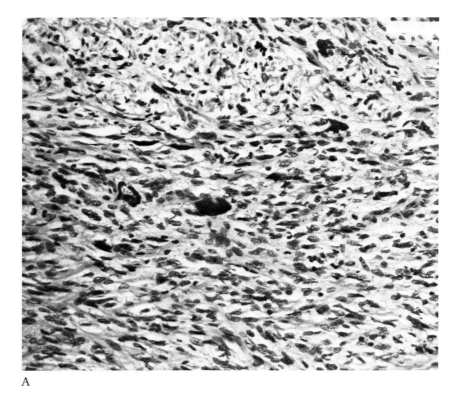

A

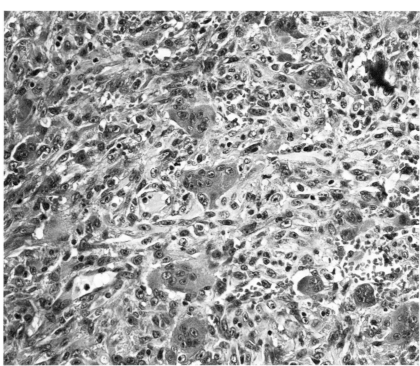

B

Fig. **20-8.** *Malignant fibrous histiocytoma.*
A. *A storiform pattern usually can be found. The dense lymphocytic infiltrates among the spindled tumor cells are not unusual. (×160)*
B. *Extremely bizarre and pleomorphic cytologic features and numerous atypical mitoses are common. (×256)*

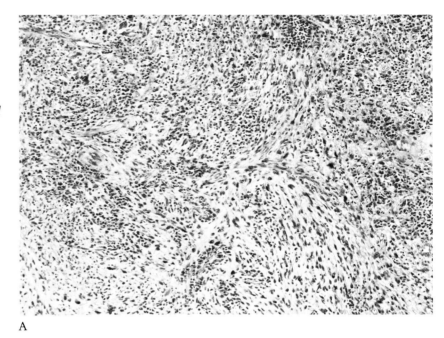

A

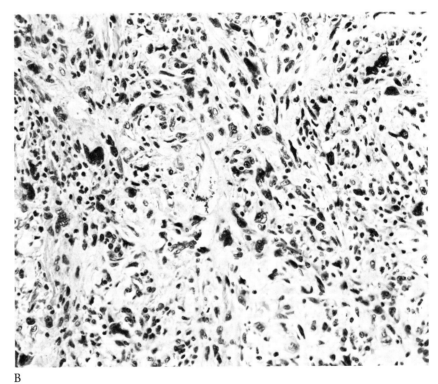

B

XII. Epithelioid cell sarcoma

1. Epithelioid and spindle-shaped cells with eosinophilic cytoplasm palisade about a zone of altered "necrobiotic" collagen
2. Variable nuclear pleomorphism with frequent and prominent mitoses
3. Spindle-shaped and epithelioid cells associated with a variably hyalinized stroma

Differential diagnosis:
    Palisading granulomas
    Infectious granulomas with fibrosis

Areas of necrosis may exhibit calcification.

XIII. Granular cell tumor (Fig. 20-9)

1. Epidermal hyperplasia, often marked, with increased melanin in basal layer
2. Distinctive, large, polygonal tumor cells with abundant, **pale eosinophilic granular cytoplasm:** small, dark, centrally placed nuclei; and usually distinct cytoplasmic membrane
3. Cells may be arranged in sheets or cords or individually dispersed between collagen or muscle fibers

The cytoplasmic granules are PAS-positive and diastase-resistant and also stain with colloidal iron and PTAH

Differential diagnosis:
    Xanthoma
    Lepromatous leprosy

Granular cell tumors occur commonly in the tongue

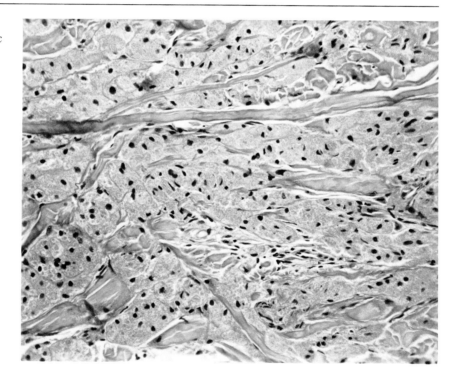

Fig. **20-9.** *Granular cell tumor. Polygonal cells with eosinophilic granular cytoplasm and small, dark nuclei are present within the dermis, infiltrating among collagen bundles. (×256)*

XIV. Pyogenic granuloma	1. Thin, often ulcerated epidermis, which may form a lateral collarette 2. Proliferation of capillaries with variable endothelial swelling and variable ectasia 3. Acute inflammation and stromal edema commonly associated with epidermal ulceration	Lesions are often elevated above the surface of the normal adjacent skin and may even be pedunculated
XV. Hemangioma		
A. Capillary (Fig. 20-10)	1. Overlying epidermis normal or flattened 2. Dermal proliferation of **capillary-sized, endothelial cell–lined** vessels	Depending on clinical features such as the age of the lesion and the patient's age when the lesion developed, these vessels may be thin-walled (mature juvenile capillary hemangioma, cherry hemangioma, nevus flammeus) or lined and surrounded by plump endothelial cells (immature juvenile capillary hemangioma)
B. Cavernous	Deep, dermal and/or subcutaneous proliferation of large, irregular, blood-filled vascular spaces lined by a single layer of endothelial cells surrounded by fibromuscular tissue	
XVI. Angiokeratoma (Fig. 20-11)	1. Exophytic structure composed of hyperkeratosis overlying epidermal hyperplasia and closely apposed, dilated, thin-walled capillary spaces 2. Blood and sometimes thrombus fills the capillaries 3. Dermal collagen appears normal	Differential diagnosis: Lymphangioma circumscriptum Chronic radiodermatitis
XVII. Lymphangioma circumscriptum (Fig. 20-12)	1. Epidermis appears thin, normal, or hyperplastic 2. Numerous dilated lymphatic channels are present in the upper dermis, usually in close approximation to the epidermis 3. Lymphatic channels in this area of the dermis have extremely thin walls lined by a single layer of endothelial cells; valves also may be observed 4. Within the lymphatic channels is lymph and/or blood 5. Communication with deep, thick-walled vessels is common but may not be apparent on histologic section	Differential diagnosis: Angiokeratoma Chronic radiodermatitis

Fig. **20-10.** *Hemangioma. (×100)*

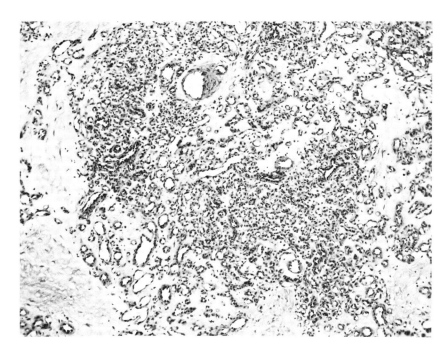

Fig. **20-11.** *Angiokeratoma. A proliferation of ectatic capillaries is capped by mildly acanthotic epidermis. (×160)*

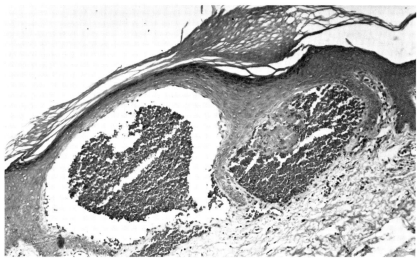

Fig. **20-12.** *Lymphangioma circumscriptum. Numerous thin-walled, dilated lymphatic channels with valves are located high in the dermis, apparently pushing up the epidermis. (×27)*

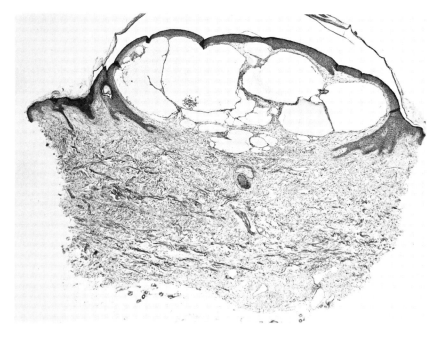

XVIII. Hemangiopericytoma

1. Epidermis normal
2. Dermal proliferation of spindle-shaped or oval pericytes surrounding numerous vessels
3. Pericytes may exhibit pleomorphism

Reticulum stain demarcates endothelial cells and vessel wall from proliferating pericytes

Differential diagnosis:
Glomus tumor
Hemangioendothelioma
Hemangioendotheliosarcoma

XIX. Glomus tumor (Fig. 20-13)

1. Small, endothelial cell–lined vessels surrounded by dense proliferation of glomus cells
2. **Glomus cells** are distinctive, large, polygonal cells with clear or faintly eosinophilic cytoplasm, distinct cell walls, and large, round basophilic nuclei
3. Areas of mucoid degeneration often present
4. Fibrous capsule present

Glomus tumors usually present as solitary, painful lesions on the digits

Bodian stain reveals numerous nerve fibers in the perivascular stroma

XX. Glomangioma (multiple glomus tumors)

1. Circumscribed but not encapsulated tumors
2. Many large, blood-filled, endothelial cell–lined vascular channels
3. Variable numbers of glomus cells surround vascular channels

The presence of glomus cells around the vessels differentiates a glomangioma from a hemangioma; Bodian stain negative

XXI. Kaposi's sarcoma (Fig. 20-14)

1. Proliferation of spindle cells arranged in irregular fascicles
2. **Erythrocyte-filled slits** form between spindle cells; these channels characteristically are *not* lined by endothelial cells
3. Proliferation of capillaries with prominent endothelial cells
4. **Extravasated erythrocytes with variable hemosiderin deposition**
5. Variable mononuclear cell infiltrate
6. Fibrosis

Early lesions often difficult to differentiate from stasis dermatitis or granulation tissue

Differential diagnosis:
Fibrosarcoma
Spindle cell squamous carcinoma
Hemangiopericytoma
Angiosarcoma
Melanoma, desmoplastic type
Dermatofibroma, sclerosing hemangioma type

Fig. **20-13.** *Glomus tumor. Numerous cells with bland, homogeneous nuclei surround these vascular spaces. (×100) See also Figure 1-4, glomus cells.*

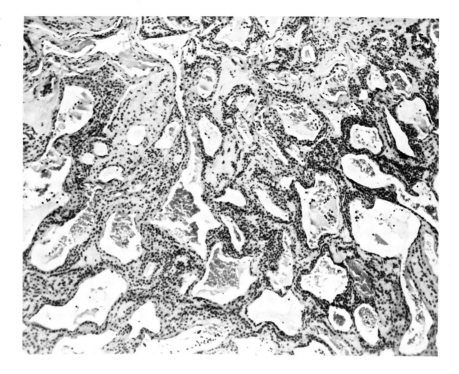

Fig. **20-14.** *Kaposi's sarcoma. Irregular bands of spindle cells with atypical hyperchromatic nuclei, poorly defined vascular spaces lined by atypical endothelial cells, and erythrocytes in slit-like openings are characteristic. (×400)*

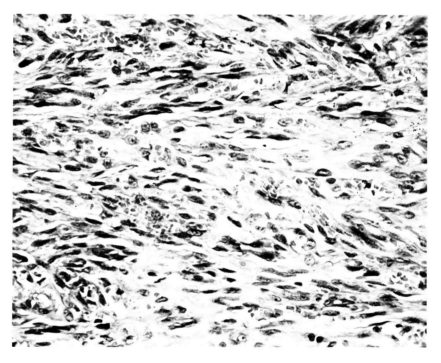

Fig. **20-15.** *Stasis dermatitis. Dermal fibrosis and thick-walled vessels (A,B) with numerous hemosiderin-laden microphages (B) are typical. (A, ×160; B, ×400)*

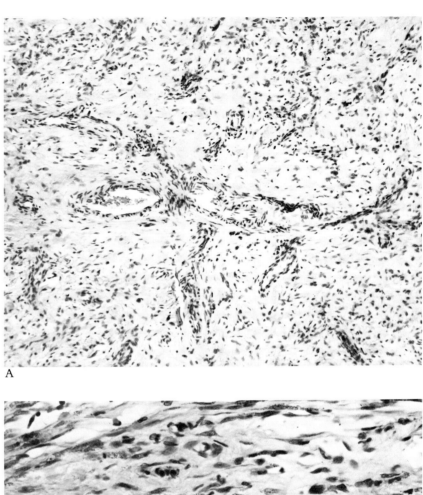

A

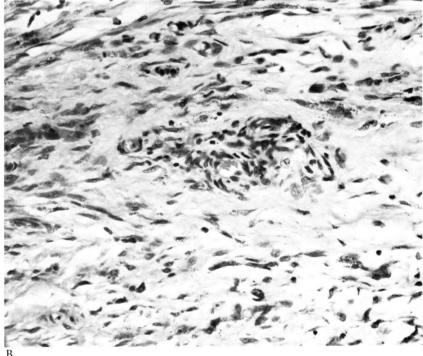

B

XXII. Stasis dermatitis, late stage (Fig. 20-15)

1. Flattened to atrophic epidermis, occasionally with spongiosis
2. **Focal proliferation of capillaries** throughout papillary and reticular dermis
3. **Thickened vessel walls**
4. Dermal **fibrosis**
5. **Hemorrhage and hemosiderin deposition** common
6. Variable mononuclear cell infiltrate

See also Ch. 14, I.B.7

XXIII. Metastatic carcinoma (Fig. 20-16)

1. Malignant tumor cells with hyperchromatic, large nuclei infiltrate and displace collagen bundles
2. Some tumors are associated with a fibroblastic (desmoplastic) response
3. Metastases frequently but not always exhibit histologic similarities to the primary tumor

Fig. **20-16.** *Adenocarcinoma of the breast metastatic to skin. Nests of tumor cells with hyperchromatic nuclei dissect between collagen bundles. (×160)*

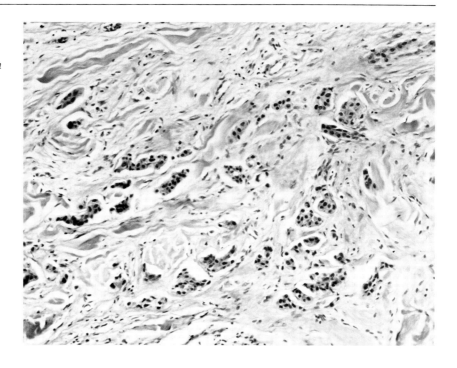

Suggested Reading
Hypertrophic Scar and Keloid

Linares, H. A., Kischer, C. W., Dobrkovsky, M., et al. The histiotypic organization of the hypertrophic scar in humans. *J. Invest. Dermatol.* 59:323, 1972.
Linares, H. A., and Larson, D. L. Early differential diagnosis between hypertrophic and nonhypertrophic healing. *J. Invest. Dermatol.* 62:514, 1974.

Connective-Tissue Nevus

Raque, C. J., and Wood, M. G. Connective-tissue nevus. *Arch. Dermatol.* 102:390, 1970.
Schorr, W. F., Optiz, J. M., and Reyes, C. N. The connective tissue nevus–osteopoikilosis syndrome. *Arch. Dermatol.* 106:208, 1972.

Neurofibroma

Brasfield, R. D., and Das Gupta, T. K. Von Recklinghausen's disease: A clinicopathological study. *Ann. Surg.* 175:86, 1972.
Crowe, F. W., Schull, . J., and Neel, J. V. *A Clinical, Pathological and Genetic Study of Multiple Neurofibromatosis.* Springfield, Ill.: Thomas, 1956.
Reed, R. J. Cutaneous manifestations of neural crest disorders (neurocristopathies). *Int. J. Dermatol.* 16:807, 1977.

Neuroma

Reed, R. J., Fine, R. M., and Meltzer, H. D. Palisaded, encapsulated neuromas of the skin. *Arch. Dermatol.* 106:865, 1972.

Neurilemmoma

Das Guptas, T. K., Brasfield, R. D., Strong, E. W., et al. Benign solitary schwannomas (neurilemmomas). *Cancer* 24:355, 1969.

Leiomyoma

Fisher, W. C., and Helwig, E. B. Leiomyomas of the skin. *Arch. Dermatol.* 88:510, 1963.

Dermatofibroma

Goette, D. K., and Helwig, E. B. Basal cell carcinomas and basal cell carcinomalike changes overlying dermatofibromas. *Arch. Dermatol.* 111:589, 1975.
Rentiers, P. L., and Montgomery, H. Nodular subepidermal fibrosis (dermatofibroma versus histiocytoma). *Arch. Dermatol. Syphilol.* 59:568, 1949.

Dermatofibrosarcoma Protuberans

Hashimoto, K., Brownstein, M. H., and Jakobiec, F. A. Dermatofibrosarcoma protuberans. *Arch. Dermatol.* 110:874, 1974.
Taylor, H. B., and Helwig, E. B. Dermatofibrosarcoma protuberans: A study of 115 cases. *Cancer* 15:717, 1962.

Desmoid Tumor

Gonatas, N. K. Extra-abdominal desmoid tumors: Report of six cases. *Arch. Pathol.* 71:214, 1961.
Weary, P. E., Linthicum, A., Cawley, E. P., et al. Gardner's syndrome. A family group study and review. *Arch. Dermatol.* 90:20, 1964.

Fibrosarcoma

Gentele, H. Malignant, fibroblastic tumors of the skin. *Acta Derm. Venereol. (Stockh.)* 31 (Suppl. 27):1, 1951.
Pritchard, D. J., Soule, E. H., Taylor, W. F., et al. Fibrosarcoma—A clinicopathologic and statistical study of 199 tumors of the soft tissues of the extremities and trunk. *Cancer* 33:888, 1974.

Epithelioid Cell Sarcoma

Frable, W. J., Kay, S., Lawrence, W., et al. Epithelioid sarcoma. *Arch. Pathol.* 95:8, 1973.
Santiago, H., Feinerman, L. K., and Lattes, R. Epithelioid sarcoma. A clinical and pathologic study of nine cases. *Hum. Pathol.* 3:133, 1972.

Granular Cell Tumor

Alkek, D. S., Johnson, W. C., and Graham, J. H. Granular cell myoblastoma: A histological and enzymatic study. *Arch. Dermatol.* 98:543, 1968.
Armin, A., Connelly, E. M., and Rowden, G. An immunoperoxidase investigation of S-100 protein in granular cell myoblastomas: Evidence for Schwann cell derivation. *Am. J. Clin. Pathol.* 79:37, 1983.

Pyogenic Granuloma	Hare, P. J. Granuloma pyogenicum. *Br. J. Dermatol.* 83:513, 1970. Zaynoun, S. T., Juljulian, H. H., and Kurban, A. K. Pyogenic granuloma with multiple satellites. *Arch. Dermatol.* 109:689, 1974.
Hemangiopericytoma	Angervall, L., Kindblom, L. G., Nielsen, J. M., et al. Hemangiopericytoma: A clinicopathologic, angiographic and microangiographic study. *Cancer* 42:2412, 1978. O'Brien, P., and Brasfield, R. D. Hemangiopericytoma. *Cancer* 18:249, 1965.
Glomus Tumor and Glomangioma	Gordon, B., and Hyman, A. B. Multiple nontender glomus tumors. *Arch. Dermatol.* 83:640, 1961. Pepper, M. C., Laubenheimer, R., and Cripps, D. J. Multiple glomus tumors. *J. Cutan. Pathol.* 4:244, 1977.
Kaposi's Sarcoma	Cox, F. H., and Helwig, E. B. Kaposi's sarcoma. *Cancer* 12:289, 1959. Harwood, A. R., Osoba, D., Hofstader, S. L., et al. Kaposi's sarcoma in recipients of renal transplants. *Am. J. Med.* 67:759, 1979. Hymes, K. B., Cheung, T., Greene, J. B., et al. Kaposi's sarcoma in homosexual men—a report of eight cases. *Lancet* 2:598, 1981. O'Connell, K. M. Kaposi's sarcoma: Histopathological study of 159 cases from Malawi. *J. Clin. Pathol.* 30:687, 1977. O'Connell, K. M. Kaposi's sarcoma in lymph nodes: Histological study of lesions from 16 cases in Malawi. *J. Clin. Pathol.* 30:696, 1977. Templeton, A. C. Studies in Kaposi's sarcoma. *Cancer* 30:854, 1972.
General	Enzinger, F. M., and Weiss, S. W. *Soft Tissue Tumors.* St. Louis: Mosby, 1983. Harkin, J. C., and Reed, R. J. *Tumors of the Peripheral Nervous System.* Washington, D.C.: Armed Forces Institute of Pathology, 1969. Mackenzie, D. H. *The Differential Diagnosis of Fibroblastic Disorders.* Oxford: Blackwell, 1970. Russell, D. S., and Rubinstein, L. J. *Pathology of Tumors of the Nervous System* (3d ed.). Baltimore: Williams & Wilkins, 1971. Stout, A. P., and Lattes, R. *Tumors of the Soft Tissues* (revised ed.). Washington, D.C.: Armed Forces Institute of Pathology, 1983.

Chapter 21

Cysts in the Dermis

I. Epidermal inclusion cyst
II. Pilar cyst
III. Steatocystoma
IV. Dermoid cyst
V. Hidrocystoma
   A. Eccrine
   B. Apocrine
VI. Vellus hair cyst
VII. Ganglion cyst

The Reactive Process and the Disease	Histopathology	Comments
I. Epidermal inclusion cyst (Figs. 21-1, 21-2A)	1. Cyst wall lined with normal epidermis, including a **granular layer** 2. Cyst contains eosinophilic, often laminated, keratinous material 3. Rupture of cyst results in inflammatory infiltrate with multinucleate foreign-body giant cells	See Table 21-1 for comparison of histologic features of dermal cysts Very small epidermal inclusion cysts are called *milia* The presence of a granular cell layer and visible intercellular bridges are features that distinguish an epidermal inclusion cyst from a pilar cyst
II. Pilar cyst (Figs. 21-1, 21-2B)	1. Cyst wall composed of eosinophilic keratinocytes which do not form a granular layer 2. Cell borders indistinct; **no visible intercellular bridges** 3. Cyst contains amorphous eosinophilic material and parakeratotic nuclear remnants 4. Focal calcification of cyst contents may occur	Pilar and epidermal inclusion cysts are indistinguishable clinically
III. Steatocystoma (Fig. 21-2C)	1. Folded, or convoluted, cyst wall composed of keratinocytes with peripheral palisading basal cells and no apparent intracellular bridges 2. Amorphous eosinophilic keratin layer centrally 3. Cyst may contain hair 4. Characteristically, **sebaceous gland lobules** are present adjacent to or within the cyst wall	
IV. Dermoid cyst	1. Cyst wall lined by epidermis with mature appendages (hair follicles, sebaceous glands, and rarely apocrine glands) 2. Cyst cavity usually contains hair	These lesions, which occur most commonly on the face, often are present at birth

Fig. **21-1.** *Comparison of epidermal inclusion and pilar cysts. In the former, cells flatten as they mature and form a granular layer with recognizable squames (*left*). In the pilar cyst, the more rounded cells mature without a granular layer and form a solid-appearing keratin product (*right*).*

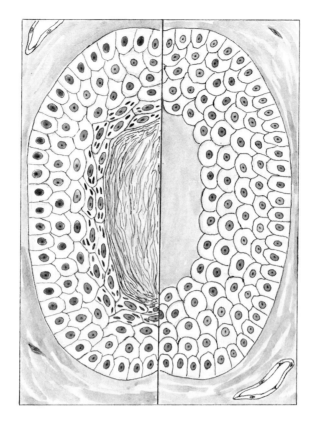

Table **21-1.** *Histologic Features Differentiating Cysts in the Dermis*

	Epidermal Inclusion Cyst	Pilar Cyst	Steatocystoma	Dermoid Cyst	Hidrocystoma	Vellus Hair Cyst	Ganglion
Cyst wall	Normal epidermis; granular layer present	Peripherally palisading eosinophilic cells with no visible intercellular bridges; no granular layer present	Convoluted or wavy wall composed of basophilic cells without visible intercellular bridges; eosinophilic cuticle centrally	Normal epidermis	Cuboidal (eccrine) or columnar (apocrine) cells; decapitation secretion of columnar cells observed	Normal epidermis	Dense, fibrous connective tissue
Cyst contents	Laminated, eosinophilic, keratinous material	Homogeneous, eosinophilic, amorphous material	Hairs may be present	May contain hair	Granular, amorphous, pale, eosinophilic material	Laminated, eosinophilic, keratinous material; numerous small vellus hairs	Myxoid, slightly basophilic, amorphous material
Appendages adjacent to or within	None	None	Sebaceous glands adjacent to or within cyst wall	Mature pilosebaceous units attach to cyst wall and open into lumen	None	Hair follicle occasionally attached to cyst wall	None
Other		Focal calcification of cyst contents common		Subcutaneous location	Outer layer of myoepithelial cells		

Fig. **21-2.** *Epidermal cysts.*
A. *Epidermal inclusion cyst.*
   (×256)
B. *Pilar cyst. (×256)*
C. *Steatocystoma. The folded*
   wall of the cyst is lined by
   stratified squamous
   epithelium, and sebaceous
   glands open into the lumen.
   (×64)
D. *Vellus hair cyst. The appear-*
   ance is similar to that of epi-
   dermal inclusion cyst, but the
   lumen contains numerous vel-
   lus hairs. (×160)

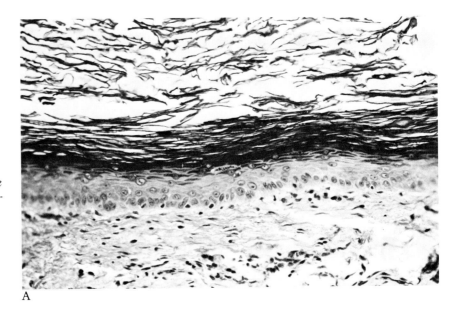

A

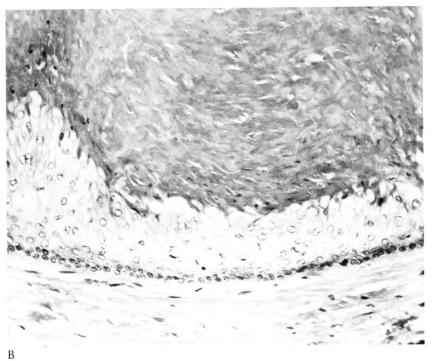

B

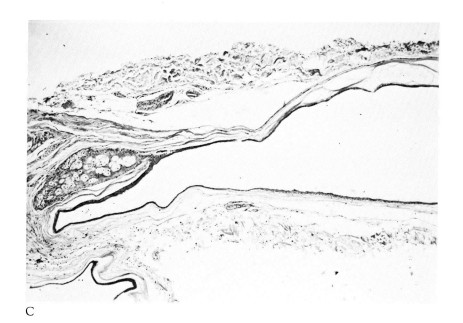

C

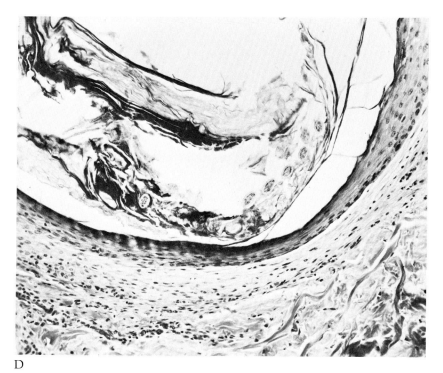

D

Fig. **21-3.** *Hidrocystoma, proba-bly eccrine. (A, approximately ×10; B, approximately ×400)*

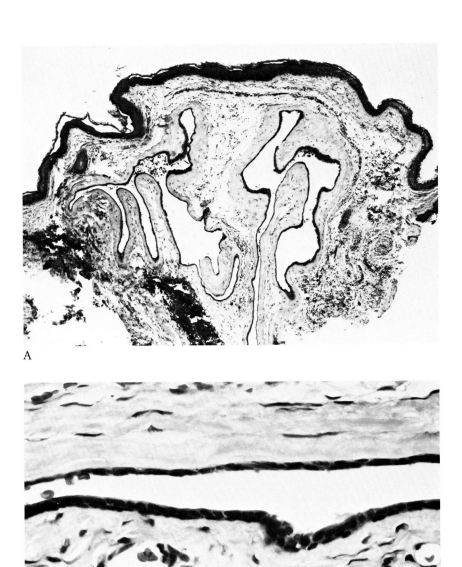

A

B

V. Hidrocystoma

    A. Eccrine (Fig. 21-3)

        1. Unilocular or multilocular intradermal cyst

        2. Cyst wall composed of one or two layers of cuboidal or flattened, eccrine epithelial cells

    B. Apocrine

        1. Large cystic spaces within the dermis

        2. Papillary projections into lumen

        3. Cyst wall composed of one or more layers of columnar cells, which exhibit "decapitation" secretion

        4. Myoepithelial cells are located peripheral to the columnar cells

        5. Loose stroma around cyst often contains extravasated erythrocytes

This lesion often presents clinically as a slowly enlarging gray or bluish, soft cystic nodule on the scalp or face

VI. Vellus hair cyst (Fig. 21-2D)

        1. Small cyst in middle dermis lined with normal epidermis

        2. Cyst contains eosinophilic, laminated keratinous material and numerous small vellus hairs

        3. Hair follicle occasionally attached to cyst wall

The presence of multiple small hairs within the cyst differentiates this lesion from an epidermal inclusion cyst

VII. Ganglion cyst (Fig. 21-4)

        1. Cystic space or spaces filled with myxoid material and surrounded by fibrous wall

        2. Located in proximity to synovium, joint capsule, or other dense collagenous tissue

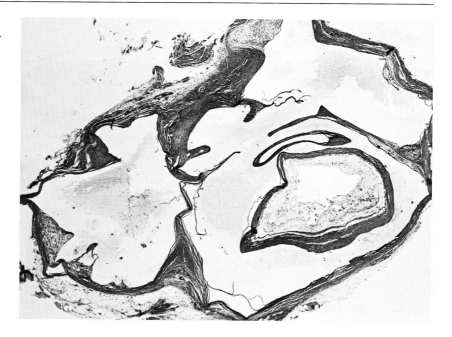

Fig. **21-4.** *Ganglion cyst. Mucoid material is present within a multilocular cyst, the walls of which are composed of fibrous tissue, probably related to joint capsule or tendon (×22).*

Suggested Reading
Epidermal Inclusion and Pilar Cysts

McGavran, M. H., and Binnington, B. Keratinous cysts of the skin: Identification and differentiation of pilar cysts from epidermal cysts. *Arch. Dermatol.* 94:499, 1966.

Rahbari, H. Epidermoid cysts with seborrheic verruca-like cyst walls. *Arch. Dermatol.* 118:326, 1982.

Steatocystoma

Brownstein, M. H. Steatocystoma simplex. A solitary steatocystoma. *Arch. Dermatol.* 118:409, 1982.

Marley, W. M., Buntin, D. M., and Chesney, T. M. Steatocystoma multiplex limited to the scalp. *Arch. Dermatol.* 117:673, 1981.

Schiff, B. L., Kern, A.B., and Ronchese, F. Steatocystoma multiplex. *Arch. Dermatol.* 77:516, 1958.

Dermoid Cyst

Brownstein, M. H., and Helwig, E. B. Subcutaneous dermoid cysts. *Arch. Dermatol.* 107:237, 1973.

Hidrocystoma

Smith, J. D., and Chernosky, M. E. Hidrocystomas. *Arch. Dermatol.* 108:676, 1973.

Smith, J. D., and Chernosky, M. E. Apocrine hydrocystoma (cystadenoma). *Arch. Dermatol.* 109:700, 1974.

Vellus Hair Cyst

Esterly, N. B., Fretzin, D. F., and Pinkus, H. Eruptive vellous hair cysts. *Arch. Dermatol.* 113:500, 1977.

Lee, S., and Kim, J-G. Eruptive vellus hair cyst. Clinical and histologic finding. *Arch. Dermatol.* 115:744, 1979.

Stiefler, R. E., and Bergfeld, W. F. Eruptive vellus hair cysts—An inherited disorder. *J. Am. Acad. Dermatol.* 3:425, 1980.

Part **V**

Appendages

Chapter 22

Disorders of the
Pilosebaceous Unit

I. Inflammatory reactions
  A. Follicular eczema
  B. Folliculitis
    1. Acute superficial
    2. Acute deep
    3. Chronic deep
  C. Perforating folliculitis
  D. Majocchi's granuloma
  E. Alopecia mucinosa
  F. Pityriasis rubra pilaris (PRP)
  G. Lupus erythematosus
  H. Lichen planopilaris
  I. Pseudopalade of Broque
  J. Alopecia areata
II. Hyperplasia and neoplasms
  A. Nevus sebaceus
    1. Childhood
    2. Adolescent and adult
  B. Sebaceous hyperplasia
  C. Sebaceous adenoma
  D. Sebaceous epithelioma
  E. Sebaceous carcinoma
  F. Trichofolliculoma
  G. Pilar tumor
  H. Trichilemmoma
  I. Trichoepithelioma
  J. Pilomatrixoma (calcifying epithelioma of Malherbe)

The Reactive Process and the Disease	Histopathology	Comments
I. Inflammatory reactions		
A. Follicular eczema	1. **Spongiosis** prominent, sometimes exclusively in follicular epithelium 2. Migration of lymphocytes and histiocytes into follicle	Differential diagnosis: alopecia mucinosa
B. Folliculitis		
1. Acute superficial	1. Subcorneal pustule present at follicular orifice 2. Perifollicular neutrophilic infiltration usually present	
2. Acute deep	1. Perifollicular abscess associated with destruction of follicle wall and sebaceous gland	
3. Chronic deep	1. Intrafollicular abscess frequently present 2. Perifollicular infiltrate of neutrophils, lymphocytes, histiocytes, plasma cells, and foreign-body giant cells 3. Variable fibrosis, sometimes even keloid formation	This type of folliculitis commonly affects the beard area (folliculitis barbae) and/or scalp (folliculitis decalvans, folliculitis keloidalis nuchae)
C. Perforating folliculitis	1. Dilated hair follicle filled with keratin, parakeratotic cells and sometimes degenerated collagen, and brightly eosinophilic elastic fibers 2. A curled-up hair is often present within the mass of material described above 3. Perforation of follicular epithelium occurs in the upper one-third of the follicle where brightly eosinophilic fibers bridge the wall	Differential diagnosis: Kyrle's disease Elastosis perforans serpiginosa Reactive perforating collagenosis
D. Majocchi's granuloma (Fig. 22-1)	1. Hyperkeratosis and variable epidermal hyperplasia 2. Dense, perifollicular and intrafollicular, lymphohistiocytic and eosinophilic infiltrate 3. Giant cells occasionally present, especially if follicle has ruptured 4. Septate hyphae present within hair, follicle, and/or perifollicular infiltrate	Organisms best visualized with special stains (see Appendix)

Fig. **22-1.** *Majocchi's granuloma. An acutely inflamed pilosebaceous follicle has ruptured, spilling its inflammatory contents including hyphal forms into the dermis (A), which apparently elicits a further inflammatory response. The hair and keratinaceous material contain numerous hyphal forms (B). (A, ×100; B, ×640)*

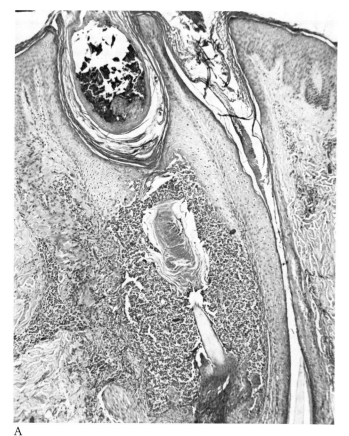

A

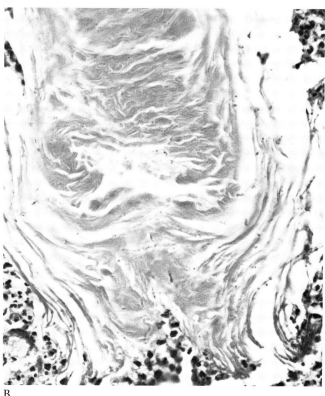

B

E. Alopecia mucinosa (Fig. 22-2)	1. **Mucin deposition** between epithelial cells results in a reticulate appearance to portions of the **hair follicle and sebaceous glands**	Mucin demonstrated with colloidal iron, Giemsa, or alcian blue stains
	2. Extent of inflammation variable; infiltrate composed of lymphocytes, histiocytes, and occasional eosinophils	Twenty percent of cases with adult-onset alopecia mucinosa are associated with mycosis fungoides; in these cases atypical mononuclear cells ("mycosis cells") are present in the infiltrate
F. Pityriasis rubra pilaris (PRP)	1. Hyperkeratosis and spotty parakeratosis	The histology of pityriasis rubra pilaris may be indistinguishable from that of psoriasis or chronic eczematous dermatitis
	2. Perifollicular psoriasiform hyperplasia	
	3. Focal "shoulder" parakeratosis sometimes present at follicular opening	
	4. Mild perivascular mononuclear cell infiltrate	See also Ch. 4, I.F
	5. Vascular ectasia	
G. Lupus erythematosus (see Fig. 9-3)	Follicular plugging seen in addition to other characteristic changes	See also Ch. 7, VI; Ch. 9, I.D, II.D; Ch. 10, III; Ch. 14, I.B.1
H. Lichen planopilaris	1. Follicular plug	
	2. Around lower one-third of follicle there is a bandlike, "hugging" mononuclear cell infiltrate	
	3. Dermal fibrosis and absence of hair follicles and sebaceous glands characteristic of end-stage lesions	
I. Pseudopalade of Broque (Fig. 22-3)	1. Epidermis normal	
	2. Sebaceous glands absent	
	3. Hair follicle changes vary with stage of disease	
	4. Perifollicular mononuclear cell infiltration about the upper portion of the hair	
	5. Thinning of follicular epithelium	
	6. Replacement of follicular epithelium by fibrous tissue is late finding	Special stains for elastic tissue highlight the fibrous tracts of advanced pseudopalade
	7. Plugging of follicles is common	

Fig. **22-2.** *Alopecia mucinosa. This pilosebaceous unit exhibits mucinous degeneration. Alcian blue stains (to demonstrate the presence of acid mucopolysaccharides) are positive and help to exclude the diagnosis of follicular eczema. (×160)*

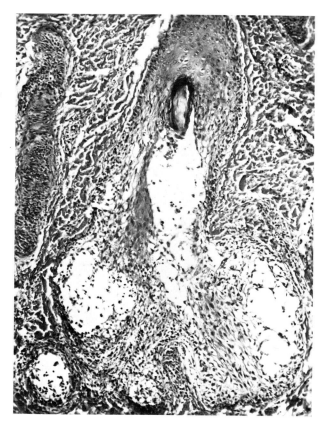

Fig. **22-3.** *Pseudopalade of Broque. In the two hairs at left and center, there is atrophy of follicular epithelium with perifollicular fibrosis in the region of the isthmus. Note also the atrophy and absence of sebaceous glands. The pilosebaceous unit at the right appears less affected. (approximately ×14)*

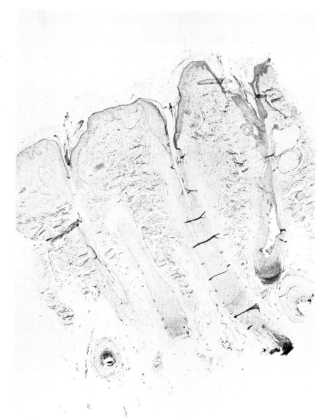

J. Alopecia areata
(Fig. 22-4)

1. Normal epidermis
2. Dermis does not exhibit scarring
3. Histology of hair follicle
varies with stage of disease
4. Early or active lesions exhibit
lymphocytic infiltration of
and around bulb of small anagen hairs; this appearance has
been likened to a swarm of
bees
5. Sebaceous glands are present
6. Fibrous root sheath of the
hair follicle is present below
anagen hair
7. Older lesions exhibit small
anagen hairs only; telogen
and catagen hairs are absent

II. Hyperplasia and neoplasms

    A. Nevus sebaceus

        1. Childhood

Incompletely differentiated
pilosebaceous structures with
cords and buds of undifferentiated cells

Fig. **22-4.** *Alopecia areata. The lymphocytic infiltrate involving the lower portion of the hair follicle ("swarm of bees") is characteristic. (×256)*

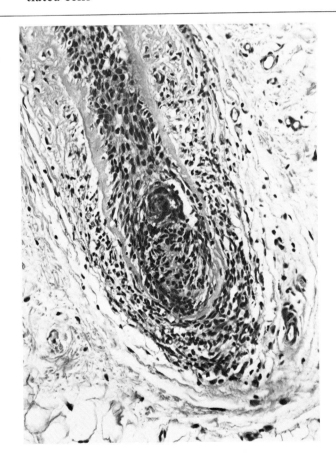

Fig. **22-5.** *Nevus sebaceus. Papillary epidermal hyperplasia, sebaceous hyperplasia, and numerous ectopic apocrine glands constitute the features of this hamartomatous disorder. Before puberty, these features may be less well developed (B, ×24).*

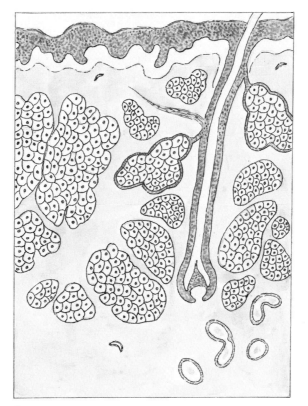

A

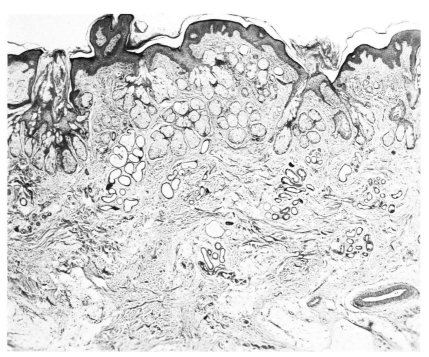

B

2. Adolescent and adult (Fig. 22-5)

1. Hyperkeratosis and **papillomatosis**
2. Large numbers of mature or nearly mature **sebaceous glands** which may open directly to the surface rather than into a follicle
3. Small hair follicles
4. **Ectopic apocrine glands** in lower dermis

B. Sebaceous hyperplasia

One or more enlarged sebaceous glands, each composed of numerous lobules grouped around a central sebaceous duct

C. Sebaceous adenoma (Fig. 22-6)

1. Circumscribed lesion
2. Multiple lobules, irregular in shape and size, containing two types of cells:
   a. **Mature sebaceous cells** are located at the center of lobules, surrounded by:
   b. Undifferentiated germinative cells, indistinguishable from basal cells

Mature sebaceous cells usually predominate; a tumor with many basaloid cells and a few sebaceous cells is more likely to be a basal cell carcinoma with sebaceous differentiation or a sebaceous epithelioma

D. Sebaceous epithelioma (Fig. 22-7)

1. Epidermis may appear normal or ulcerated
2. **Poorly circumscribed** proliferation of predominantly **basaloid cells** with focal differentiation toward sebaceous cells

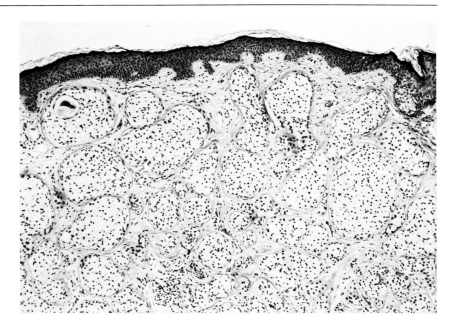

Fig. **22-6.** *Sebaceous adenoma. Nests of benign sebaceous cells are present throughout the dermis without any relationship to pilar structures. (×100)*

Fig. **22-7.** *Sebaceous epithelioma. This tumor is composed of numerous sebaceous cells and generous numbers of less differentiated basaloid cells. (×100)*

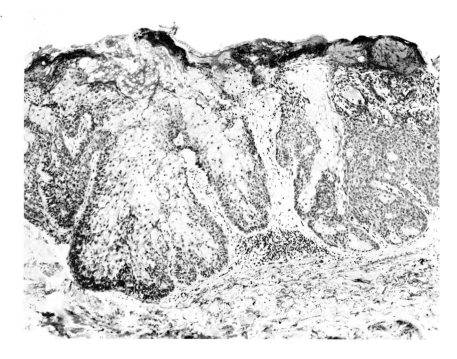

Fig. **22-8.** *Sebaceous carcinoma. Irregular masses of sebaceous cells with pleomorphic hyperchromatic nuclei replace normal dermal structures. (×250)*

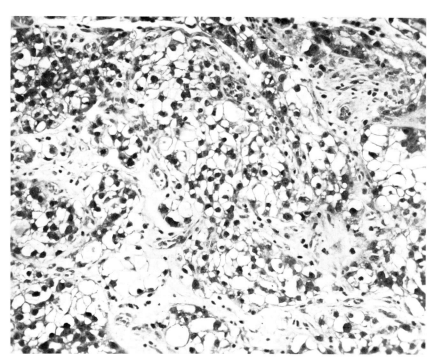

E. Sebaceous carcinoma (Fig. 22-8)

1. Overlying epidermis may be normal
2. Tumor composed of irregular aggregates of basaloid cells and atypical sebaceous cells with foamy cytoplasm and large hyperchromatic nuclei
3. Numerous mitoses

F. Trichofolliculoma

1. **Large cystic spaces,** lined with squamous epithelium and containing keratinous material and hair shafts **surrounded** by groups of small hair follicles containing hair or keratin
2. Stroma rich with fibroblasts

G. Pilar tumor

1. Interlacing strands and lobules of squamous epithelium surround central keratinaceous areas
2. Some nuclear anaplasia, squamous eddy or pearl formation, and individual cell keratinization
3. Circumscribed
4. Calcification common

This tumor is most commonly located on the scalp

H. Trichilemmoma (Fig. 22-9)

1. Platelike or small lobular proliferation of epithelial cells connected to overlying epidermis or hair follicle
2. Centrally located cells have **pale-staining or clear cytoplasm**
3. Peripheral cells exhibit **palisading**

Differentiation toward glycogen-rich, clear cells as seen in outer root sheath of the hair follicle

Fig. **22-9.** *Trichilemmoma.*
A. *Continuity with the epidermis and/or hair follicle is usually apparent in these tumors, composed of cells with clear and eosinophilic (keratinizing) cytoplasm. Palisading of cells at the periphery of the tumor is usually present. (×160)*
B. *Cytologic features and a small hair are more apparent at this higher magnification. (×400)*

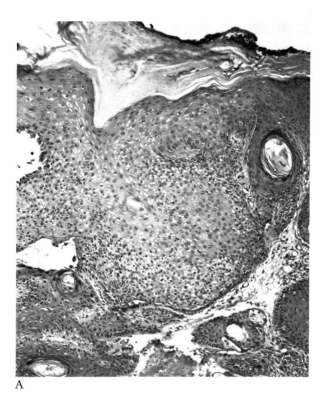

A

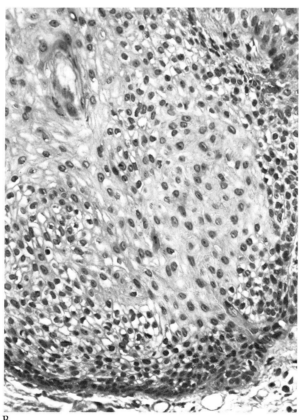

B

I. Trichoepithelioma
(Fig. 22-10)

1. Circumscribed tumor
2. **Horn cysts** with fully keratinized center surrounded by flattened basophilic cells
3. Reticulate or solid aggregates of basaloid cells with surrounding **cellular stroma**
4. Foreign-body giant cells and calcium deposits may be present
5. Melanin may be present within horn cysts and surrounding cells

Differential diagnosis: basal cell carcinoma

Desmoplastic trichoepithelioma is composed of variable numbers of horn cysts and very thin strands of basaloid cells separated by fibrous stroma

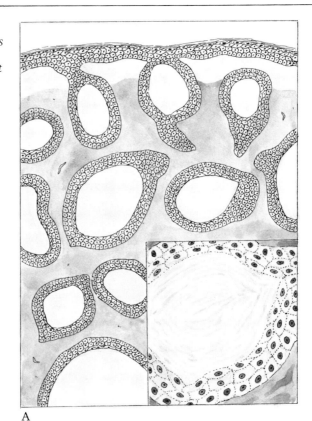

Fig. **22-10.** *Trichoepithelioma. Basaloid cells forming horn cysts (A and B) and/or abortive hair follicles (B and C) are prominent histologic features. (B, ×100; C, ×160)*

A

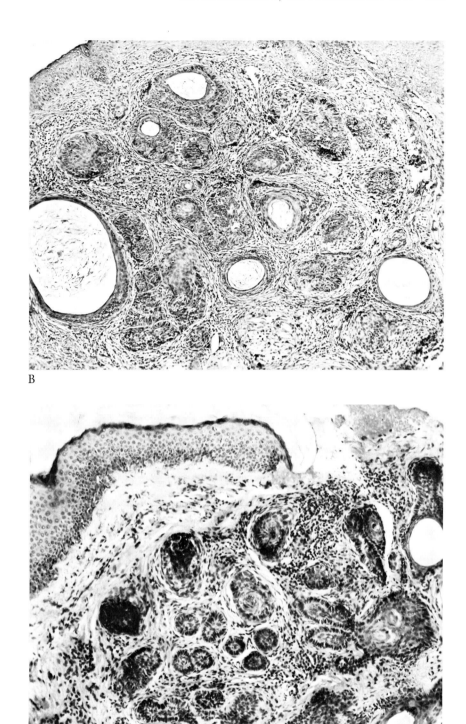

B

C

J. Pilomatrixoma (calcifying epithelioma of Malherbe) (Fig. 22-11)

1. Circumscribed tumor located in the dermis, sometimes surrounded by a connective-tissue capsule
2. Irregular islands of cells made up of:
   a. *Basophilic cells*—cells with scanty cytoplasm, indistinct cell borders, and dark, round nuclei
   b. *Ghost cells*—pale, dead cells with retained nuclear outlines (see Fig. 2-6)
3. Fibroblastic and inflammatory stroma, sometimes with foreign-body giant cells
4. Calcification often present; ossification occasionally occurs

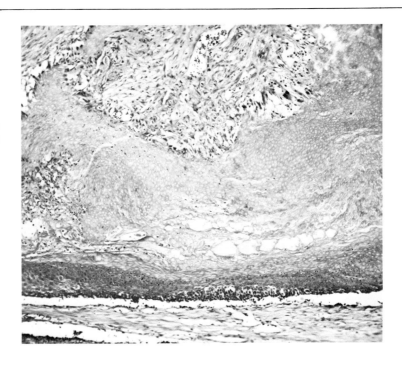

Fig. **22-11.** *Pilomatrixoma (calcifying epithelioma of Malherbe). Basaloid cells (here seen as a thin rim of darkly stained cells located near the base of the micrograph) and ghost cells (mummified cells with negative nuclear images located above the basaloid cells) are the distinctive components of this tumor. The amount of foreign-body inflammation (above the ghost cells), calcification, and fibrous stroma is variable. (×100)*

Suggested Reading
Inflammatory Reactions

Ofuji, S., and Uehara, M. Follicular eruptions of atopic dermatitis. *Arch. Dermatol.* 107:54, 1973.

Pseudopalade of Broque

Gay Prieto, J. Pseudopalade of Broque: Its relationship to some forms of cicatricial alopecias and to lichen planus. *J. Invest. Dermatol.* 24:323, 1955.
Pinkus, H. Differential pattern of elastic fibers in scarring and nonscarring alopecias. *J. Cutan. Pathol.* 5:93, 1968.
Ronchese, F. Pseudopalade. *Arch. Dermatol.* 82:336, 1960.

Alopecia Areata

Mehregan, A. H. Histopathology of alopecias. *Cutis* 21:249, 1978.
Pierard, G. E., and de la Brassinne, M. Cellular activity in the dermis surrounding the hair bulb in alopecia areata. *J. Cutan. Pathol.* 2:240, 1975.
Van Scott, E. J. Morphologic changes in pilosebaceous units and anagen hairs in alopecia areata. *J. Invest. Dermatol.* 31:35, 1958.

Hyperplasias and Neoplasms

Brownstein, M. H., and Shapiro, L. Trichilemmoma: Analysis of 40 new cases. *Arch. Dermatol.* 107:866, 1973.
Forbis, R., and Helwig, E. B. Pilomatrixoma (calcifying epithelioma). *Arch. Dermatol.* 83:606, 1961.
Gray, H. R., and Helwig, E. B. Trichofolliculoma. *Arch. Dermatol.* 86:619, 1962.
Hashimoto, K., and Lever, W. F. *Appendage Tumors of the Skin.* Springfield, Ill.: Thomas, 1968.
Headington, J. T. Tumors of the hair follicle. *Am. J. Pathol.* 85:480, 1976.
Mochlenbeck, F. Pilomatrixoma (calcifying epithelioma). *Arch. Dermatol.* 108:532, 1973.

Chapter 23

Disorders of the
Sweat Glands

I. Inflammatory reactions
  A. Miliaria
    1. Crystallina
    2. Rubra
    3. Profunda
  B. Fox-Fordyce disease (apocrine miliaria)
  C. Hidradenitis suppurativa
  D. Necrosis of eccrine glands: coma bulla
II. Hyperplasias and neoplasms
  A. Syringoma
  B. Clear cell hidradenoma
  C. Eccrine spiradenoma
  D. Eccrine poroma
  E. Cutaneous mixed tumor
  F. Syringocystadenoma papilliferum
  G. Hidradenoma papilliferum
  H. Cylindroma

The Reactive Process and the Disease	Histopathology	Comments
I. Inflammatory reactions		
A. Miliaria		
1. Crystallina	1. Subcorneal vesicle with slight spongiosis of the upper portion of the intraepidermal eccrine duct 2. Mild lymphohistocytic infiltrate present about and within affected ducts	
2. Rubra	1. Prominent spongiosis and vesiculation of the intraepidermal and superficial dermal eccrine duct 2. Moderate perivenular lymphohistiocytic infiltrate that extends into the affected epidermis	
3. Profunda	1. Intraepidermal intraductal hyperkeratosis 2. Spongiosis of intraepidermal duct and upper dermal duct 3. Rupture of intradermal sweat duct below dermoepidermal junction with marked lymphohistiocytic infiltration of adjacent dermis	
B. Fox-Fordyce disease (apocrine miliaria)	1. Acute inflammation of apocrine glands associated with acute and chronic inflammation of the adjacent dermis and subcutaneous fat 2. Entrapment of secretion with dilation of apocrine glands 3. Chronic inflammation is associated with scarring in persistent lesions	Chronic lesions may exhibit only fibrosis and inflammation, without evidence of residual apocrine glands
C. Hidradenitis suppurativa (Fig. 23-1)	1. Polymorphous infiltrate throughout the dermis, with acute inflammation of apocrine glands 2. In late stages, inflammation around apocrine glands may be scant and fibrosis may be prominent	
D. Necrosis of eccrine glands: coma bulla (Fig. 23-2)	See also Ch. 5, II.J, IV.P	

Fig. **23-1.** *Hidradenitis sup-purativa. Acute and chronic in-flammation in and about these apocrine glands is characteristic of early lesions. Fibrosis super-venes in end-stage or chronic dis-ease. (×100)*

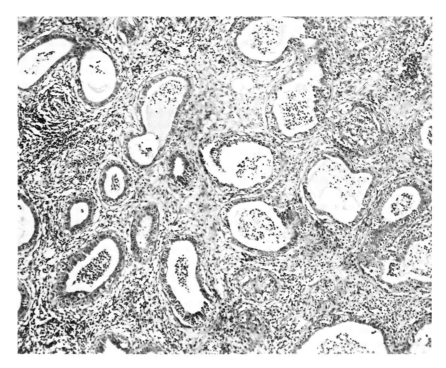

Fig. **23-2.** *Coma bulla (pressure necrosis). These eccrine glands exhibit nuclear pyknosis and cy-toplasmic dissolution, which are changes of early necrosis. Note also the congested capillaries. The overlying epidermis had sloughed. (×400)*

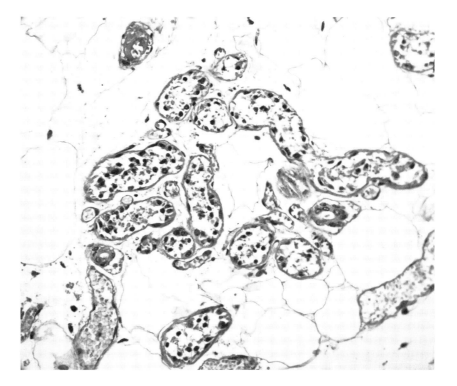

II. Hyperplasias and neoplasms

A. Syringoma (Fig. 23-3)

1. Ducts, small cysts, and nests or strands of epithelial cells
2. Ducts and cysts lined with two layers of flat or cuboidal cells with eosinophilic or pale cytoplasm
3. Cysts may contain keratin or amorphous material
4. Ducts and epithelial structures often have "tails," which give them the appearance of a **comma, or tadpole**
5. Fibrous stroma in upper and mid dermis

Syringomas usually present as multiple flesh-colored to yellowish papules around the eyes, or less commonly on the trunk

B. Clear cell hidradenoma (Fig. 23-4)

1. This circumscribed tumor is located in the dermis, frequently extending to subcutaneous fat; epidermal connection is variable
2. Tumor is composed of **multiple lobules of epithelial cells with ducts and cystic spaces**
3. Two cell types in solid portions consist of:
   a. Large polygonal cells with **clear cytoplasm** and round nucleus
   b. Spindle and polygonal cells with eosinophilic cytoplasm and fusiform nuclei
4. Lumen of ducts lined by cuboidal or columnar cells
5. Ducts with PAS-positive inner hyaline cuticle may be seen
6. Cystic spaces, which may be quite large, contain eosinophilic amorphous material

Clear cell hidradenoma presents as a solitary, cystic, or nodular lesion on the face or trunk; the overlying epidermis may be smooth or ulcerated

Clear cells contain abundant glycogen, which is PAS-positive and diastase-digestible

Differential diagnosis:
  Metastatic renal cell carcinoma
  Sebaceous adenoma
  Trichilemmoma

Fig. **23-3.** *Syringoma. Tubules with tortuous configurations (when viewed in one plane of section) exhibit the irregular shapes seen in this micrograph. Some tubules allegedly resemble tadpoles (arrow). (×160)*

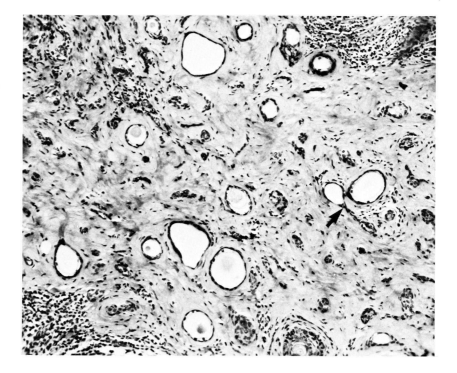

Fig. **23-4.** *Clear cell hidradenoma. Basophilic and clear cells in large dermal masses with occasional ductlike spaces compose this tumor. Considerable variation in the number of clear cells present in this tumor is the rule but at times they may be absent. (×100)*

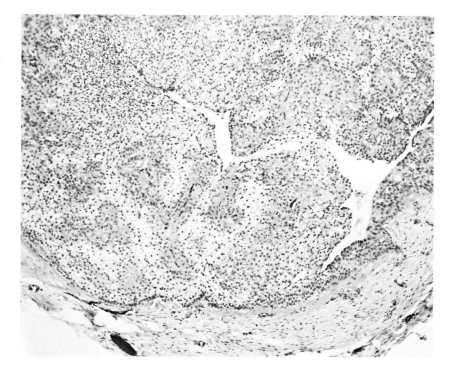

C. Eccrine spiradenoma (Fig. 23-5)

1. Normal epidermis
2. One or more well-circumscribed basophilic "balls" in the middle to lower reticular dermis
3. Tumor often composed of two distinct cell types:
   a. **Small cells** with scant clear cytoplasm and a round, dark, nucleus are located peripherally
   b. **Larger cells** with more abundant cytoplasm and a pale nucleus are located within the lobules and form anastomosing cords
4. The larger pale cells sometimes form small ducts lined by a PAS-positive, diastase-resistant, thin hyaline cuticle
5. Edematous stroma may contain many ectatic blood and lymph vessels

Eccrine spiradenomas present as painful, tender, red to blue nodules; they are *not* found on the palms, soles, axillae, or perineum

Fig. **23-5.** *Eccrine spiradenoma.*
A. *The scanning picture is that of "blue balls in the dermis." (×160)*
B. *Two cell types can be recognized within the balls. Large cells forming ribbons and sometimes ducts are surrounded by smaller cells with dark nuclei and clear cytoplasm. (×640)*

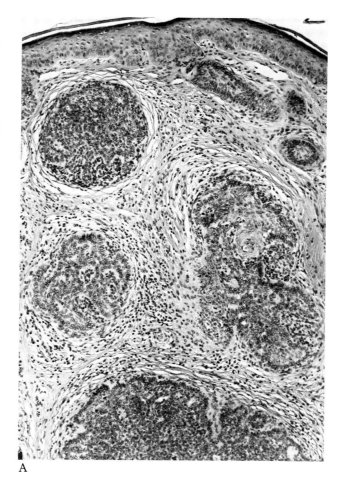

A

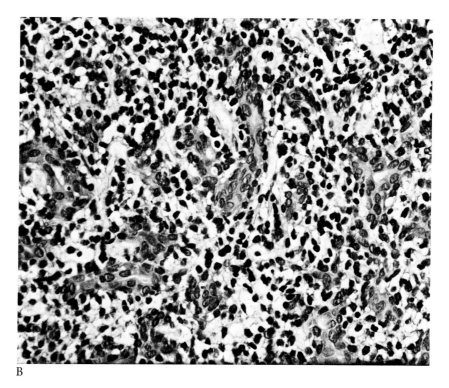

B

D. Eccrine poroma
(Fig. 23-6)

1. **Wide, anastomosing tracts of cells extend from epidermis** into the dermis
2. Basaloid or keratinizing tumor cells are uniform, small, and cuboidal, sometimes with intercellular bridges
3. Lumens of small ducts lined with PAS-positive hyaline cuticle
4. Melanocytes and melanin usually absent

Eccrine poromas characteristically present as a solitary nodule on the plantar surface of the foot

E. Cutaneous mixed tumor (Fig. 23-7)

1. Normal epidermis
2. One or more dermal nodules composed of:
   a. Sheets, cords, and nests of epithelial cells
   b. Cuboidal cells that form tubular structures of varying size
3. Surrounding stroma may be fibrous, myxomatous, **cartilagenous,** and/or hyalinized

The cutaneous mixed tumor is a solitary nodule most commonly located on the head or neck

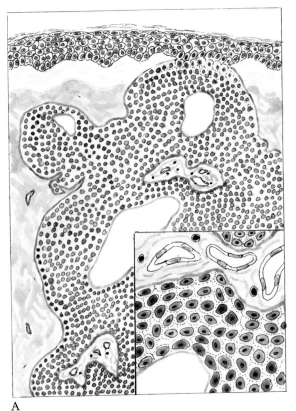
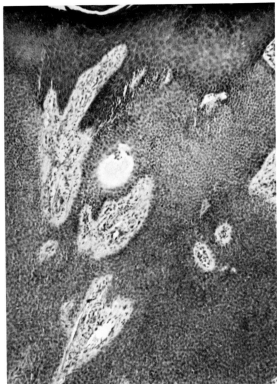

A   B

Fig. **23-6.** *Eccrine poroma.*
A. *Uniform, small epithelial cells in anastomosing bands connect to the epidermis.* Inset: *The glycogen-rich cytoplasm of these cells is PAS-positive and diastase-sensitive.*
B. *Photomicrograph for comparison. (approximately ×160)*

Fig. **23-7.** *Mixed tumor of the skin. Basaloid cells form a net-like pattern with numerous luminal spaces (A) and are closely associated with fibrous stroma, portions of which appear cartilaginous (B). (A, ×45; B, ×256)*

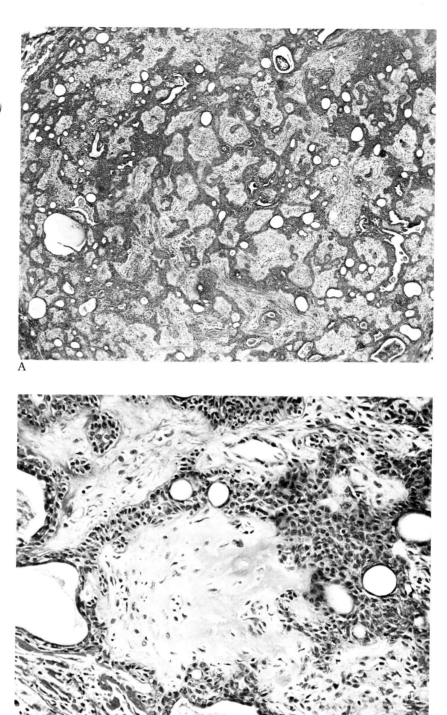

A

B

F. Syringocystadenoma
papilliferum (Fig. 23-8)

1. Papillomatosis of epidermis with one or more porelike openings communicating with the dermal portion of the tumor
2. Beneath the porelike structure is a cystic, epithelial-lined invagination with papillary projections
3. **Papillary projections** are lined with:
   a. An outer (paraluminal) layer of columnar cells
   b. An inner (basal) layer of cuboidal cells
4. Columnar cells often exhibit decapitation secretion
5. Fibrous stroma contains numerous **plasma cells**

Most of these lesions arise in association with a nevus sebaceus and so are most commonly found on the head

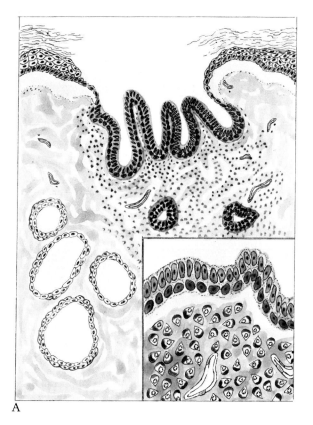

A

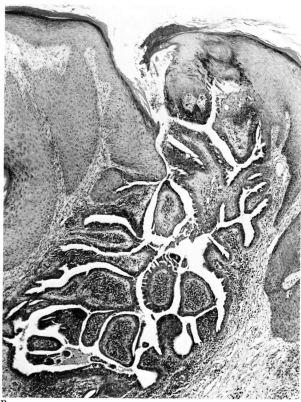

B

Fig. **23-8.** *Syringocystadenoma papilliferum. This tumor exhibits the configuration of a papillary cystadenoma and communicates with the surface (A and B). The papillae are lined by a double layer of cells, and the stroma of the tumor characteristically contains numerous plasma cells (A, inset, and C). (B, ×160; C, ×400)*

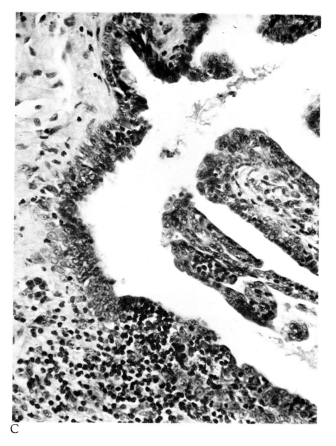

C

G. Hidradenoma papil-
liferum (Fig. 23-9)

1. One or more encapsulated intradermal nodules
2. Nodules composed of cystic
   spaces with complex folds
   and papillary projections, resulting in a delicate, mazelike
   appearance
3. Cystic spaces are lined by:
   a. A paraluminal layer of co-
      lumnar cells with decapita-
      tion secretion
   b. A peripheral (basal) layer of
      cuboidal or flat cells some-
      times
4. Stroma characteristically de-
   void of inflammatory cells

This hidradenoma typically presents as a slow-growing nodule
on the vulva

Fig. **23-9.** *Hidradenoma papilliferum. This tumor is composed of anastomosing ducts (A) lined by basophilic cuboidal to columnar cells resting upon a layer of myoepithelial cells (B). It usually occurs on the vulva. (A, ×64; B, ×400)*

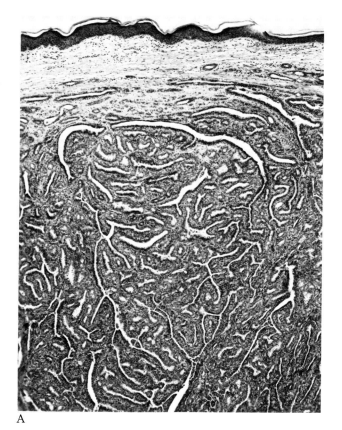

A

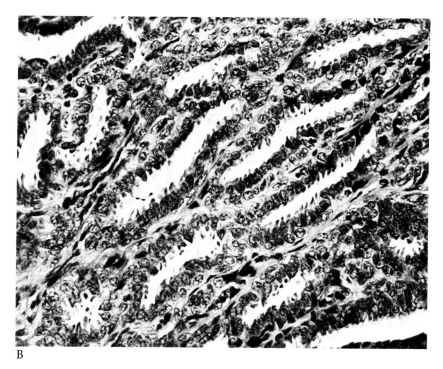

B

H. Cylindroma (Fig. 23-10)

1. One or more intradermal, small, basophilic nodules of varying size
2. Each nodule surrounded and outlined by an **eosinophilic hyaline band**
3. The nodules lie in close approximation to each other and give a **jigsaw puzzle** appearance
4. Tumor nodules are composed of:
   a. Peripheral small cells with scant cytoplasm and a densely basophilic nucleus
   b. Central large cells with pale eosinophilic cytoplasm and a larger pale nucleus
5. Tubular lumens containing amorphous eosinophilic material may be present within the islands
6. Droplets of glassy eosinophilic hyaline material often deposited between cells

A cylindroma may be present as one or more flesh-colored to pink, firm nodules, usually on the head and neck; multiple lesions on the scalp may produce the "turban tumor"

The hyaline band around tumor islands and the eosinophilic hyaline droplets are PAS-positive and diastase-resistant

Fig. **23-10.** *Cylindroma. Cell nests within the dermis, each surrounded by a hyaline sheath, fit together like a jigsaw puzzle. Darker cells are frequently located at the periphery of the nests, while lighter cells sit centrally. (B, ×160)*

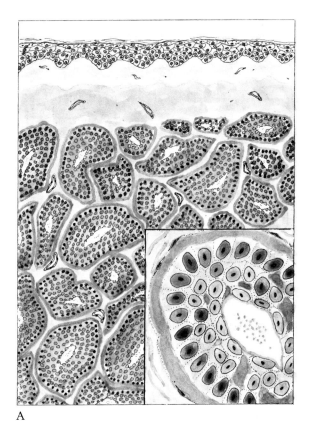

A

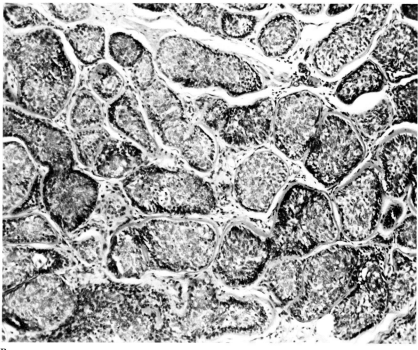

B

Suggested Reading

Hashimoto, K., and Lever, W. F. *Appendage Tumors of the Skin.* Springfield, Ill.: Thomas, 1968.

Mehregan, A. H., and Rahbari, H. Benign epithelial tumors of the skin. IV: Benign apocrine gland tumors. *Cutis* 21:53, 1978.

Mehregan, A. H., and Rahbari, H. Benign epithelial tumors of the skin. V: Benign eccrine gland tumors. *Cutis* 23:573, 1979.

Shelly, W. B., and Cohn, M. M. Pathogenesis of hidradenitis suppurative in man: Experimental and histologic observations. *Arch. Dermatol.* 72:502, 1955.

Shelly, W. B., and Horvath, P. N. Experimental miliaria in man. *J. Invest. Dermatol.* 11:193, 1950.

Winklemann, P. K., and Muller, S. Sweat gland tumors. *Arch. Dermatol.* 89:827, 1964.

Part **VI**

Panniculus

Chapter 24

Inflammation of the Panniculus

I. Predominantly septal inflammation
    A. Erythema nodosum
        1. Early lesion
        2. Late lesion
    B. Migratory panniculitis of Vilanova and Piñol
II. Predominantly lobular inflammation
    A. Weber-Christian disease
        1. Early phase
        2. Subacute phase
        3. Late phase
    B. Panniculitis associated with pancreatitis or pancreatic carcinoma
    C. Injection granuloma
    D. Cold panniculitis
        1. Early lesion
        2. Late (48 hours) lesion
    E. Sclerema neonatorum
III. Combined septal, lobular, and vascular inflammation
    A. Erythema induratum
IV. Disorders that may affect the panniculus

The Reactive Process and the Disease	Histopathology	Comments
I. Predominantly septal inflammation		
A. Erythema nodosum	1. **Septal edema** with variable, **polymorphous, inflammatory infiltrate** composed of lymphocytes, histiocytes, epithelioid cells, Langhans giant cells, neutrophils, and occasional eosinophils	Dermal perivenular lymphocytic infiltrate frequently observed
1. Early lesion (Fig. 24-1)	2. Fibrin exudate in septum	Differential diagnosis of septal panniculitis:
	3. Extravasation of erythrocytes may be observed	Erythema nodosum
	4. Venulitis with fibrinoid necrosis common	Migratory panniculitis of Vilanova and Piñol
	5. Paraseptal, perivenular lymphocytic infiltrate (Miescher's nodules)	Necrobiosis lipoidica
2. Late lesion	Late lesions exhibit septal fibrosis with rare focal paraseptal fat necrosis	

Fig. **24-1.** *Erythema nodosum.*
A. Septal disease with sparing of lobules is characteristic. The septa may exhibit edema, acute and chronic inflammation, and multinucleate giant cells as well as fibrosis, depending on the stage of the lesion. Large-vessel vasculitis and large granulomas are absent usually. Mild inflammation may be seen in the dermis overlying the lesion.
B. This micrograph illustrates the septal nature of the disease and the relative lobular sparing. (×160)
C. This higher magnification illustrates edema, lymphohistiocytic infiltrates with some angiocentricity, and multinucleate giant cells. (×256)

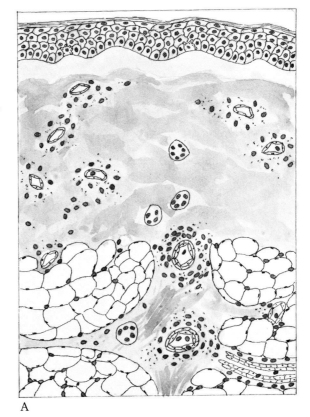

A

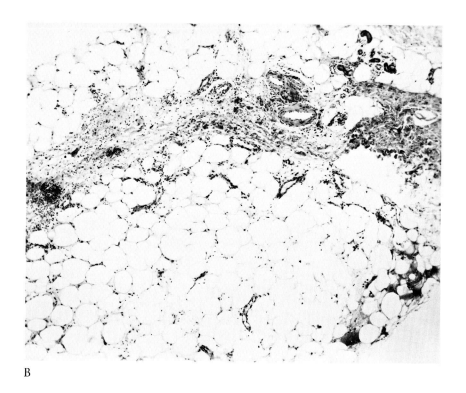

B

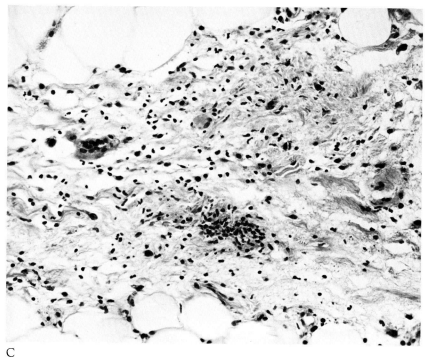

C

B. Migratory panniculitis of Vilanova and Piñol	Septal changes similar to those seen in the late lesions of erythema nodosum with marked vessel proliferation	Migratory panniculitis is probably a variant of erythema nodosum
II. Predominantly lobular inflammation		
A. Weber-Christian disease		
1. Early phase	Neutrophilic infiltration of lobules with marked focal lobular necrosis and abscess formation; septa spared	Lipogranuloma of Rothman-Makai probably a variant
2. Subacute phase	Numerous lipophages and lipogranulomas throughout lobule	
3. Late phase	Lobular fibrosis with fat necrosis and chronic inflammatory cells; septal fibrosis also occurs	
B. Panniculitis associated with pancreatitis or pancreatic carcinoma (Fig. 24-2)	1. Fat necrosis with abnormally large "ghost," or "shadow," cells in lobule 2. **Ghost cells** have poorly defined walls and no nuclei 3. Granular basophilic material (calcium) may be present in area of necrosis 4. Variable infiltrate composed of neutrophils, lymphocytes, histiocytes, foam cells, and giant multinucleate cells	
C. Injection granuloma (Fig. 24-3)	1. **"Swiss cheese"** microcystic spaces of variable size 2. Marked **fat necrosis** 3. Focal, prominent, chronic, and foreign-body inflammation	
D. Cold panniculitis		
1. Early lesion	Nonspecific lobular inflammation	
2. Late (48 hours) lesion	Cystic spaces of variable size surrounded by acute and chronic inflammatory cells	

Fig. **24-2.** *Panniculitis secondary to pancreatitis or pancreatic carcinoma. This highly magnified micrograph exhibits the characteristically ghostlike outlines of anuclear necrotic lipocytes. Calcium deposits are present at the base of this micrograph as a dense linear band. (×400)*

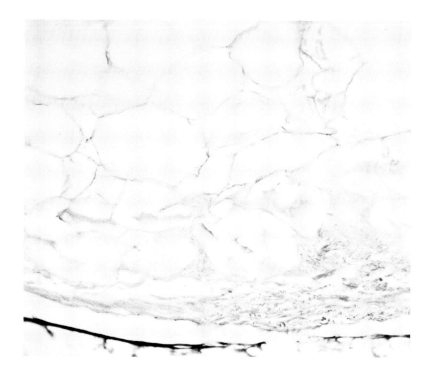

Fig. **24-3.** *Injection granuloma. Irregular ("Swiss cheese") spaces with marked, acute and chronic inflammation are characteristic. (×160)*

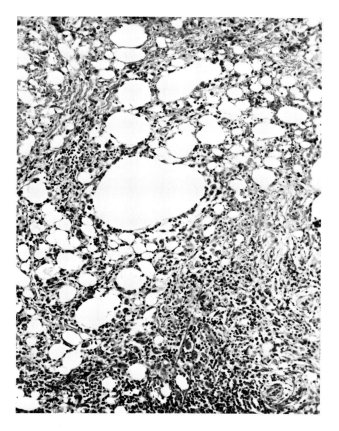

E. Sclerema neonatorum

1. Prominent fat necrosis
2. Lipophages with **needlelike clefts** in cytoplasm
3. Zones of necrosis surrounded by acute and chronic inflammatory cells
4. Broad fibrous septa usually present

Needlelike clefts also seen in subcutaneous fat necrosis of the newborn and poststeroid withdrawal panniculitis; no calcification present

III. Combined septal, lobular, and vascular inflammation

A. Erythema induratum (Fig. 24-4)

1. Epidermal ulceration may be present
2. Caseation necrosis (i.e., granular necrosis of collagen and fat) is helpful when present but frequently is absent
3. Granulomas associated with a polymorphous infiltrate, including epithelioid histiocytes and multinucleate giant cells, are present adjacent to necrotic areas
4. Necrotizing vasculitis of large and small vessels may be observed
5. Fibrosis overshadows the above findings in the late stages

Differential diagnosis:
   Nodular vasculitis (probably a variant of erythema induratum)
   Syphilitic gumma
   Scrofuloderma
   Subcutaneous mycotic abscesses

Stains for acid-fast bacilli should be examined but are rarely positive

IV. Disorders that may affect the panniculus

Inflammation of the panniculus may also occur in:
   Sarcoidosis
   Lupus erythematosus
   Granuloma annulare
   Rheumatoid nodule
   Necrobiosis lipoidica
   Scleroderma
   Periarteritis nodosa
   Blunt trauma
   Leprosy
   Deep fungal infection
   Light eruption
   Insect bite reaction
   Drug eruption

The characteristic features of these disorders, however, usually occur in the dermis (for example, epithelioid cell granulomas in sarcoidosis)

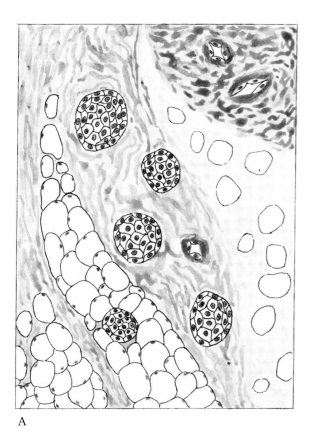

A

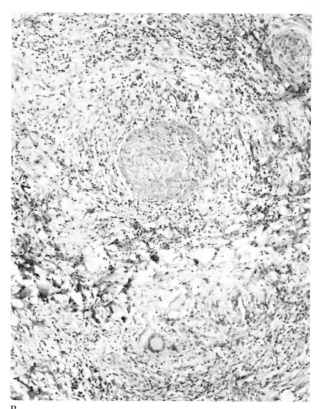

B

Fig. **24-4.** *Erythema induratum.*
A. *This panniculitis is character-*
ized by inflammation of both
lobules and septa and the
presence of granulomas (center) *and necrotizing vasculitis*
(upper right).
B. *Vasculitis of small- and*
medium-sized vessels (upper
right and center); *an inflam-*
matory infiltrate including
neutrophils, lymphocytes, his-
tiocytes, and multinucleate
giant cells; and fibrosis.
(×160)

Suggested Reading
Panniculitis

Case records of the Massachusetts General Hospital. Weekly clinicopathological exercises. Case 17-1982. Fever and subcutaneous masses in an elderly man. *N. Engl. J. Med.* 306:1035, 1982.

Duncan, W. C., Freeman, R. G., and Heaton, C. L. Cold panniculitis. *Arch. Dermatol.* 94:722, 1966.

Fine, R. M., and Meltzer, H. D. Chronic erythema nodosum. *Arch. Dermatol.* 100:33, 1969.

Förström, L., and Winkelmann, R. K. Acute panniculitis: A clinical and histopathologic study of 34 cases. *Arch. Dermatol.* 113:909, 1977.

Gordon, H. Erythema nodosum: A review of one hundred and fifty cases. *Br. J. Dermatol.* 73:393, 1961.

Horsfield, G. I., and Yardley, H. J. Sclerema neonatorum. *J. Invest. Dermatol.* 44:326, 1965.

Hughes, P. S. H., Apisarnthanarax, P., and Mullins, J. F. Subcutaneous fat necrosis associated with pancreatic disease. *Arch. Dermatol.* 111:506, 1975.

MacDonald, A., and Feiwel, M. A review of the concept of Weber-Christian panniculitis with a report of five cases. *Br. J. Dermatol.* 80:355, 1968.

Perry, H. O., and Winkelmann, R. K. Subacute nodular migratory panniculitis. *Arch. Dermatol.* 89:170, 1964.

Potts, D. E., Mass, M. F., and Iseman, M. D. Syndrome of pancreatic disease, subcutaneous fat necrosis and polyserositis: Case report and review of literature. *Am. J. Med.* 58:417, 1975.

Reed, R. J., Clark, W. H., and Mihm, M. C. Disorders of the panniculus adiposus. *Hum. Pathol.* 4:219, 1973.

Sanderson, T. L., Moskowitz, L., Hensley, G. T., et al. Disseminated *Mycobacterium avium-intracellulare* infection appearing as a panniculitis. *Arch. Pathol. Lab. Med.* 106:112, 1982.

Williams, H. J., Samuelson, C. O., and Zone, J. J. Nodular nonsuppurative panniculitis associated with jejunoileal bypass surgery. *Arch. Dermatol.* 115:1091, 1979.

Winkelmann, R. K. Panniculitis in connective tissue disease. *Arch. Dermatol.* 119:336, 1983.

Chapter 25

Hyperplasia and Neoplasms of the Panniculus

I. Benign
   A. Lipoma
   B. Hibernoma
II. Malignant
   A. Liposarcoma

The Reactive Process and the Disease	Histopathology	Comments
I. Benign		
A. Lipoma (Fig. 25-1)	Proliferation of mature fat cells within thin connective-tissue capsule	Fibrous tissue proliferation produces *fibrolipomas;* capillary proliferation results in *angiolipomas*
B. Hibernoma	Encapsulated proliferation of immature fat cells with vacuolated cytoplasm and central nucleus	These tumors are grossly brown on cut section; the fat is doubly refractile when examined with polarized light
II. Malignant		
A. Liposarcoma (Fig. 25-2)	1. Lower dermis and subcutaneous fat infiltrated by malignant fat cells 2. Tumor cells are large, vacuolated, lipid-laden cells with pyknotic atypical nuclei 3. Malignant cells variably admixed with normal-appearing fat cells 4. Tumor cells may assume a myxoid appearance (myxoid liposarcoma) 5. Tumor cells may appear extremely pleomorphic and undifferentiated (pleomorphic liposarcoma)	The differential diagnosis includes lipoblastoma

Fig. **25-1.** *Lipoma. This proliferation of cytologically benign lipocytes is delimited by a fibrous capsule. (×160)*

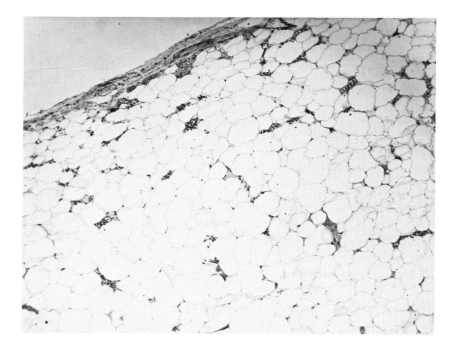

Fig. **25-2.** *Liposarcoma, well differentiated. These lipocytes with extremely large and bizarre nuclei are typical of this disorder (×400)*

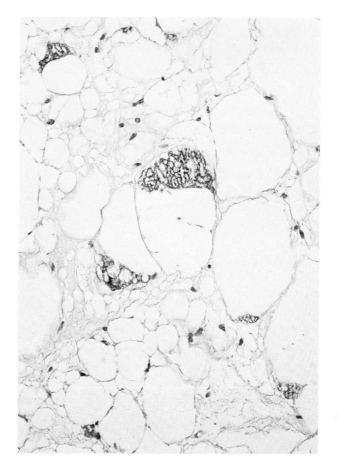

Suggested Reading

Arbabi, L., and Warhol, M. J. Pleomorphic liposarcoma following radiotherapy for breast carcinoma. *Cancer* 49:878, 1982.

Bolen, J. W., and Thorning, D. Benign lipoblastoma and myxoid liposarcoma: A comparative light- and electron-microscopic study. *Am. J. Surg. Pathol.* 4:163, 1980.

Enzinger, F. M., and Weiss, S. W. *Soft Tissue Tumors.* St. Louis: Mosby, 1983.

Shmookler, B. M., and Enzinger, F. M. Pleomorphic lipoma: A benign tumor simulating liposarcoma. A clinicopathologic analysis of 48 cases. *Cancer* 47:126, 1981.

Snover, D. C., Sumner, H. W., and Dehner, L. P. Variability of histologic pattern in recurrent soft tissue sarcomas originally diagnosed as liposarcoma. *Cancer* 49:1005, 1982.

Appendix

*Special Stains
Used in
Dermatopathology*

Material to Be Demonstrated	Stains	Results
Actinomyces	Brown-Brenn Gram-Weigert MacCallum-Goodpasture	Organism: blue
Acid mucopolysaccharides (AMPS)	Alcian blue at pH 4.5 Colloidal iron Crystal violet Toluidine blue	AMPS: light blue AMPS: blue to light green AMPS: metachromatic magenta AMPS: metachromatic magenta

Amyloid	Congo red
	Congo red and polarized light
	
	Crystal violet
		Amyloid: pale pink to red
		Amyloid: red with green
		  birefringence
		Amyloid: purplish red
		  (metachromasia)

Bacteria	Brown-Brenn Gram-Weigert MacCallum-Goodpasture	Gram-positive bacteria: blue Gram-negative bacteria: red
Basement membrane	Periodic acid-Schiff (PAS) Jones methenamine silver	Basement membrane: red Basement membrane: black
Blood cells	Giemsa	Erythrocytes: red Leukocytes: cytoplasm, light blue; nucleus, dark blue
Blood vessel walls	Verhoeff elastic Periodic acid-Schiff (PAS) Gomori's aldehyde fuchsin	Elastic membrane: black Basement membrane: red Elastic fibers, mucin: deep purple
Calcium	Alizarin red-S Von Kossa	Calcium: orange-red Calcium salts: black
Collagen	Mallory aniline blue Masson trichrome Van Gieson Movat's pentachrome	Collagen: blue Elastic fibers: pale yellow Mature collagen, mucin: green Keratin, nuclei, muscle fibers, nerve fibers: dark red Mature collagen: red Muscle, nerves: yellow Collagen, reticular fibers: yellow Nuclei, elastic fibers: black Muscle: red Ground substance, mucin: blue Fibrinoid: intense red
Cryptococcus	Alcian blue Mucicarmine Periodic acid-Schiff (PAS)	Capsule: blue Capsule: red Cell wall of organism: red
Donovan bodies	Giemsa Warthin-Starry	Organism: blue Organism: black
Elastic fibers	Verhoeff–van Gieson Weigert's resorcin-fuchsin Acid orcein	Elastic fibers: blue-black to black Elastic fibers: violet to purple Elastic fibers: dark brown
Fat	*See* lipid	
Fibrin	Phosphotungstic acid- hematoxylin (PTAH)	Fibrin: deep blue
Fungi	Gomori methenamine silver (GMS) Periodic acid-Schiff (PAS) *See* Actinomyces, Cryptococcus, Histoplasma	Fungus walls: black Fungus: red

Glycogen	Best's carmine
	Periodic acid-Schiff with and
	  without diastase digestion
		Glycogen: pink to red
		Glycogen is PAS-positive (pink)
		  before but not after diastase
		  digestion

Hemosiderin	*See* iron	
Histoplasma capsulatum	Giemsa	Organism: reddish blue

Material to be Demonstrated	Stains	Results
Hyaline droplets	Periodic acid-Schiff (PAS)	Hyaline: pink
Leishmania bodies	Giemsa	Organism: reddish blue
Iron	Perl's potassium ferrocyanide Prussian blue Turnbull blue Gomori's iron reaction	Iron: blue
Lipids: frozen sections of fresh or formalin-fixed tissue	Oil-red O Sudan Black B Scharlack R	Fat: orange to bright red Fat: black Fat: bright red
Mast cells	Giemsa Toluidine blue	Metachromatic granules: magenta and blue
Melanin	Fontana-Masson	Melanin: black granules
Mucin	Mucicarmine (*See also* acid mucopolysaccharides *and* mucoprotein)	Mucin: red

Mucoprotein
  With acid
    mucopolysaccharides
 	
  With neutral
    mucopolysaccharides
	
	Alcian blue
	Toluidine blue
	Mucicarmine
	Colloidal iron
	Periodic acid-Schiff (PAS) with diastase digestion
		
		Mucin: blue
		Mucin: magenta
		Mucin: red
		Mucin: blue to light green
		Mucin: pink; no change after diastase digestion

Muscle	Masson trichrome Phosphotungstic acid-hematoxylin (PTAH)	Muscle: red Collagen: green Muscle: blue to purple

Mycobacteria	Acid-fast stains:
	  Ziehl-Neelsen
	  Putt-Fite
	  Kinyoun's carbol fuchsin
	  Wade-Fite
		Mycobacteria: bright red
		
		This modification is favored for the demonstration of *M. leprae*

Nerve	Bodian Osmium tetroxide	Axons: black Myelin: black

Nocardia	Gram stains:
	  Brown-Brenn
	  Gram-Weigert
	  MacCallum-Goodpasture
	Gomori methenamine silver (GMS)
	Acid-fast stains:
	  Ziehl-Neelsen
	  Putt-Fite
		
		Organism: irregularly blue
		
		Organism: black
		
		Organism: bright red

Plasma cell	Giemsa Methyl green-pyronin (MGP)	Cytoplasm: blue Cytoplasm: red
Reticulum fibers	Foot Wilder Gridley	Reticulum fibers, melanin, nerves: black Collagen: rose red Reticulum fibers: black
Rickettsia	Giemsa	Organism: blue to violet
Spirochetes	Levaditi Warthin-Starry Dieterle	Organism: black

Suggested Reading

Bancroft, J. D., and Stevens, A. *Theory and Practice of Histologic Techniques.* New York: Churchill Livingstone, 1977.

Clark, G. *Staining Procedures* (2d ed.). Baltimore, Md.: Williams & Wilkins, 1973.

Graham, J. H., Johnson, W. C., and Helwig, E. B. (Eds.). *Dermal Pathology.* Hagerstown, Md.: Harper & Row, 1972.

Lillie, R. W. *Histopathologic Technic and Practical Histochemistry* (3d ed.). New York: McGraw-Hill, 1965.

Luna, L. G. *Manual of Histologic Staining Methods of the Armed Forces Institute of Pathology* (3d ed.). New York: McGraw-Hill, 1968.

Preece, A. *A Manual for Histologic Technicians* (3d ed.). London: J&A Churchill, 1972.

Sheehan, D. C., and Hrapchak, B. B. *Theory and Practice of Histotechnology.* St. Louis: Mosby, 1973.

Index

Index